Anticancer Spices

Anticancer Spices
Dietary Input to Health

edited by
Hardeep Singh Tuli

JENNY STANFORD
PUBLISHING

Published by

Jenny Stanford Publishing Pte. Ltd.
101 Thomson Road
#06-01, United Square
Singapore 307591

Email: editorial@jennystanford.com
Web: www.jennystanford.com

British Library Cataloguing-in-Publication Data
A catalogue record for this book is available from the British Library.

Anticancer Spices: Dietary Input to Health

ISBN 978-981-5129-28-1 (Hardcover)
ISBN 978-1-003-53466-2 (eBook)

Contents

Preface

Every year, millions of people worldwide die due to the rising frequency of cancer disorders. New anticancer medications and treatment approaches are being created with a huge amount of academic work and funding because cancer is one of the leading causes of disease-related death. However, it appears that focusing on the characteristics of cancer is a more sensible method for creating and developing effective anticancer medications and treatment modalities. Humankind has already used a variety of spices to flavor the food for centuries. However, the chemistry and potential health benefits of these herbs have become clearer only rather recently. Numerous studies performed over the past decades have revealed several advantageous properties of bioactive constituents of different spices, including their anticancer effects. In this edited collection, diverse types of anticancer activities of compounds derived from some well-known spices are summarized, describing the anticancer mechanisms behind their action and highlighting molecular targets and cellular signaling pathways. In this way, the reader will be acquainted with the potential anticancer activities of agents contained in laurel, oregano, thyme, rosemary, basil, dill, parsley, and several other common spices. These molecular entities could probably be considered as lead structures for further design of more efficient anticancer drugs in the future.

Hardeep Singh Tuli

Chapter 1

Introduction to Spices, Sources, and Chemistry

Priti Giri,[a] Deepika Sharma,[a] Ravi Kumar Goswami,[b]
Anamika Singh,[c] Pratibha Kumari,[d] Hardeep Singh Tuli,[e]
and Tejveer Singh[a,f]

[a]Translational Oncology Laboratory, Department of Zoology,
Hansraj College, University of Delhi, Delhi, India
[b]Department of Zoology, Hindu College, University of Delhi, Delhi, India
[c]Department of Botany, Maitreyi College, University of Delhi, Delhi, India
[d]Department of Botany, Daulat Ram College, University of Delhi, Delhi, India
[e]Department of Biosciences and Technology,
Maharishi Markandeshwar (Deemed to be University), Mullana, Ambala, India
[f]Division of Cyclotron and Radiopharmaceutical Sciences,
Institute of Nuclear Medicine and Allied Science, DRDO, New Delhi, India

tej6875@gmail.com, tejveer@hrc.du.ac.in

1.1   Introduction

Spices are products of plants, and they are typically aromatic and spicy. It has been suggested that the existence of various essential oil types in these plants gives rise to these properties (Achinewu et al., 1995; Iwu, 1993). Specifically used for flavoring, seasoning, coloring, and preserving food goods, these naturally fragmented dried plant components include seeds, bark, roots, flowers, and

Anticancer Spices: Dietary Input to Health
Edited by Hardeep Singh Tuli
Copyright © 2025 Jenny Stanford Publishing Pte. Ltd.
ISBN 978-981-5129-28-1 (Hardcover), 978-1-003-53466-2 (eBook)
www.jennystanford.com

fruits (Singh et al., 2021). Thousands of different are used all over the world to color, flavor, and preserve culinary food products. These species are used and preferred in different ways depending on the locale. Therefore, it appears challenging to combine all the spices in one shot. In accordance with Indian law, the Spices Board is authorized to regulate 52 different spices; however, the International Organization for Standardization (ISO) list includes 109 different spices. India is properly known as the "land of spices" because it is the home to many different types of spices. The majority of the time, spices are used sparingly and primarily for food preservation, flavoring, and coloration, but they also have a wealth of health advantages (Kunnumakkara et al., 2018; Sachan et al., 2018). The trans-border trade in areas such as India, Ceylon, China, Indonesia, East and West Africa, and the West Indies is heavily reliant on spices. It is crucial to preserve conventional biological legacy knowledge and investigate new resources. Traditional and ethnic knowledge has been crucial in the development of original concepts for natural resource conservation. Due to their beneficial anti-oxidant, anti-microbial, and antibiotic properties, spices are also utilized in medicine. Some of the spices are high in potassium, iron, vitamins, and trace metals. India, which has a long history of producing species, is home to about 60 different types of them. It has been established that tribes employed spices as herbal ethnomedicine to cure a variety of common illnesses, including boils, fever, intestinal disorders, piles, indigestion, diarrhea, vomiting, asthma, heart ailments, headaches, leukoderma, bold disorders, piles, and bug bites (Babu et al., 2013; Mathew, 2013). One of the most promising anticancer treatments is thought to be a spice. Spices are regarded as one of the most promising anticancer treatments because of their inverse relationship to oncological incidences such as inappropriate cell proliferation, irregular cell cycle, cell cycle arrest, faulty apoptosis, damage to healthy tissues, and tumor-initiating signaling pathways (Perez-Ortiz et al., 2020; Kammath et al., 2021). The efficacy of spices in the manufacture of folklore medicines for treating common illnesses and reviving overall health has been established by numerous research for millennia.

The pharmacological properties of spices are rendered by their active compounds (Sachan et al., 2018).

Alkaloids, phenols, phenylpropanoids, flavonoids, terpenoids, anthocyanins, fibers, sugar, fat, protein, ash, calcium, iron, vitamin B, vitamin C, gum, essential oils, carotene, and many more substances make up their composition. They can satisfy their dietary needs and are a good source of sodium and fat. As a result, they help people reduce their intake of salt and sugar (Balasubramanian et al., 2016). Spices are often regarded as the primary source of nutraceuticals and are a rich source of beneficial dietary bioactive (Srinivasan, 2017).

Numerous pharmacological effects of dietary spices, including antioxidant, antimicrobial, antidiabetic, wound healing, anti-inflammatory, and immunomodulatory properties have been thoroughly documented. The anticancer effectiveness of spices is mostly due to all these pharmacological potentials. Many spices such as *Curcuma longa* (Turmeric), *Cinnamomum verum* (Cinnamon), *Nigella sativa* (Black cumin), *Cuminum cyminum* (Cumin), *Zingiber officinale* (Ginger), *Trigonella foenum-graecum* (Fenugreek), *Allium sativum* (Garlic), *Crocus sativus* (Saffron), *Piper nigrum* (Black pepper), and *Capsicum annum* (Chili powder) are well documented for their anticancer and other property (Zheng et al., 2016).

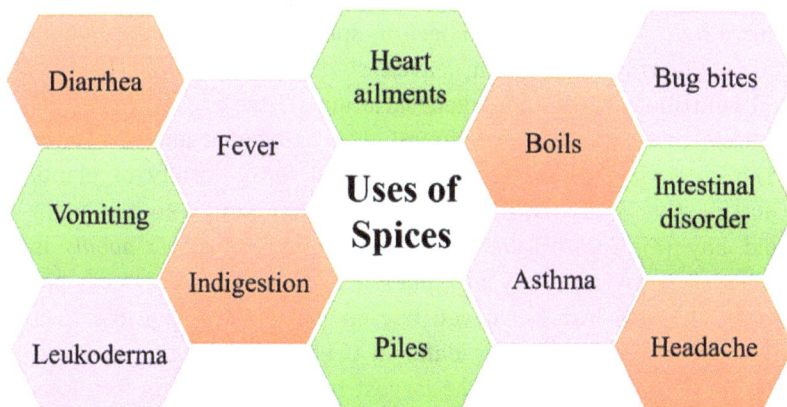

Figure 1.1 Bubble diagram showing the traditional uses of spices in treating various ailments.

Various bioactive compounds including curcumin, sulfur compounds, 6-gingerol, thymoquinone, eugenol, and capsaicin have been extensively studied for their potential to fight cancer. A single plant can be used to cure different ailments besides cancer, as evidenced by the diverse ethnomedicinal uses of spices (Fig. 1.1). The bioactive properties of spices were used to represent the potential anticancer effects of a single phytocompound (Srinivasan, 2017). Therefore, the present study summarizes the source, chemistry, and medicinal properties of bay leaf and parsley.

1.2 *Laurus* sp. (Bay Leaf)

The origin of bay leaf is probably in South Asia, from where it spread to Asia Minor and the rest of the world. *Laurus nobilis* is an evergreen perennial plant in the Lauraceae family. It has been used for over a thousand years and is an essential part of many recipes and ceremonies from the past (Parthasarathy et al., 2008). The Southern Mediterranean region, Eastern Asia's subtropics and tropics, South and North America, the Balkans, and Asia Minor are the native habitats of 24,00–25,00 species that make up the genus *Laurus*. The significant degree of variance among species is partially due to the uncertainty surrounding an exact number of species. Morphology, flower color, growth environment, leaves, stems, and chemical contents all contribute to the observed variation. There are two types of laurels that are commonly found: *Laurus azorica* and *L. nobilis*. The common term "bay laurel" is used for a variety of plants outside the genus *Laurus* including the bay rum tree and plain old bay (*Pimenta racemosa*) (Akgül et al., 1989). *L. nobilis* is referred to by a variety of names. It is referred to as teejh pat in Urdu, bay leaf or sweet bay in English, waraq ghaar in Arabic, lorbeer in German, dafni in Greek and teejpatta in Hindi (Choudhary et al., 2014). The largest bay leaf collection locations for export are in the Aegean and Eastern Mediterranean regions (Nurbas and Bal, 2005).

1.2.1   Chemical Composition

Bay leaf has very few calories because it only contains traces of lipids (i.e., a small amount is present). It is also renowned as a good and important source of numerous nutrients including vitamin A, 54 calories, 1–1.2 g protein, 12–13 g carbs, a trace of fat, 1–1.5 mg of iron (Fe), 51–53 mg of calcium (Ca), 2000–3000 IU of vitamin A, 14–15 mg of vitamin C, and a negligible quantity of potassium are contained in one ounce of bay leaf. Dietary fibers are abundant in bay seeds. Eugenol (11–12%), methyl eugenol (9–12%), and elemicin (1–12%) are chemicals in bay leaves that are important for the spicy aroma of bay leaves and are used as important determinants of bay leaf quality (Biondi et al., 1993). The essential oils range from 0.8% to 3% in leaves and from 0.6% to 10% in dry bay fruits.

1.2.2   Traditional and Pharmaceutical Uses of Bay Leaves

Bay tea enhances the flavor of food and is used to treat stomachaches, lung congestion, colds, and sore throat. Rheumatism and neuralgia are both treated with bay leaf poultices. Bay leaf is used to cure headaches by placing it under headbands or in the nostrils. It has historically been used to treat gastrointestinal issues such as poor digestion, flatulence, eructation, and epigastric bloating (Elmastas et al., 2006). As well as adding flavor and taste, bay leaves have additional health advantages (Fig. 1.2).

1.2.2.1   Wound healing activity

It was established that *L. nobilis* was more effective at healing wounds than *Allamanda* aqueous extract. The wound healing activity was measured using a variety of excision and incision wound healing activities. Tensile strength, granulation tissue weights, pace of wound closure, length of epithelialization, histology of the granulation tissue, and hydroxyproline concentration of the granulation tissue were among the factors that were examined in order to gauge the wound healing activity. The amount of hydroxyproline, the weight of the granulation tissue, and the pace of wound contraction were all shown to be rather high in animals given bay leaves. Comparatively to animals treated with *Allamanda cathartica,* those given bay leaves displayed more inflammatory cells and less collagen (Nayak et al., 2006).

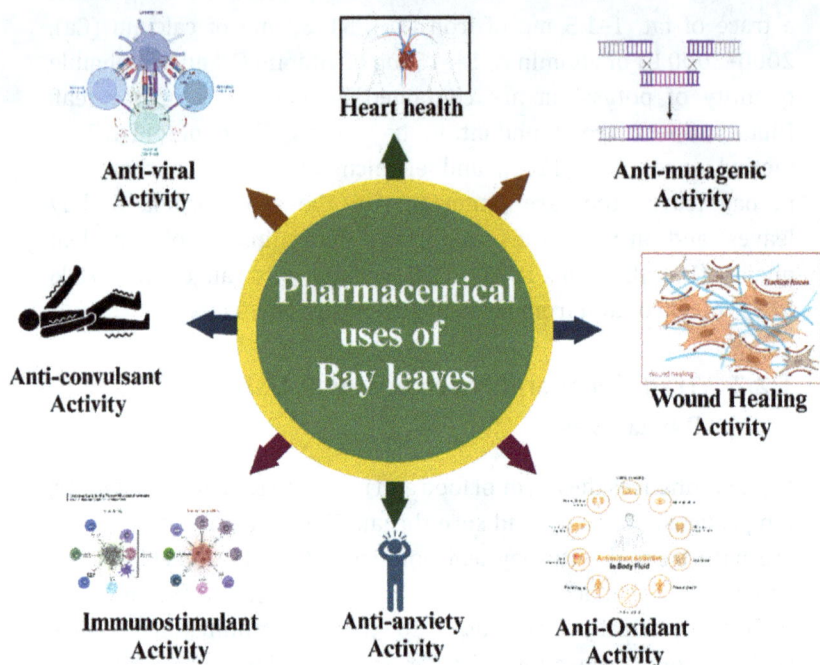

Figure 1.2 Pharmaceutical uses of bay leaf.

1.2.2.2 Antioxidant activity

L. nobilis ethanol extract shows potent antioxidant properties. Superoxide anion radical, hydrogen peroxide radical, and free radical scavenging were evaluated to determine the antioxidant activity (Sayyah et al., 2003).

1.2.2.3 Anticonvulsant activity

In mice, the essential oil from *L. nobilis* leaves exhibited anti-convulsant properties. This activity is brought on by essential oil components such as eugenol, pinene, and methyl eugenol (Sayyah et al., 2002).

1.2.2.4   Antimutagenic activity

Bay leaf ethyl acetate extract contains the experimentally confirmed and chromatographically purified antimutagen 3-kaempferol p-coumarate. The Trp-P-2 metabolically activated form was mutagenically changed into its essential carcinogenic form, which resulted in antimutagenicity (Samejima et al., 1998).

1.2.2.5   Immunostimulant activity

Immunostimulant effects of powder of bay leaf were detected on rainbow trout by giving them dietary constituents. Various diets were fed to three groups of rainbow trout. After 21 days, nonspecific immunological measures were investigated and demonstrated immunostimulant activities, including phagocytosis in blood leukocytes, extra- or intra-cellular respiratory burst activities, lysozymes, and protein levels (Bilen and Bulut, 2010).

1.2.2.6   Antiviral activity

Beta-ocimene, 1,8-cineol, alpha-pinene, and beta-pinene components of *L. nobilis* essential oil have been shown to have an inhibitory effect against SARS-CoV and HSV-1 replication. With an IC50 value of 120 mg/mL and a selectivity index of 4.16, essential oil exhibits this action (Bilen and Bulut, 2010).

1.3   *Petroselinum* sp. (Parsley)

Parsley is a biennial aromatic plant in the Apiaceae family. Since Hippocrates first used it as a diuretic, this medicinal herb has been utilized extensively in the Mediterranean region for more than 2000 years, firstly by Ancient Greeks in religious rituals. Parsley was brought to Central Europe by The Romans introduced parsley to central Europe and Charles the Great's legislation made its growth here mandatory around 795CE. In addition to its medical applications, parsley is now used as a spice in omelets, salads, sauces, and soups, and for producing herb butter as well as a compliment to many other foods. Nowadays, it is now grown throughout the world, including the Mediterranean region (Teuscher et al., 2006).

1.3.1 Chemical Composition of Parsley

A variety of metabolites, including phenylpropanoids, monoterpenes, sesquiterpenes, alcohols, aldehydes, ketones, and aromatic compounds, are mixed together to form essential oil (Teuscher et al., 2006; Farzaei et al., 2013). The application of parsley essential oil in the food, pharmaceutical, cosmetics, and chemical industries is best known (Marín et al., 2016).

1.3.1.1 Leaf essential oil

The predominant chemical components of 0.02–0.9% of essential oil found in parsley leaves are phenylpropanoids (up to 80%) followed by monoterpenes. Sesquiterpenes can be found in tiny concentrations of up to 4%. The smell is caused by phenylpropanoids and monoterpenes (Teuscher et al., 2006). Odor contributing chemicals, found in small amounts, are also: methyl-2-methylbutanoate, oct-1-en-3-one, (Z)-1,5-octadiene-3-one, 2-(p-tolyl) propan-2-ol, 2-isopropyl-3-methoxypyrazine, 2-sec-butyl-3-methoxypyrazine, (Z)-6-decenal, (E, E)-2,4-decadienal, myrcene, linalool, citronellol, and β-ionone (Teuscher et al., 2006). In addition to these components, parsley essential oil also contains aldehydes (phenylacetaldehyde, hexanal, benzaldehyde), aromatic compounds (toluene, m- and/or p-xylene), ethers (2-pentylfuran), alcohols ((Z)-hex-3-en1-ol), and ketones (cryptone) (Farzaei et al., 2013).

As a result of 3-methyl-2,4-nonanedione developing during the drying processes of the laves, a hay-like odor arises. Parsley leaf taste is similar to cabbage. Due to the presence of dimethyl sulfide, methylpropane, and 2- and 3-methylbutanal, the taste of parsley leaves taste is comparable to that of cabbage (Teuscher et al., 2006). The main chemical components in parsley leaves are flavonoids. Other flavonoid components, besides apiin, which is also present in the roots and fruits, include glycosides such as luteolin 7-apiosylglucoside, apigenin 7-glucoside, isorhamnetin 3,7-diglucoside and 6"-acetylapiin, and aglycones quercetin and kaempferol (Teuscher et al., 2006; Farzaei et al., 2013; Fernandes et al., 2020; Hozayen et al., 2016).

The glycosides of luteolin, isorhamnetin, and apigenin with arabinose, rhamnose, and glucose as well as those of kaempferol chrysoeriol and naringin with naringenin are all found in parsley aqueous extract (Farzaei et al., 2013; Hozayen et al., 2016; Epifanio et al., 2020). Additionally, 0.2% of furanocoumarins (oxypeucetanin, bergaptene, psoralen, and others) are found in parsley leaves (Teuscher et al., 2006; Fernandes et al., 2020). In fresh parsley leaves, vitamin C concentration ranges from 0.12% to 0.4% (Teuscher et al., 2006). The highest concentration of ascorbic acid is found in the cultivated flat leaf of *P. crispum* ssp. *Foliosum*, followed by α- and γ-tocopherol. The form of flat-leaf parsley has the highest concentration of γ-tocopherol and total tocopherol. Variations in the source of α-tocopherol and vitamin E can have a big impact in relation to the antioxidative activity of this plant (Fernandes et al., 2020).

Additionally, the parsley leaf includes sugar like apiose, which is mostly flavonoid glycosides (Farzaei et al., 2013). In the aqueous extract of parsley leaves, sucrose, glucose, rhamnose, mannose, arabinose, and mannitol were found (Hozayen et al., 2016). There are also carotenoids, including lutein, violaxanthin, and neoxanthin as well as β-carotene (Farzaei et al., 2013; Fernandes et al., 2020). Among polyacetylenes, falcarinol, falcarindiol, falcarinone, and falcarinolone are recognized.

1.3.1.2 Root essential oil

The essential oil content and composition of *P. crispum* ssp. *foliosum* and *P. crispum* ssp. *tuberosum* roots differ slightly. The roots of *P. crispum* ssp. *tuberosum* contain 0.1–0.3% of essential oil. *P. crispum* ssp. *foliosum* roots contain 0.20–0.75% essential oil (Wichtl et al., 2002; Teuscher et al., 2006). The primary ingredients of roots are Furanocoumarins (oxypeucetanin, bergaptene, xanthotoxin, and others) (Teuscher et al., 2006, Fernandes et al., 2020). Phtalides such as (Z)-ligustilide, senkyunolide, and butylphtalide have been demonstrated to contribute to odor in parsley roots in lower amounts (Wichtl et al., 2002; Teuscher et al., 2006). Falcarinol, falcarindiol, falcarinone, and falcarinolone are the most common polyacetylenes found in parsley root (Teuscher et al., 2006; Heber et al., 2007; Wichtl et al., 2002).

1.3.2 Ethnomedicinal Uses of Parsley

Petroselinum crispum seeds are used for gastrointestinal disorders, inflammation, halitosis, kidney stones, and amenorrhea in traditional Iranian medicine. These seeds are also said to be antimicrobial, antiseptic, astringent, gastronomic, antidote, antispasmodic, carminative, digestive, and sedative (Behtash et al., 2006; Moazedi et al., 2007; Tonkaboni et al., 2007; Aghili et al., 2009). Additionally, leaves are used as a food flavoring, antitussive, and treatment for gastrointestinal disorders, exanthema, dermatitis, alphosis, macula, headcool, sniffle, vision performance, hemorrhoid, kidney stone, diuretic, and otitis (Tonkaboni et al., 2007; Aghili et al., 2009; Eddouks et al., 2002; Jouad et al., 2001; Benítez et al., 2010).

In ethnomedicine of other nations, these leaves also have anticoagulant and abortifacient properties and are beneficial for treating conditions like lumbago, eczema, nosebleeds, amenorrhea, dysmenorrhea, kidney stones, prostatitis, hypertension, hyperuricemia, constipation, odontalgia, pain, baldness, urinary tract disease, fluid retention, and urinary tract infections.

The active components in parsley are also responsible for a wide range of beneficial effects, including hepatoprotective, antidiabetic, and analgesic properties, in addition to the well-known diuretic and antispasmodic actions. The active ingredients in parsley leaves are primarily responsible for anti-inflammatory, anti-anemic, antihyperlipidemic, anticancer, antihypertensive, anticoagulant, and immunosuppressive actions (Fig. 1.3).

Additionally, parsley formulations contain antibacterial, estrogenic, hypouricemic, and antioxidant properties (Fernandes et al., 2020). Moreover, parsley formulations contain antibacterial, estrogenic, hypouricemic, and antioxidant properties. The seeds are beneficial for treating gastritis and shown diuretic and carminative activity (Jouad et al., 2001; Eddouks et al., 2002; Bolkent et al., 2004; Aghili et al., 2009; Benítez et al., 2010; Montesano et al., 2012; Savikin, 2013; Aljanaby et al., 2013; El Rabey et al., 2017).

(A)

(B)

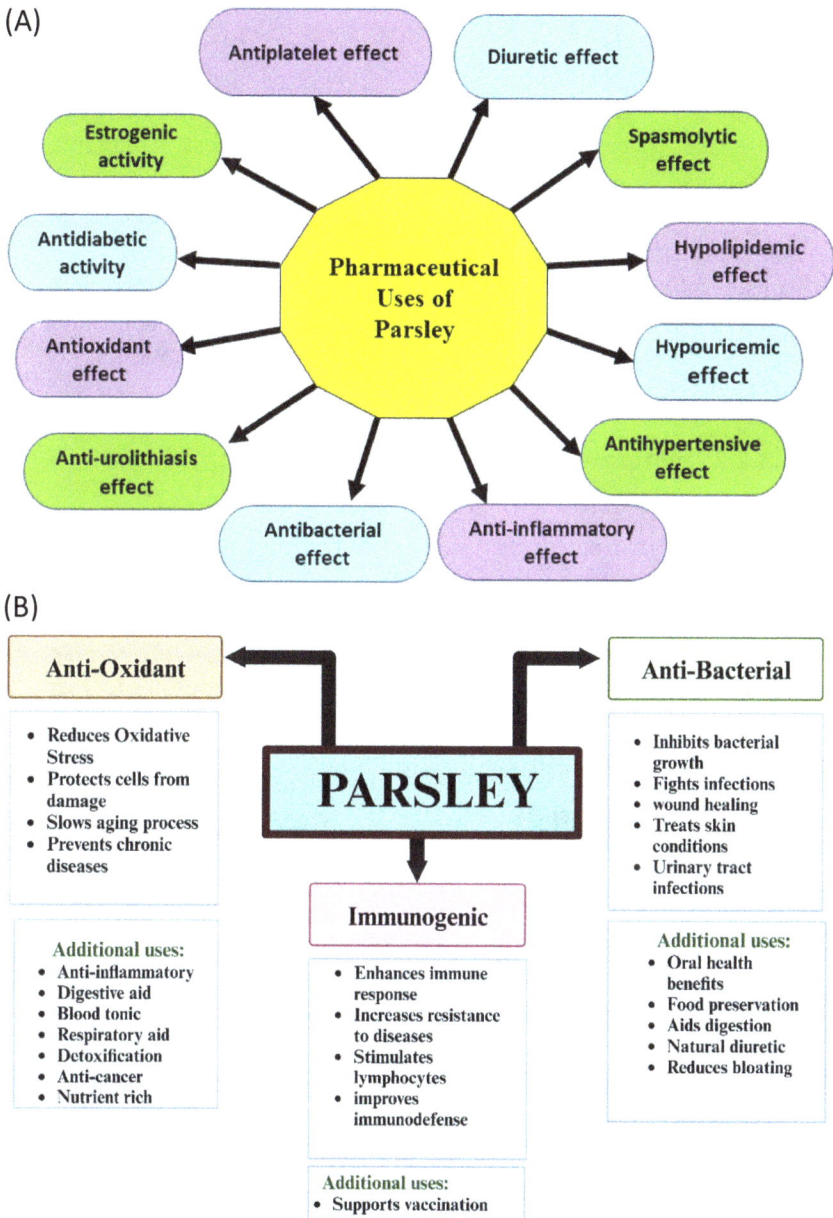

Figure 1.3 Pharmaceutical uses of parsley (A) and the various effects of parsley (B).

1.3.2.1 Estrogenic activity

Methanol extract from the aerial parts of parsley exhibits proliferative activity (estrogenic action), similar to soybean isoflavone glycoside, in estrogen-dependent breast carcinoma cell lines. The flavonoid glycoside 6″-acetylapiin, aglycones apigenin, diosmetin, and kaempferol are principally responsible for this action. Furthermore, oral treatment of the extract can considerably increase the amount of uterine mass that is lost following a mouse ovariectomy; this action is due to apiin and apigenin (Teuscher et al., 2006; Hozayen et al., 2016; Yoshikawa et al., 2000).

1.3.2.2 Antiplatelet effect

Apigenin and cosmosin are the active ingredients in aqueous parsley leaf extract, which exhibits a potent antiplatelet action *in vitro* (Chaves et al., 2011). ADP, collagen, and thrombin-induced aggregation are all inhibited by kaempferol and apigenin aglycones, which were previously integrated into human platelets (Gadi et al., 2012). Aqueous extract given orally to rats prevents aggregation *in vivo* and greatly reduces bleeding time ex vivo (Gadi et al., 2009).

1.3.2.3 Diuretic effect

Due to the irritating effect of the essential oil and flavonoids on renal parenchyma, it has been demonstrated *in vivo* in mice and rats that parsley fruit has a diuretic effect (Teuscher et al., 2006; Kovačević and Farmakognozije, 2004; Wichtl et al., 2002). Aqueous extract of parsley fruit also increases water intake and urine flow while inhibiting kidney Na^+/K^+-ATPase activity, with cortex ATPase showing a stronger inhibitory effect (94.7% compared to 55% inhibition of medullary ATPase), according to *in vivo* experiments. K^+ and Na^+ are less likely to be reabsorbed from the tubular lumen as a result of this inhibition; water follows these ions and has a diuretic effect (Kreydiyyeh and Usta, 2002).

1.3.2.4 Spasmolytic effect

Parsley's fruit, root, and herb are used in dishes that have a spasmolytic effect. Apiol and myristicin, two components of essential oils, predominantly affect the uterus (Wichtl et al., 2002). By inhibiting voltage-dependent Ca^{2+} channels, *P. crispum* fruit extract's ethanol inhibits the concentration that KCl and $CaCl_2$ cause in isolated rat ileum. Additionally, constricted isolated rat ileum generated both spontaneously and by acetylcholine exhibits a spasmolytic action in response to aqueous and ethanol extracts of the aerial portions. These two effects are both dose-dependent (Moazedi et al., 2007; Branković et al., 2010). Additionally, parsley root functions as a moderate spasmodic (Kovačević and Farmakognozije, 2004).

1.3.2.5 Anti-urolithiasis effect

Several *in vivo* investigations on rats with induced urolithiasis examined the anti-urolithiasis activity of parsley, and the outcomes were consistent. The aqueous extract of *P. crispum* aerial parts and roots decreased serum urea and uric acid levels and elevated serum Mg^{2+} levels in ethylene glycol (EG)-induced urolithiasis. The aqueous extract of *P. crispum* roots and aerial parts reduced the amount of calcium oxalate deposits in rats fed EG (Nirumand et al., 2018).

1.3.2.6 Hypouricemic effect

Aqueous parsley leaf extract had an impact on mice with oxonate-induced hyperuricemia in a vivo study, and different techniques were used to show this. Blood urea nitrogen (BUN), aspartate transaminase (AST), and alanine transaminase (ALT), as well as the activity of serum and hepatic xanthine oxidase (an enzyme responsible for uric acid production), are all significantly reduced as a result of using this extract (Soliman et al., 2020).

1.3.2.7 Antioxidant effect

Inhibiting several biochemical processes in the human body, phenolic compounds, especially flavonoids, can act as H-donors to free radicals, preventing cell damage and having a good impact on atherosclerosis chronic degenerative, neurodegenerative changes, and the consequences of aging (Epifanio et al., 2020). Flavonoids were most abundant in parsley extracts produced from leaves (Wichtl et al., 2002).

1.3.2.8 Anti-inflammatory effect

A water-methanol extract of the parsley herb, which is high in flavonoids and other polyphenols, was studied *in vitro* for its anti-inflammatory properties. The quantity of total polyphenols was not linked with any of the effects of parsley extract, indicating the importance of flavonoids in the anti-inflammatory action. In comparison to diclofenac-sodium as a benchmark parsley extract exhibits a high capacity for eliminating nitric oxide (NO) free radicals, a significant anti-denaturation action protein, and a high potential for membrane stabilization (Derouicha et al., 2020).

1.3.2.9 Antibacterial effect

The growth of *Escherichia coli, Listeria monocytogenes, L. innocua,* and *Erwinia carotovora* is inhibited by freeze-dried parsley leaves (in concentrations ranging from 0.12% to 8%); however, *Pseudomonas fragi* is unaffected. The existence of furanocoumarins may be responsible for this impact (Teuscher et al., 2006). *Bacillus subtilis* and *E. coli* are both susceptible to the antibacterial effects of methanol and aqueous leaf and stem extracts. Another element that contributes to this effect is furanocoumarins. While leaf extracts are more effective in harming both bacteria's cells, stem extracts have a better growth-inhibiting effect on both bacteria (Wong et al., 2009). *In vitro* antibacterial activity against *Pseudomonas aeruginosa, Staphylococcus epidermidis, S. aureus,* and *Saccharomyces cerevisiae* is also demonstrated by methanol leaf extract (Ojala et al., 2000). *Lactobacillus plantarum* and *Leuconostoc mesenteroides* cannot grow when ethanol leaf extract is used (Farzaei et al., 2013).

1.3.2.10 Hypolipidemic effect

In rats fed a high-fat, high-cholesterol diet, the hypolipidemic impact of a 20% methanol extract of parsley fruit was proven in real time. An 8-week administration of the aforementioned parsley extract significantly increased the level of high-density lipoprotein (HDL) cholesterol in the blood, while lowering the total cholesterol, triglycerides, low-density lipoprotein (LDL) cholesterol, and very low-density lipoprotein (VLDL) cholesterol in hypercholesterolemic (El Rabey et al., 2017).

1.3.2.11   Antihypertensive effect

The antihypertensive effect of parsley aerial part aqueous extract on rats with normal blood pressure and N-nitro-l-arginine methyl ether (L-NAME) induced hypertension was studied *in vivo* after a single application, application of parsley extract (acute treatment), and repeated applications of the same extract (sub-chronic treatment). A drop in systolic, diastolic, and mean blood pressure was observed after one dosage of the aqueous extract in hypertensive rats, but not in normotensive rats. With repeated treatment, both groups had a decrease in arterial blood pressure in hypertensive people experiencing a higher hypotensive impact (Ajebli et al., 2009; Farzaei et al., 2013).

1.3.2.12   Antidiabetic activity

Several research have been done to look at the anti-diabetic effectiveness of aqueous parsley leaf extract. The extract lowers blood glucose levels, serum ALP levels, and ALT levels, and exhibits hepatoprotective and cardioprotective effects in rats with streptozotocin-induced diabetes. Since no morphological changes in the pancreas have been seen after treatment with parsley leaf extract, the antihyperglycemic effect is instead due to the presence of flavonoids, phenolic components, and ascorbic acid as well as their antioxidant function (Farzaei et al., 2013).

1.4   Conclusions and Future Prospects

Further research on spices is required using modern analytical methods and pharmaceutical approaches in order to get a deeper understanding. This chapter will probably add something to the fascinating plant's possible therapeutic uses. A further study on spices should concentrate on identifying the bioactive ingredients for long-term therapeutical usage of this priceless medicinal plant. Combining spices with other synthetic medications or medicinal plants increases the effectiveness through beneficial interactions. This is a demand for more investigation into the creation of combination medications that increase therapeutical efficacy by combining active pharmaceutical compounds with plant extracts from spices. The therapeutical efficacy of nanomaterials against various medical disorders, particularly microbial infections, was seen to be improved by the modification of nanoparticles utilizing the spices plant extract for medical uses, but the work is still in its infancy. Therefore, more research is advised to ensure the sustainable use of spices as potential medicinal plants to create healthier communities all over the world. Combination medications boost therapeutic efficacy by combining potent pharmaceutical compounds with plant extracts from spices.

Acknowledgments

Dr. TS would like to acknowledge ICMR-DHR, the Government of India (ICMR-DHR Young Scientist Fellowship, F.NO: R. 12014/29/2022/HR), and the college Research and Development Cell (RDC) Scheme (File no. HRC/ RDC/2021/RP/13). We are thankful to CSIR for CSIR NET JRF fellowship to DS (Reference no. Sept/06/22(1)EU-V).

Author Contributions

Conceptualization, methodology, validation, writing review: P.G., D.S., R.K.G., and T.S.; formal analysis: A.S. and P.K. All authors have read and agreed to the published version of the manuscript.

Declarations

Ethics approval: Not applicable.

Consent to participate: Not applicable.

Consent for publication: All authors have their consent to publish.

Competing interests: The authors declare no competing interests.

References

Achinewu SC, Aniena MI, Obomanu FG. Studies on spices of food value in the South Eastern of Nigeria 1: Antioxidants properties. *J. African Med. Plants,* 1995, 18: 135–139.

Aghili MH, Makhzan-al-Advia, Rahimi R, Shams Ardekani MR, Farjadmand F (editors). Tehran: Tehran University of Medical Sciences, 2009, 329–330.

Ajebli M, Eddouks M. Antihypertensive activity of Petroselinum crispum through inhibition of vascular calcium channels in rats. *J Ethnopharmacol.,* 2019, 242: 112039.

Akgül A., Kivanc M., Bayrak A. Chemical composition and antimicrobial effect of Turkish laurel leaf oil. *Journal of Essential Oil Research,* 1989, 1: 277–280.

Aljanaby AAJJ. Antibacterial activity of an aqueous extract of petroselinum crispum leaves against pathogenic bacteria isolated from patients with burns infections in Al-najaf Governorate, Iraq. *Res Chem Intermed.,* 2013, 39 (8): 3709–3714.

Babu N, Srivastava SK, Agarwal S. Traditional storage practices of spices and condiments in Odisha. *Indian J Trad Know,* 2013, 12 (3): 518–523.

Balasubramanian S., Roselin P., Singh K.K., Zachariah J., Saxena S.N. Postharvest processing and benefits of black pepper, coriander, cinnamon, fenugreek, and turmeric spices. *Crit. Rev. Food Sci. Nutr.,* 2016, 56: 1585–1607. https:// doi.org/10.1080/10408398.2012.75 9901.

Behtash N, Kargarzadeh F, Shafaroudi H. Analgesic effects of seed extract from Petroselinum crispum (tagetes minuta) in animal models. *Toxicol Lett,* 2008, 180 (Suppl 5): S127–S128.

Benítez G, González-Tejero MR, Molero-Mesa J. Pharmaceutical ethnobotany in the western part of Granada province (southern Spain): Ethnopharmacological synthesis. *J Ethnopharmacol,* 2010, 129 (1): 87–105.

Bilen S., Bulut M. Effects of laurel (Laurus nobilis) on the non-specific immune responses of rainbow trout (Oncorhynchus mykiss, Walbaum). *Journal of Animal and Veterinary Advances,* 2010, 9: 1275–1279.

Biondi D., Cianci P., Geraci C., Ruberto G., Piattelli M. Antimicrobial activity and chemical composition of essential oils from Sicilian aromatic plants. *Flavour and Fragrance Journal,* 1993, 8: 331–337.

Bolkent S, Yanardag R, Ozsoy-Sacan O, et al. Effects of parsley (Petroselinum crispum) on the liver of diabetic rats: A morphological and biochemical study. *Phytother Res.*, 2004, 18 (12): 996–999.

Branković S, Kitić D, Radenković M, Ivetić V, Veljković S, Nešić M. Relaxant activity of aqueous and ethanol extracts of parsley (Petroselinum crispum (Mill) Nym. ex A. W Hill, Apiaceae) on isolated ileum of rat. *Med Pregl.*, 2010, 63(7–8): 475–8.

Chaves DS, Frattani FS, Assafim M, de Almeida AP, de Zingali RB, Costa SS. Phenolic chemical composition of Petroselinum crispum extract and its effect on haemostasis. *Nat Prod Commun.*, 2011, 6(7): 961–4.

Choudhary D., Kala S., Todaria N., Dasgupta S., Kollmair M. Effects of harvesting on productivity of bay leaf tree (Cinnamomum tamala Nees & Eberm): Case from Udayapur district of Nepal. *Journal of Forestry Research*, 2014, 25: 163–170.

Derouicha M, Bouhlali EDT, Hmidani A, Bammouc M, Bourkhis B, Sellamc K, et al. Assessment of total polyphenols, flavonoids and anti-inflammatory potential of three Apiaceae species grown in the Southeast of Morocco. *Sci Afr.*, 2020, 9: e00507.

Eddouks M, Maghrani M, Lemhadri A, et al. Ethnopharmacological survey of medicinal plants used for the treatment of diabetes mellitus, hypertension and cardiac diseases in the south-east region of Morocco (Tafilalet). *J Ethnopharmacol*, 2002, 82(2–3): 97–103.

El Rabey HA, Al-Seeni MN, Al-Ghamdi HB. Comparison between the hypolipidemic activity of parsley and carob in hyper-cholesterolemic male rats. *BioMed Res Int.*, 2017, 2017: 1–10. doi: 10.1155/2017/3098745.

Elmastas M., Gülcin I., Isildak Ö., Küfrevioglu Ö., Ibaoglu K., Aboul-Enein H. Radical scavenging activity and antioxidant capacity of bay leaf extracts. *Journal of the Iranian Chemical Society*, 2006, 3: 258–266.

Epifanio NMM, Cavalcanti LRI, Santos KF, Duarte PSC, Kachlicki P, Ożarowski M, et al. Chemical characterization and *in vivo* antioxidant activity of parsley (Petroselinum crispum) aqueous extract. *Food Funct.*, 2020, 11: 5346–56.

Farzaei MH, Abbasabadi Z, Ardekani MRS, Rahimi R, Farzaei F. Parsley: A review of ethnopharmacology, phytochemistry and biological activities. *J Tradit Chin Med.*, 2013, 33(6): 815–26.

Fernandes A, Polyzos N, Petropoulos SA, Pinela J, Ardohain E, Moreira G, et al. Phytochemical composition and nutritional value of pot-grown turnip-rooted and plain and curly-leafed parsley cultivars. *Agronomy*, 2020, 10: 1416–15.

Gadi D, Bnouham M, Aziz M, Ziyyat A, Legssyer A, Bruel A, et al. Flavonoids purified from parsley inhibit human blood platelet aggregation and adhesion to collagen under flow. *J Complement Integr Med.*, 2012, 9 (Article 19).

Gadi D, Bnouham M, Aziz M, Ziyyat A, Legssyer A, Legrand C, et al. Parsley extract inhibits *in vitro* and ex vivo platelet aggregation and prolongs bleeding time in rats. *J Ethnopharmacol.*, 2009, 125(1): 170–4.

Heber D. *PDR for Herbal Medicines*, 4th ed., Thomson Healthcare Inc., 2007, p. 1026.

Hozayen WG, El-Desouky MA, Soliman HA, Ahmed RR, Khaliefa AK. Antiosteoporotic effect of Petroselinum crispum, Ocimum basilicum and Cichorium intybus L. in glucocorticoid-induced osteoporosis in rats. *BMC Comp Alt Med.*, 2016, 16: 165.

Iwu M.M. *Handbook of African Medicinal Plants*, Boca Raton CKC Press, Free Enterprise Publishers, Lagos, 1993, p. 435.

Jouad H, Haloui M, Rhiouani H, et al. Ethnobotanical survey of medicinal plants used for the treatment of diabetes, cardiac and renal diseases in the North centre region of Morocco (Fez-Boulemane). *J Ethnopharmacol.*, 2001, 77 (2–3): 175–182.

Kammath A.J., Nair B., Nath L.R. Curry versus cancer: Potential of some selected culinary spices against cancer with *in vitro*, *in vivo*, and human trials evidences. *J. Food Biochem.*, 2021, 45: e13285. https://doi.org/10.1111/jfbc.13285.

Kovačević N. *Osnovi farmakognozije*, 3rd ed. Beograd: Srpska školska knjiga, 2004, p. 408.

Kreydiyyeh SI, Usta J. Diuretic effect and mechanism of action of parsley. *J Ethnopharmacol.*, 2002, 79: 353–7.

Kunnumakkara A.B., Sailo B.L., Banik K., Harsha C., Prasad S., Gupta S.C., Aggarwal B.B. Chronic diseases, inflammation, and spices: How are they linked? *J. Transl. Med.*, 2018, 16: 1–25. https://doi.org/10.1186/s12967-018-1381-2.

Marín I, Sayas-Barberá E, Viuda-Martos M, Navarro C, Sendra E. Chemical composition, antioxidant and antimicrobial activity of essential oils from organic fennel, parsley, and lavender from Spain. *Foods*, 2016, 5: 18.

Mathew J. Indigenous aromatic and spice plants described in van rheed's hortus indici malabarici. *Indian J Appl Res.*, 2013, 3(11): 30–33.

Moazedi AA, Mirzaie DN, Seyyednejad SM, et al. Spasmolytic effect of Petroselinum crispum (Parsley) on rat's ileum at different calcium chloride concentrations. *Pak J Biol Sci.*, 2007, 10(22): 4036–4042.

Montesano V, Negro D, Sarli G, et al. Notes about the uses of plants by one of the last healers in the Basilicata Region (South Italy). *J Ethnobiol Ethnomed*, 2012, 8: 15.

Nayak S., Nalabothu P., Sandiford S., Bhogadi V., Adogwa A. Evaluation of wound healing activity of Allamanda cathartica. L. and Laurus nobilis. L. extracts on rats. *BMC Complementary and Alternative Medicine*, 2006, 6: 1.

Nirumand MC, Hajialyani M, Rahimi R, Farzaei MH, Zingue S, Nabavi SM, et al. Dietary plants for the prevention and management of kidney stones: Preclinical and clinical evidence and molecular mechanisms. *Int J Mol Sci.*, 2018, 19: 765.

Nurbas M., Bal Y. Recovery of fixed and volatile oils from Laurus nobilis L. fruit and leaves by solvent extraction method. *Journal of Engineering and Architectural Faculty of Eskisehir,* Osmangazi University, 2005.

Ojala T, Remes S, Haansuu P, Vuorela H, Hiltunen R, Haahtela K, et al. Antimicrobial activity of some coumarin containing herbal plants growing in Finland. *J Ethnopharmacol.*, 2000, 73(1–2): 299–305.

Parthasarathy V.A., Chempakam B., Zachariah T.J. *Chemistry of Spices*, Cabi, 2008.

Perez-Ortiz J.M., Galan-Moya E.M., de la Cruz-Morcillo M.A., Rodriguez J.F., Gracia I., Garcia M.T., Redondo-Calvo F.J. Cost effective use of a thiosulfinate-enriched Allium sativum extract in combination with chemotherapy in colon cancer. *Int. J. Math. Stat.*, 2020, 21: 2766. https://doi.org/10.3390/ijms21082766.

Sachan A.K., Kumar S., Kumari K., Singh D. Medicinal uses of spices used in our traditional culture: Worldwide. *JMPS*, 2018, 6: 116–122.

Samejima K., Kanazawa K., Ashida H., Danno G.-i. Bay laurel contains antimutagenic kaempferol coumarate acting against the dietary carcinogen 3-amino-1-methyl-5 H-pyrido [4, 3-b] indole (Trp-P-2). *Journal of Agricultural and Food Chemistry*, 1998, 46: 4864e4868.

Savikin K, Zdunic G, Menkovic N, et al. Ethnobotanical study on traditional use of medicinal plants in South-Western Serbia, Zlatibor district. *J Ethnopharmacol*, 2013, 146 (3): 803–810.

Sayyah M., Saroukhani G., Peirovi A., Kamalinejad M. Analgesic and anti-inflammatory activity of the leaf essential oil of Laurus nobilis Linn. *Phytotherapy Research*, 2003, 17: 733–736.

Sayyah M., Valizadeh J., Kamalinejad M. Anticonvulsant activity of the leaf essential oil of Laurus nobilis against pentylenetetrazole-and maximal electroshock-induced seizures. *Phytomedicine*, 2002, 9: 212–216.

Singh N., Rao A.S., Nandal A., Kumar S., Yadav S.S., Ganaie S.A., Narasimhan B. Phytochemical and pharmacological review of Cinnamomum verum J. Presl-a versatile spice used in food and nutrition. *Food Chem.* 2021, 338: 127773. https://doi.org/ 10.1016/j.foodchem.2020.127773.

Soliman MM, Nassan MA, Aldhahrani A, Althobaiti F, Mohamed WA. Molecular and histopathological study on the ameliorative impacts of petroselinum crispum and apium graveolens against experimental hyperuricemia. *Sci Rep.*, 2020, 10: 9512.

Srinivasan K. Antimutagenic and cancer preventive potential of culinary spices and their bioactive compounds. *PharmaNutrition*, 2017, 5: 89–102. https://doi.org/ 10.1016/j.phanu.2017.06.001.

Teuscher E, Bauermann U, Werner M. *Medicinal Spices: A Handbook of Culinary Herbs, Spices, Spice Mixtures and Their Essential Oils*, Florida: Medpharm Scientific Publishers, Stuttgart, CRC Press, Taylor and Francis Group, 2006, p. 460.

Tonkaboni MM. Tohfeh-al-Momenin Rahimi R, Shams Ardekani MR, Farjadmand F (editors). Tehran: Shahid Beheshti University of Medical Sciences, 2007, 129.

Wichtl M. *Teedrogen und Phytopharmaka Ein Handbuch fur die Praxis auf wissenschaftlicher Grundlage*, 4th ed., Stuttgart: Wissenschaftliche Verlagsgesellschaft, 2002, p. 441–8.

Wong PYY, Kitts DD. Studies on the dual antioxidant and antibacterial properties of parsley (Petroselinum crispum) and cilantro (Coriandrum sativum) extracts. *Food Chem.*, 2006, 97(3): 505–15.

Yoshikawa M, Uemura T, Shimoda H, Kishi A, Kawahara Y, Matsuda H. Medicinal foodstuffs. XVIII. Phytoestrogens from the aerial part of Petroselinum crispum MIll. (Parsley) and structures of 6″-acetylapiin and a new monoterpene glycoside, petroside. *Chem Pharm Bull (Tokyo)*, 2000, 48(7): 1039–44.

Zhang L., Bai Y., Yang Y. Thymoquinone chemosensitizes colon cancer cells through inhibition of NF-κB. *Oncol. Lett.*, 2016, 12: 2840–2845. https://doi.org/10.3892/ol.2016.4971.

Chapter 2

Quantification and Identification Tools of Major Bioactive Moieties in Spices

Vivek Sheel Jaswal,[a] Kusham Lata,[a] Manish Kumar,[a] and Surinder Paul[b]

[a]*Department of Chemistry & Chemical Sciences*
Central University of Himachal Pradesh, Dharamshala, Himachal Pradesh, India
[b]*Department of Physics and Astronomical Science*
Central University of Himachal Pradesh, Dharamshala, Himachal Pradesh, India

chemsheel@gmail.com

Spices are obtained from natural sources, often plants, and can be used whole or crushed while cooking. In addition to their role in enhancing food quality, they also provide health advantages. The identification and quantification give an overview of spices from several categories, such as flavonoids and polyphenolics, as well as qualitative and quantitative guidelines for providing their quality and safety using modern analytical technology and methodologies. The role of quantitative analytical approaches is highlighted in this chapter.

Anticancer Spices: Dietary Input to Health
Edited by Hardeep Singh Tuli
Copyright © 2025 Jenny Stanford Publishing Pte. Ltd.
ISBN 978-981-5129-28-1 (Hardcover), 978-1-003-53466-2 (eBook)
www.jennystanford.com

2.1 Introduction

Any part of a plant that is predominantly used for flavoring or coloring food is referred to as a spice. It may include seeds, fruits, roots, bark, or other parts of a plant. Sometimes, these are also used for medicinal, religious, and cosmetic purposes. There are different types of spices that are widely used throughout the world. The majority of spices are dried. For ease, spices can be made into powder. Since whole dried spices can be bought and stored in larger quantities and have the longest shelf lives, they are more affordable per serving. The flavor of fresh spices, like ginger, is generally superior to that of their dried counterparts, but they are more expensive and have a much shorter shelf life. For instance, turmeric is one spice that is usually purchased in ground form and is not always available fresh. In 2019, there was little clinical proof that ingesting spices affected people's health. Around 75% of the world's spice production comes from India. The spice trade historically evolved across the Indian subcontinent, as well as in East Asia and the Middle East, and this is represented culturally in their food. The demand for spices in Europe throughout the early modern era was one of the economic and cultural factors that encouraged travel [1].

The main bioactive moieties found in spices are phenolics, terpenoids, flavonoids, and alkaloids. They are thought to be the source of their therapeutic and medical effects. There are many analytical techniques that can be used to measure and identify these bioactive compounds in spices. Common techniques are:

1. **Basic analytical procedure also referred to as high-performance liquid chromatography (HPLC):** It is a typical technique to recognize, quantify, and identify the bioactive elements found in various kinds of spices. This type of chromatography divides a mixture into its constituent parts depending on their chemical properties and presents a chromatogram that can be used for the identification and quantification of particular substances [2].

2. **Gas chromatography-mass spectrometry (GC-MS):** It is an effective method for identifying and measuring volatile bioactive components in spices. This type of chromatography

separates and identifies components according to their boiling point [2].

3. **Fourier transform-infrared spectroscopy (FT-IR):** It is also a very important non-destructive method that reveals details about the functional groups a chemical contains. On the basis of its distinctive infrared spectra, it can be used to identify and measure particular bioactive substances in spices [2].

4. **Nuclear magnetic resonance spectroscopy (NMR):** It is an effective method for determining the structures of the bioactive substances found in spices. It gives details on the atoms' chemical surroundings within molecules and can be utilized to work out the structure of certain substances.

5. **Ultra-performance liquid chromatography (UPLC):** It is an innovative technique that offers quick and high-resolution chemical separation. It can be applied for detecting and measuring bioactive substances in spices [2].

2.2 Spices and Their Chemical Composition

2.2.1 Black Pepper

Black pepper or *Piper nigrum* has held a prominent and distinctive place because of its distinctive pungency and flavor. Black pepper is the most significant and widely used spice worldwide. It is also known as the "King of Spices." The pungency and flavor of pepper are what make it valuable, and they are caused by the substance piperine (Fig. 2.1). It is a volatile essential oil and a

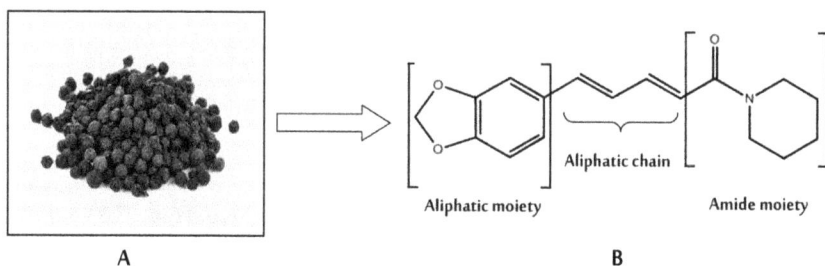

Figure 2.1 (A) Image of black pepper and (B) Structure of piperene.

naturally occurring alkaloid. Different Piperaceae plants have different amounts of piperine. The most abundant alkaloid in peppers is piperine, which presents sarmentine, pinene, terpenes, limonene, camphene, isoquercetin, and piperidine [3].

2.2.2 Cinnamon

The perennial tree used in tropical medicine known as cinnamon (*Cinnamomum zeylanicum*, *Cinnamomum verum*, and *Cinnamon cassia*) belongs to the Lauraceae family. It ranks among the most important spices that people consume every day. Cinnamon contains a variety of substances in addition to essential oils, such as cinnamaldehyde, cinnamic acid, and cinnamate (Fig. 2.2). The bark of numerous species of cinnamon spices is used in both ancient and modern treatments, as well as in food preparation. Cinnamaldehyde and trans-cinnamaldehyde (Cin), which are contained in the essential oil and contribute to the flavor and many biological activities of cinnamon, are very significant components of the spice [4].

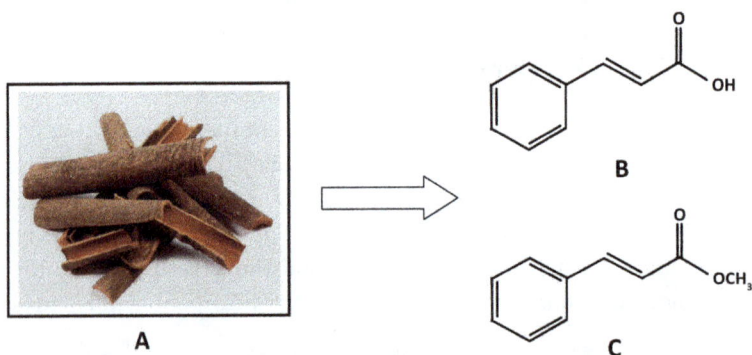

Figure 2.2 (A) Image of cinnamon, (B) Structure of cinnamic acid, and (C) Structure of cinnamate.

2.2.3 Clove

Syzygium aromaticum, commonly known as clove (Fig. 2.3), is a moderate evergreen tree that is a member of the Myrtaceae family. It originated on the Maluku Islands in Indonesia and is also widely cultivated in other parts of the world [5]. The phenolic chemicals flavonoids, hydroxybenzoic acids, hydroxyl cinnamic acids, and hydroxy phenylpropenes are all abundant in clove. Eugenol, the primary bioactive component of clove, is found in high concentrations per 100 g of fresh plant material (9,381.70 to 14,650.00 mg), making up the majority of the clove's bioactive compounds [6]. Another significant phenolic acid that may be found in cloves is gallic acid, which is also present in large concentrations in the fresh material (783.50 mg/100 g) along with other gallic acid derivatives including hydrolysable tannins, which have massive concentrations of 2,375.8 mg/100 g. Clove also contains the phenolic acids caffeic, ferulic, ellagic, and salicylic. It also includes trace levels of flavonoids such as quercetin, kaempferol, and their glycosylated derivatives. Additionally, clove has a large amount of essential oil, with flower buds containing up to 18% of the total amount. Clove essential oil contains 89% eugenol on average, while eugenol acetate and caryophyllene make up 5–15%. Humulene, which can present clove's essential oil in amounts up to 2.1%, is another significant component. In small proportions, clove essential oil also contains the following volatile substances: pinene, farnesol, 2-heptanone, benzaldehyde, limonene, and ethyl hexanoate [7].

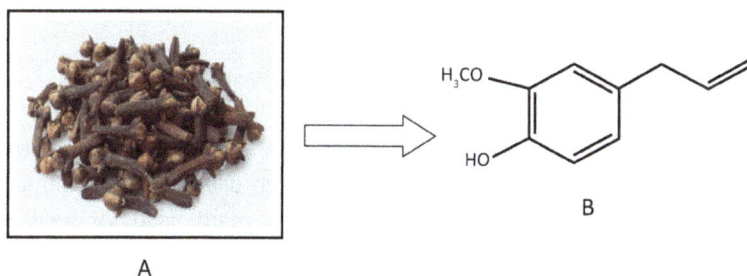

A

B

Figure 2.3 (A) Image of clove and (B) Chemical structure of eugenol [8].

2.2.4 Cumin

The herb *Cuminum cyminum*, which is native to South Asia and the Eastern Mediterranean and is a member of the parsley family Apiaceae, is what produces cumin seeds. The oblong, yellow-gray seeds of cumin are in form (Fig. 2.4). Since ancient times, cumin seeds have played a significant role in Indian cooking, appearing in a variety of dishes such as soups and kormas as well as in several spice blends. Aside from food, it has numerous applications in traditional medicine. Cumin seeds have tremendous medical benefits in India's Ayurvedic School of Medicine, notably for digestive issues. The principal volatile components of this spice are cymene, cumin aldehyde, and terpenoids. The main chemical that contributes to odor is cumin aldehyde. The substituted pyrazines 2-methoxy-3-sec-butylpyrazine, 2-ethoxy-3-isopropylpyrazine, and 2-methoxy-3-methylpyrazine are additional important fragrance components in roast cumin. Safranal, p-cymene, terpinene, and pinene are additional constituents [9].

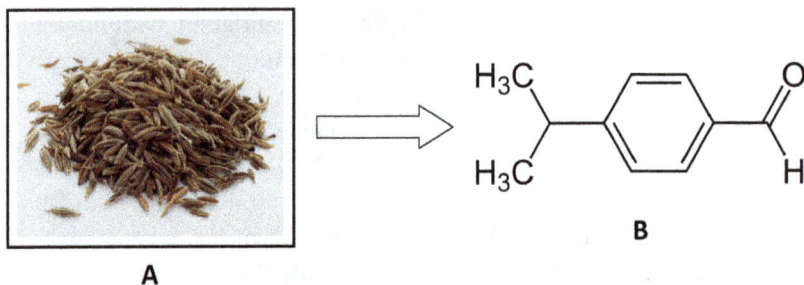

Figure 2.4 (A) Image of cumin and (B) Structure of cumin aldehyde.

2.2.5 Fenugreek

Trigonella foenum-graecum, often known as Methi belongs to the legume family and is an important herb used in conventional medicine. Fenugreek is the oldest herb or plant used for health purposes, it is grown commercially in India, Nepal, Pakistan, France, Egypt, Afghanistan, Iran, Turkey, Spain, Morocco, North Africa, and Argentina [10]. Among the bioactive compounds isolated from fenugreek seeds (Fig. 2.5) are saponins like fenugreekine and diosgenin, alkaloids, amino acids, and flavonoids, some of which act as insulin secretogogues (such as 4-hydroxy isoleucine and arginine), mucilaginous fibers, coumarins, nicotinic acid, and other minerals and vitamins. In addition to their amazing biological effects on enzymes and some cell types, flavonoids also exhibit antibacterial, antifungal, antiviral, antimalarial, antioxidant, anti-inflammatory, and anticarcinogenic capabilities. They also protect against allergies.

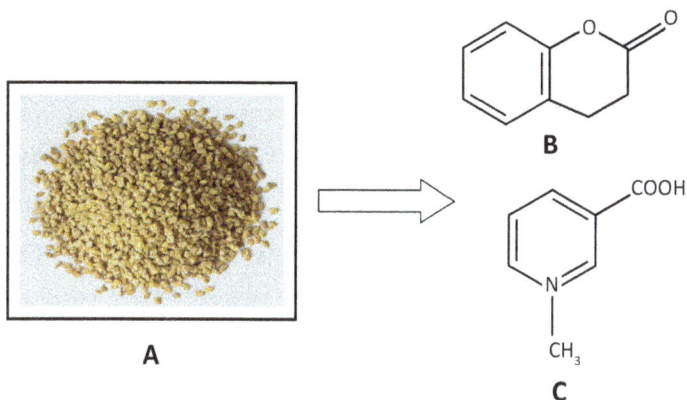

Figure 2.5 (A) Seeds of fenugreek, (B) Structure of coumarin, and (C) Structure of trigonelline.

The Elite-1 included a Perkin Elmer GC Claurus 500 system and gas chromatograph with a 30 m by 0.25 mm ID silica capillary column with a mass spectrometer (GC/MS). The GC/MS analysis of this sample was carried out using a 1 Mdf, constructed entirely of dimethylpolysiloxane. An electron ionization device with a 70 eV ionization energy was used for GC/MS detection. Helium gas (99.999%) was used as the carrier gas, with an injection volume of 2 L and a constant flow rate of 1 mL/min (split ratio of 10:1). The oven is preheated to 110 °C (isothermal for 2 minutes), then the temperature rises by 10 °C per minute to 200 °C, declines by 5 °C per minute to 280 °C, and finally remains at 280 °C for 9 minutes. With a 0.5-second scan interval, mass spectra were collected on fragments with sizes ranging from 45 to 450 Da. The GC lasted 36 minutes in total. Through a comparison of the average peak areas of each component to the total areas, we were able to determine the proportional percentage amount of each component. The software used to manage mass spectra and chromatograms was called TurboMass Ver5.2.0 [11].

2.2.6 Ginger

Spices like ginger (*Zingiber officinale* Roscoe) are well-liked and well-known. When compared to other chemical compounds, ginger has higher concentrations of phenolic compounds, polysaccharides, terpenes, organic acids, lipids, and raw fibers. Ginger, which belongs to the Zingiberaceae family and the genus Zingiber, has a long history of usage in cooking and as an herbal remedy. This spice contains phenolic and terpene compounds, among other active ingredients. Mostly gingerols, shogaols, and paradols make up ginger's phenolic compounds. In fresh ginger, the most prevalent polyphenols are gingerols, which comprise 6-, 8-, and 10-gingerol (Fig. 2.6). Storing or heating transforms gingerols into shogaols. Paradols form when shogaols are hydrogenated. The phenolic substances quercetin, zingerone, gingerenone-A, and 6-dehydrogingerdione are also found in ginger. Additionally, ginger contains terpenes that are thought to be the primary components of ginger essential oils, including -bisabolene, -curcumene, -zingiberene, -farnesene, and -sesquiphellandrene. The remaining components of ginger are lipids, polysaccharides, organic acids, and raw fibers [12].

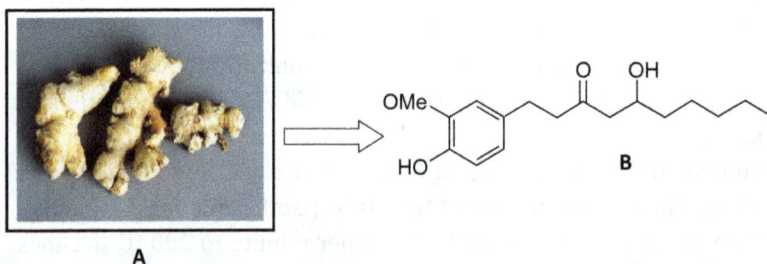

A

Figure 2.6 (A) Image of ginger and (B) Structure of [6]-gingerol.

2.2.7 Nutmeg

An annual spice from the Myristicaceae family is *Myristica fragrans*. Terpenes and phenylpropenes are the main components of nutmeg. Fats (30–40%) and essential oils (10%) are both present in nutmeg. GC-MS analysis is typically used to characterize essential oils. Nutmeg's distinct aroma is due to the presence of essential oil, which contains terpenes (pinene, sabinene, camphene, p-cymene, myrcene, and terpinene), terpene derivatives (geraniol, terpinol, and linalool), and phenylpropanes (safrole, myristicin, and elemicin) (Fig. 2.7) [13].

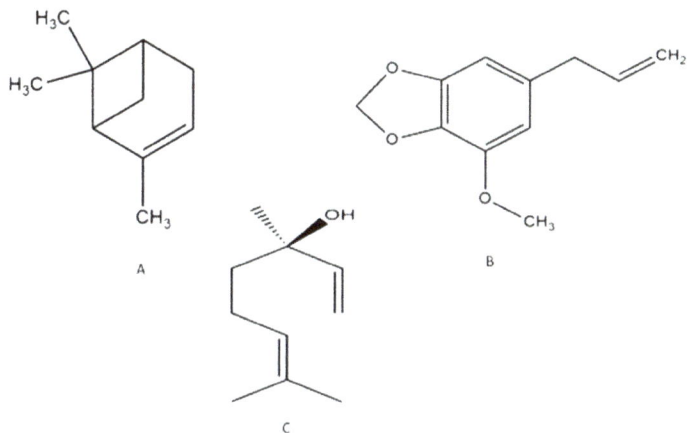

Figure 2.7 Structure of (A) alpha-pinene, (B) myristicin, and (C) linalool.

2.2.8 Turmeric

Turmeric, having the chemical formula $C_{21}H_{20}O_6$, is a polyphenol antioxidant phytochemical (Fig. 2.8). In addition to 5% volatile oil containing turmerone and zingiberene, cineole and other monoterpenes, starch, protein, high levels of vitamin A and other vitamins like vitamin C and E, as well as many carotenoids, and curcumin, it also contains 5% curcumin and curcuminoids.

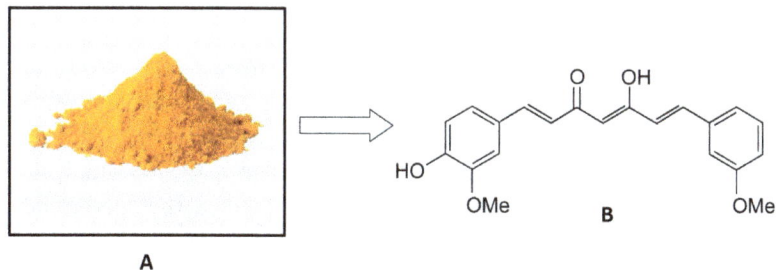

Figure 2.8 (A) Image of turmeric powder and (B) Structure of curcumin.

Curcumin is isolated and purified from crude extracts using methods such as column chromatography, high-performance liquid chromatography (HPLC), high-speed counter-current chromatography, and supercritical fluid chromatography [14].

2.2.9 Garlic

The popular spice garlic (*Allium sativum L.*) contains full of bioactive ingredients such as organic sulfides, saponins, phenolic compounds, and polysaccharides (Fig. 2.9). Bioactive substances found in garlic include polysaccharides, phenolic compounds, saponins, and organosulfur compounds. The main elements of garlic are organosulfur compounds such E/Z-ajoene, diallylthiosulfonate (allicin), diallyl disulfide (DADS), S-allyl-cysteine (SAC), diallyl trisulfide (DATS), diallyl sulfide (DAS), and S-allyl-cysteine sulfoxide (alliin) [15].

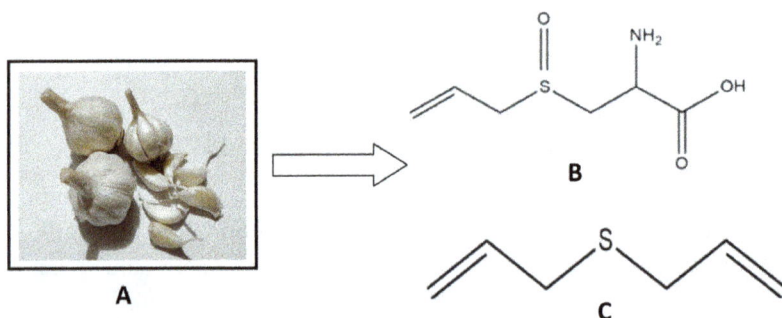

Figure 2.9 (A) Image of garlic, (B) Structure of alliin, and (C) Structure of diallyl sulfide.

2.2.10 Cardamom

The main bioactive ingredients of black and green cardamom were 1,8-cineole and terpinyl acetate, according to methodologies for identifying bioactive constituents, particularly GC-MS analysis (Fig. 2.10). The Zingiberaceae family includes the perennial herbaceous plant known as cardamom [16]. Several chromato-graphic techniques are used to characterize and quantify the bioactive components. For instance, distinct fractions of fatty acids and phytosterols, tocopherols, and lipids can all be separated using column chromatography, high-performance liquid chromatography, and gas chromatography. The primary bioactive ingredients in green and black cardamom that contribute to their pleasant and pungent scents, respectively, are 1,8-cineole (a potent antioxidant) and terpinyl acetate, according to a chromatographic investigation on cardamom phytochemicals. Among other bioactive compounds, cardamom also contains linalool acetate, sabinene, nerolidol, thujene, cymene, pinene, limonene, myrcene, and geranial. The GC-MS technique is a sophisticated analytical technique that is commonly used to evaluate physiologically active components present in cardamom phytochemicals. The following compounds were found in the green cardamom-derived sample: -terpinyl acetate (34.95%), linalool acetate (8.13%), 1,8-cineole (25.30%), limonene (2.80%), sabinene (5.48%), -terpineol (2.79%), myrcene (1.76%), -pinene (1.81%), and nerolidol [16].

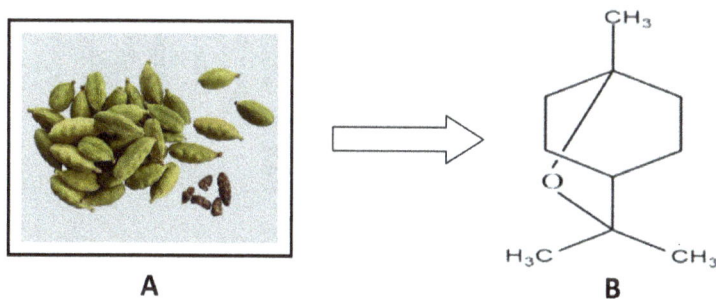

Figure 2.10 (A) Image of cardamom and (B) Structure of 1,8-cineole.

The chemical compositions, scientific names, and common names of different spices are given in Table 2.1.

2.3 Extraction

Spices contain a variety of bioactive chemicals that must be removed for maximum utilization in food preparation and the medical sector. Spice extraction requires the separation of these bioactive components depending on their solubility in various stages. Depending on the physical state of the spices, two procedures have traditionally been employed to extract bioactive components from

Table 2.1 The common names, scientific names, and chemical compositions of different spices

Sr. No.	Common name	Scientific name	Part used	Chemical composition
1.	Black pepper	*Piper nigrum*	Berry	Piperine, sarmentine, pinene, terpenes, limonene, camphene, isoquercetin, and piperidine
2.	Cinnamon	*Cinnamomum verum*	Bark	Eugenol, terpineol, limonene tannins, proanthocyanidins, linalool, pinene, safrole, catechins, benzaldehyde, and methyl eugenol
3.	Clove	*Syzygium aromaticum*	Bud	Eugenol, acetyl eugenol, isoeugenol, pinene, sesquiterpene, flavonoids, gallic acid, vanillin, and phenolic acids
4.	Cumin	*Cuminum cyminum*	Seed	
5.	Fenugreek	*Trigonella foenum-graecum*	Seed	Sesquiterpenes, terpenes, and aromatic aldehydes
6.	Ginger	*Zingiber officinale*	Root	Gingerol, zingiberon, turmeric, paradol, geranial, geraniol, borneol, linalool, zingerol, and camphene
7.	Nutmeg	*Myristica fragrans*	Seed	Catechins, caffeic acid, myricetin, lignans, and orgentin
8.	Turmeric	*Curcuma longa*	Root	Curcumins, vanillic acid, essential oils, carotene, eugenol, caffeic, protocatechuic, syringic, p-coumaric, and ascorbic acid.
9.	Garlic	*Allium sativum*	Root	Allicin, diallyl sulfide, diallyl trisulfide, diallyl disulfide, S-allyl cysteine, and allylisothiocyanate
10.	Cardamom	*Elettaria cardamomum*	Fruit	1,8-cineole, terpinyl linalool acetate, etc.

spices: solid-liquid extraction and liquid-liquid extraction. Bioactive components are partitioned between two immiscible liquids, polar and non-polar liquids such as water and chloroform, in the liquid-liquid extraction process. Solid-liquid extraction, on the other hand, involves separating the solid phase containing bioactive chemicals using solvents. Modern methods for extracting bioactive components from spices include enzyme-assisted extraction, ultrasonic and microwave-assisted extraction, supercritical fluid extraction, and pressurized liquid extraction. Modern methods for extracting bioactive components from spices include enzyme-assisted extraction, ultrasonic and microwave-assisted extraction, supercritical fluid extraction, and pressurized liquid extraction. These new procedures are less harmful to the environment, as well as more effective and cost-effective. Combinations of these procedures are also used to extract bioactive chemicals from spices. Overall, the process of removing bioactive elements from spices is the critical procedure that allows for the most effective utilization of their benefits in a variety of businesses. Modern approaches are proving to be a more sustainable and efficient way to extract spices [17].

2.4   Identification and Quantification of Bioactive Moieties Present in Spices

Using GC-MS, the total chemically active chemicals found in spices such as cinnamon, nutmeg, cardamom, and garlic were identified. However, each spice contained more than ten chemically active substances, the majority of which were volatile oils in various alpha and beta forms. They vary in terms of concentration, with some having the lowest concentrations and others having the highest concentrations. The GC-MS method of analysis has been used to identify and measure the volatile components in the spices. The amount of powdered spices utilized for the analysis was around 10 mg. A Restec RTX-5MS GC column with particular dimensions was employed in the GC-MS. Starting at 30 °C, the temperature gradient in the GC rose to 200 °C at a rate of 5 °C/min, then to 280 °C at a rate of 20 °C/min, where it stayed for

2 minutes. In split mode (1:10), helium gas was used as a carrier gas at a constant flow rate of 1.2 mL/min while the injector temperature was maintained at 230 °C. With an ion source temperature of 220 °C and an interface temperature of 260 °C, the mass detector was run in electron impact mode. By comparing the mass spectra obtained from the analysis with those in the NIST v1.7 database, chemicals were identified. The positive identification was taken into consideration when good matches (90% and above) were established. It is important to note that additional non-volatile chemicals that may be present in the spices may not be observed because this method only detects and quantifies volatile compounds. The use of HPLC to identify and measure bioactive substances in diverse plant extracts. With a UV-diode array detector and a Hypercil Gold column C18 column, the Waters 600 HPLC system was employed. To achieve the best chromatographic separation, a variety of gradient techniques were applied to a variety of samples. Using an isocratic technique using an acetonitrile and 2% acetic acid mobile phase at a flow rate of 1 mL/min for 30 minutes, and detection at 425 nm, the active components in turmeric were measured. The same mobile phases, A: 0.2% aqueous formic acid and B: methanol, with different gradients at flow rates of 0.8 mL/min and column temperatures of 24 °C, were employed for the ginger samples. Using a unique gradient, ginger was seen at 265 nm. Using a gradient program and mobile phases of 10% methanol at pH 3.5 with 0.01% formic acid and methanol, water, and acetonitrile (20:20:60) at pH 3.5 with 0.01% formic acid, curry leaf bioactive components were detected at room temperature. 1 mL/min was the constant flow rate, and 366 nm was used for detection. Curry leaf bioactive components were identified at room temperature using a gradient program and mobile phases of 10% methanol at pH 3.5 with 0.01% formic acid and methanol, water, and acetonitrile (20:20:60) at pH 3.5 with 0.01% formic acid. The constant flow rate was 1 mL/min, and the detection wavelength was 366 nm [17].

2.5 Conclusions

From the above study, it may be concluded that spices can be used whole or in crushed form while cooking. They enhance food quality and also provide many health effects. The identification and quantification of these spices provide information about different constituents and also provide information about their quality and safety while using these spices by different analytical techniques. The phytochemical and pharmacological properties of several spices as active medicinal ingredients demonstrated their utility in pharmaceutical chemistry and biomedicine. Various synthesis strategies, extraction, and detection techniques highlighted the significance of these spices in the creation of novel natural treatments.

References

1. https://www.researchgate.net/publication/363683775_Spice_ Bioactive_Compounds_Properties_Applications_and_Health_Benefits/ link/632c0c77071ea12e3651d22f/download (accessed 2023-07-13).

2. Osman, A.; Raman, V.; Ali, Z.; Chittiboyina, A.; Khan, I. Overview of Analytical Tools for the Identification of Adulterants in Commonly Traded Herbs and Spices. *J. AOAC Int.* **2019**. https://doi.org/10.5740/ jaoacint.18-0389.

3. Gorgani, L.; Mohammadi, M.; Najafpour, G.; Nikzad, M. Piperine-The Bioactive Compound of Black Pepper: From Isolation to Medicinal Formulations: Piperine Isolation from Pepper. *Comprehensive Reviews in Food Science and Food Safety* **2016**, *16*. https://doi. org/10.1111/1541-4337.12246.

4. Rao, P. V.; Gan, S. H. Cinnamon: A Multifaceted Medicinal Plant. *Evid Based Complement Alternat Med* **2014**, *2014*, 642942. https://doi. org/10.1155/2014/642942.

5. Kamatou, G. P.; Vermaak, I.; Viljoen, A. M. Eugenol--from the Remote Maluku Islands to the International Market Place: A Review of a Remarkable and Versatile Molecule. *Molecules* **2012**, *17* (6), 6953–6981. https://doi.org/10.3390/molecules17066953.

6. Neveu, V.; Perez-Jiménez, J.; Vos, F.; Crespy, V.; du Chaffaut, L.; Mennen, L.; Knox, C.; Eisner, R.; Cruz, J.; Wishart, D.; Scalbert, A. Phenol-Explorer: An Online Comprehensive Database on Polyphenol Contents in Foods. *Database* **2010**, *2010*, bap024. https://doi.org/10.1093/database/bap024.

7. Cortés-Rojas, D. F.; de Souza, C. R. F.; Oliveira, W. P. Clove (Syzygium Aromaticum): A Precious Spice. *Asian Pac J Trop Biomed* **2014**, *4* (2), 90–96. https://doi.org/10.1016/S2221-1691(14)60215-X.

8. Ulanowska, M.; Olas, B. Biological Properties and Prospects for the Application of Eugenol—A Review. *International Journal of Molecular Sciences* **2021**, *22*, 3671. https://doi.org/10.3390/ijms22073671.

9. Srinivasan, K. Cumin (Cuminum Cyminum) and Black Cumin (Nigella Sativa) Seeds: Traditional Uses, Chemical Constituents, and Nutraceutical Effects. *Food Quality and Safety* **2018**, *2*. https://doi.org/10.1093/fqsafe/fyx031.

10. Idris, S.; Mishra, A.; Khushtar, M. Recent Therapeutic Interventions of Fenugreek Seed: A Mechanistic Approach. *Drug Res (Stuttg)* **2021**, *71* (4), 180–192. https://doi.org/10.1055/a-1320-0479.

11. Priya, V.; Jananie, R. K.; Vijayalakshmi, K. GC/MS Determination of Bioactive Components of TrigonellaFoenumGrecum. *J. Chem. Pharm. Res.* **2011**, *3* (5).

12. *Bioactive Compounds and Bioactivities of Ginger (Zingiberofficinale Roscoe)* - *PMC*. https://www.ncbi.nlm.nih.gov/pmc/articles/PMC6616534/ (accessed 2023-07-13).

13. Naeem, N.; Rehman, R.; Mushtaq, A.; Ghania, B. *Nutmeg: A Review on Uses and Biological Properties.* **2016**, 107–110.

14. *Frontiers | Curcumin Extraction, Isolation, Quantification and Its Application in Functional Foods: A Review with a Focus on Immune Enhancement Activities and COVID-19*. https://www.frontiersin.org/articles/10.3389/fnut.2021.747956/full (accessed 2023-07-13).

15. Shang, A.; Cao, S.-Y.; Xu, X.-Y.; Gan, R.-Y.; Tang, G.-Y.; Corke, H.; Mavumengwana, V.; Li, H.-B. Bioactive Compounds and Biological Functions of Garlic (Allium Sativum L.). *Foods* **2019**, *8* (7), 246. https://doi.org/10.3390/foods8070246.

16. Abdullah; Ahmad, N.; Tian, W.; Zengliu, S.; Zou, Y.; Farooq, S.; Huang, Q.; Xiao, J. Recent Advances in the Extraction, Chemical Composition, Therapeutic Potential, and Delivery of Cardamom Phytochemicals.

Front. Nutr. **2022**, *9*, 1024820. https://doi.org/10.3389/fnut.2022.1024820.

17. Sepahpour, S.; Selamat, J.; Abdul Manap, M. Y.; Khatib, A.; AbdullRazis, A. F. Comparative Analysis of Chemical Composition, Antioxidant Activity and Quantitative Characterization of Some Phenolic Compounds in Selected Herbs and Spices in Different Solvent Extraction Systems. *Mol. Basel Switz.* **2018**, *23* (2), 402. https://doi.org/10.3390/molecules23020402.

Chapter 3

Worldwide Uses of Spices

Ujjawal Sharma,[a] **Ambrish Mishra,**[a] **Praveen Kumar Sahni,**[a]
Bunty Sharma,[b] **and Hardeep Singh Tuli**[b]

[a]*Department of Human Genetics and Molecular Medicine,*
School of Health Sciences, Central University of Punjab, Bathinda, Punjab, India
[b]*Department of Biosciences and Technology,*
Maharishi Markandeshwar Engineering College,
Maharishi Markandeshwar (Deemed to be University), Mullana, Ambala, India

sharmabunty097@gmail.com

3.1 Introduction

Spice refers to the desiccated fruit, seed, bark, flower, or root of an herb or plant, which is employed in minimal quantities to enhance taste, add color, or aid in preservation (Kunnumakkara et al., 2009). Spices are defined as "vegetable products or mixtures thereof, free from extraneous matter, used for flavoring, seasoning and imparting aroma to foods" by the International Organization for Standardization (ISO) (ISO 676:1995(En), Spices and Condiments — Botanical Nomenclature, n.d.).

Spices originated in warm and humid climate areas, primarily in India and Southeast Asia, and their availability was initially

Anticancer Spices: Dietary Input to Health
Edited by Hardeep Singh Tuli
Copyright © 2025 Jenny Stanford Publishing Pte. Ltd.
ISBN 978-981-5129-28-1 (Hardcover), 978-1-003-53466-2 (eBook)
www.jennystanford.com

restricted to some areas of the world (Darriet, 2007). Since ancient civilizations, spices have been used in culinary and medicinal applications due to their flavor and qualities (Parthasarathy et al., 2008). The expeditions undertaken to Africa and India, along with exploratory voyages to uncharted territories; for instance, the Spice Islands, resulted in identifying the novel species in Europe and establishing the intricate networks for the spice trade. Nowadays, India, China, Madagascar, and Indonesia dominate spice production (Elizabeth et al., 2017). The tropical spice crops that hold significant global commercial value include pepper, ginger, allspice/pimento, cardamom, cinnamon, cloves, and turmeric (UNIDO and FAO, 2005). The major exporters and importers of spices are depicted in Figs. 3.1 and 3.2.

Cancer is one of the leading causes of death in the world. Nearly 10 million cancer-related deaths were projected globally in 2020, with 19.3 million new cancer diagnoses (Sung et al., 2021). Radiation, chemotherapy, and surgery are the main ways to treat cancer. However, surgery or radiation only helps localized and small tumors. Small tumors may respond to chemotherapy alone. They may also be harmful. Thus, new, side-effect-free cancer treatments are needed. Spices may reduce nausea, vomiting, and indigestion induced by chemotherapy (Giacosa et al., 2015; IJpma et al., 2015). Numerous bioactive chemicals with diverse health benefits are present in various spices, rendering them valuable medicinal herbs in traditional folk medicine for the treatment of many diseases (Zheng et al., 2016a).

Natural bioactive substances derived from various plant sources, including spices, have received significant attention for treating various cancer types (Singh et al., 2022; Singh et al., 2022b; Kumar et al., 2023). For instance, numerous studies have demonstrated that spices contain antioxidants, including curcumin (found in turmeric), eugenol (found in cloves), and capsaicin (found in red pepper). These antioxidants have been discovered to efficiently reduce cellular oxidative stress due to their antioxidant capabilities and ability to prevent the generation of reactive oxygen species (Rubió et al., 2013; Srinivasan, 2014; Kumar et al., 2017). Certain bioactive compounds of spices, such as curcumin and thymoquinone, were found to influence inflammatory processes (Ghosh et al., 2014; Majdalawieh & Fayyad, 2015). Furthermore, spices, especially some from the genus Cinnamomum, were sometimes exploited as a source of alternate antibacterial medications (Nabavi et al., 2015). Majdalawieh and Fayyad (2015) discovered that other spice components, such as thymoquinone, exhibit immunomodulatory properties. Numerous studies have found that spices have anti-inflammatory, antioxidant, and immunomodulatory activities (Nilius & Appendino, 2013). These properties are particularly significant because of oxidative stress (Fu et al., 2011; Guo et al., 2012; Deng et al., 2012; Li et al., 2013a; Bensimon et al., 2016; Chang et al., 2016), inflammatory stress (Amara et al., 2016; Maisonneuve et al., 2016), and immunological reaction (Hegde et al., 2016; Ubillos et al., 2016), which have all been closely linked with the development, progression, and spreading of cancer (Li et al., 2013b; Li et al., 2013c; Zhou et al., 2016). As a result, there is promising potential for using spices in the prevention and treatment of cancer. Indeed, the available epidemiological and experimental evidence indicates that specific spices possess the potential to mitigate the likelihood of developing particular types of cancers (Butt et al., 2013; Fridlender et al., 2015; Park et al., 2015; Zick et al., 2015; Zheng et al., 2016a).

This chapter discusses major spices, namely, clove (*Syzygium aromaticum L.*), black cumin (*Nigella sativa*), saffron (*Crocus sativus*), black pepper (*Piper nigrum L.*), red chili pepper (*Capsicum annuum*), oregano (*Origanum vulgare*), rosemary (*Rosmarinus officinalis*), cardamom (*Elettaria cardamomum*), turmeric (*Curcuma longa*), garlic (*Allium sativum L.*), ginger (*Zingiber officinale*), cinnamon (*Cinnamomum cassia*), and coriander (*Coriandrum sativum L.*), which are used worldwide and possess significant anti-cancerous properties.

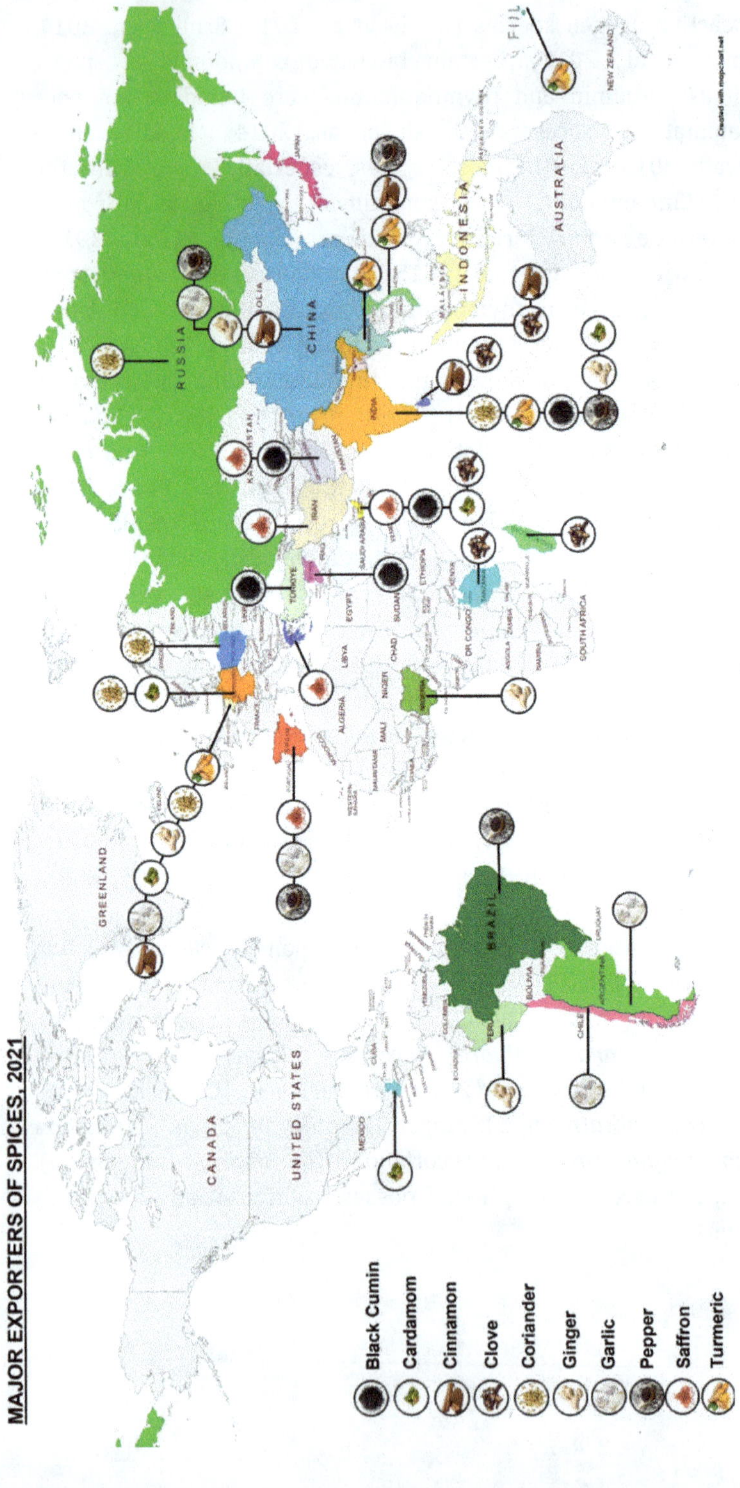

Figure 3.1 Major exporters of spices (2021).

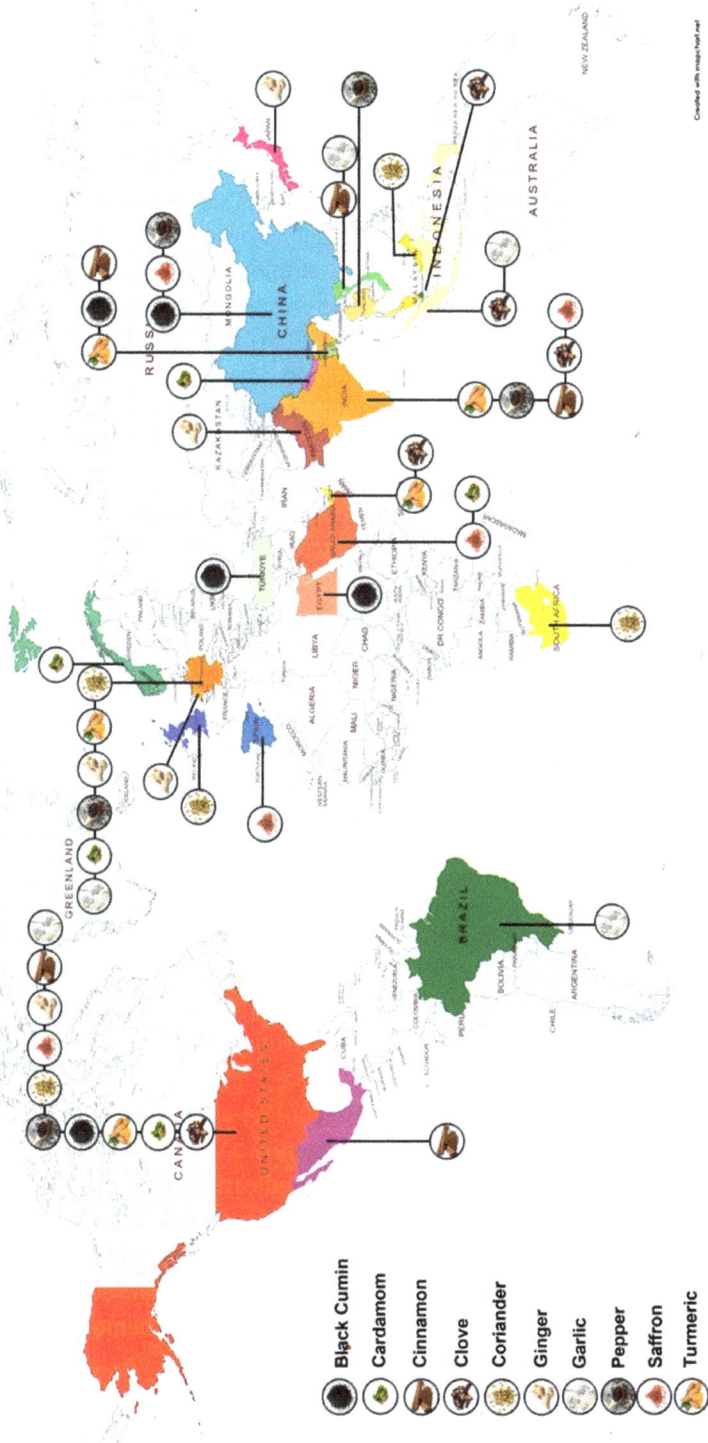

Figure 3.2 Major importers of spices (2021).

3.2 Clove

Clove (*Syzygium aromaticum L.*), a perennial spice crop that is Myrtaceae family member, is known for its wide variety of biological activities and is recognized as an essential plant in traditional medicine (Zari et al., 2021a). Due to its strong flavor and aroma, which have increased how much food people appreciate worldwide, cloves are employed as a culinary spice. When cooking, cloves can be used whole or ground to flavor a wide range of dishes, from sweet to savory (Herbst, 2001). Historically, cloves have been used in Mexican food, where they are frequently combined with cumin and Canela (cinnamon), as well as in Indian food (both North and South Indian) (Dornenburg & Page, 2003).

Clove trees are commonly cultivated in coastal areas, with a preference for elevations not exceeding 200 meters above sea level. According to Kamatou et al. (2012), the current leading countries in clove production include India, Indonesia, Sri Lanka, Malaysia, Madagascar, and Tanzania, with a specific focus on the island of Zanzibar and Brazil (Oliveira et al., 2007).

The phenolic chemicals flavonoids, hydroxybenzoic acids, hydroxycinnamic acids, and hydroxyphenyl propens are primarily found in plants, and clove is one of the key sources. Eugenol (EUG), or 4-allyl-2-methoxyphenol ($C_{10}H_{12}O_2$), is the main bioactive compound of clove (Neveu et al., 2010a). It contains several functional groups, like allyl ($-CH_2-CH=CH_2$), methoxy ($-OCH_3$), and phenol (OH). EUG is an aromatic, pale yellow liquid that exhibits partial solubility in water and significant solubility in organic solvents (Zari et al., 2021a). The concentrations of EUG in the fresh plant material range from 9.4 g to 14. 6 g per 100 g (Neveu et al., 2010b).

The biological benefits of eugenol (4-allyl-2-methoxyphenol) include its antioxidant, anticarcinogenic, antibacterial, antifungal, and insecticidal properties. This medication has no cytotoxic impacts on healthy cells, even at high doses. The Food and Drug Administration (FDA) of the United States has concluded that EUG is neither mutagenic nor carcinogenic (Nisar et al., 2021; Zari et al., 2021b). The combination of EUG and a chemo-inhibitory medication demonstrates a synergistic effect, resulting in a notable reduction in drug toxicity toward healthy cells (Gemma et al., 2001). In an *in vitro* experiment, gemcitabine's effects are enhanced by a tiny amount of EUG despite having no negative effects on healthy cells (Nisar et al., 2021). EUG has demonstrated anticancer activity against several cancer types, including lung, leukemia, colorectal, cervical, breast, gastric, prostate, skin, and colon cancers (Yi et al., 2015; Nisar et al., 2021; Petrocelli et al., 2021; Ulanowska & Olas, 2021). Several breast cancer cell types are explicitly lethal to EUG at low doses. This deadly effect is principally made possible by intensely suppressing E2F1 and its downstream antiapoptotic target while activating the intrinsic apoptotic pathway, which still functions without p53 (Al-Sharif et al., 2013). The EUG compound inhibits various oncogenes associated with breast cancer, including NF-κB and cyclin D1. Furthermore, Zari et al. (2021b) discovered that EUG had an upregulation effect on the p21WAF1 protein, a flexible inhibitor of cyclin-dependent kinases, and efficiently reduced breast cancer cell proliferation in the presence or absence of p53. A study found that eugenol had a strong antimutagenic effect on breast cancer cells, specifically the MCF-7 subtype. The inhibitory effect of EUG on MCF-7 cell proliferation is dependent on the duration and dosage of its treatment (Anuj & Sanjay, 2010; Vidhya & Devaraj, 2011).

3.3 Black Cumin

Black cumin (*Nigella sativa*) is a member of the botanical family Ranunculaceae. Western Asia, Eastern Europe, and the Middle East are among the regions where it frequently flourishes (Randhawa & Alghamdi, 2011). Despite its widespread cultivation, black cumin is claimed to be a native of the "Mediterranean region," according to literature (Dessie et al., 2020).

It is a small shrub with green leaves that taper to a point and rosaceous white flowers with a purplish tinge (Randhawa & Alghamdi, 2011). Indian, Middle Eastern, and North African curries, rice, bread, and sweets are seasoned with roasted and ground seeds (Nova et al., 2021). The Unani, Ayurvedic, Chinese, and Arabic systems of traditional medicine, as well as the traditional medicine of several Asian countries, all use the seeds of the *Nigella sativa* plant to treat and prevent illness (Randhawa & Alghamdi, 2011). It is additionally used for bread and pickles as a seasoning agent (El-Kadi & Kandil, 1986; Al-Jishi, 2000). Many researchers were inspired to separate *Nigella sativa*'s active compounds, including thymohydroquinone, thymoquinone, thymol, dithymoquinone, carvacrol, nigellicine, alpha-hederin, nigellimine-N-oxide, and nigellidine, because of the plant's varied usage in traditional medicine (Randhawa & Al-Ghamdi, 2002).

Thymoquinone (TQ), also known as 2-isopropyl-5-methyl-1,4-benzoquinone, is an important bioactive component of *Nigella sativa* seeds. It possesses powerful chemo-preventive and chemotherapeutic effects (Schneider-Stock et al., 2014). The anticancer qualities of TQ have been demonstrated in numerous studies to be effective against several cancers (Khan et al., 2011).

Research findings have indicated that TQ may function as an inhibitor of Akt. The activation (phosphorylation) of Akt can be facilitated by PI3K, thereby promoting cell survival through inhibiting apoptosis. This is accomplished by inhibiting downstream targets such as Bcl-2 family members BAD and GSK-3 (Franke & Cantley, 1997). TQ has an anti-proliferative impact on human myeloblastic leukemia HL-60 cells in cases of blood cancer, according to ElMahdy et al. (2005). TQ-containing terpene-terminated 6-alkyl residues have been discovered to induce apoptosis. The study conducted by Effenberger et al. (2010) demonstrated that the terpene-terminated 6-alkyl residues of TQ exhibited the ability to induce apoptosis of MCF-7/Topo breast carcinoma and KB-V1/Vb1 cervical carcinoma by down-regulating the androgen receptor and the transcription factor E2F-1, TQ decreased DNA synthesis, cell proliferation, and viability in malignant prostate epithelial cells (LNCaP, DU145, C4-B, and PC-3). However, these effects were not observed in non-cancerous prostate epithelial cells (BPH-1). TQ has been effective in treating both hormone-sensitive and hormone-refractory prostate cancer, according to guidelines. TQ's oral administration, which boosts the activities of glutathione transferase and quinone reductase, is responsible for its possible preventive efficacy. This makes TQ a good candidate for reducing the toxicity of liver cancer and chemical carcinogenesis (Kaseb et al., 2007; Nagi & Almakki, 2009).

3.4 Saffron

Saffron, scientifically known as *Crocus sativus*, is an Iridaceae family member. This highly valued spice is obtained by harvesting the plant's dried, deep red flower stigmas. It is widely acknowledged as one of the priciest spices in the world (Maghsoodi et al., 2012). According to Tong et al. (2015), the primary countries responsible for the majority of its distribution are Iran, Spain, China, Morocco, Greece, Italy, and India. Saffron is utilized as a chromatic and gustatory constituent in comestibles and cosmetic products, owing to its characteristic pigmentation and fragrance (Ahrazem et al., 2015; Bononi et al., 2020). Around the world, saffron is employed in many culinary creations. In Sweden, it is used to make saffron buns (known as lussekat), and it is utilized in various salty or sweet-and-salty foods in Morocco and the Italian confectionery and alcohol sectors. Saffron has been used as a fabric dye in China and India (Willard, 2002; Kafi, 2006).

The chemical study has revealed that saffron stigmas contain more than 150 different substances, including flavonoids, carotenoids, terpenoids, and alkaloids (Bathaie & Mousavi, 2010; Rahaiee et al., 2015; Broadhead et al., 2016). Between them, the most important chemicals are carotenoids since they decide the color and flavor of the spice (Gismondi et al., 2012).

Picrocrocin ($C_{16}H_{26}O_7$), Crocin ($C_{44}H_{64}O_{24}$), Crocetin ($C_{20}H_{24}O_{40}$), and Safranal ($C_{10}H_{14}O$) are the four primary chemical components of saffron (Ashktorab et al., 2019). Additionally, saffron has shown promise in the treatment of various cancers like lung, gastric, skin, colorectal, hepatic, cervical, prostate, ovarian, pancreatic, and breast (Bhandari, 2015; Shahi et al., 2016; Xing et al., 2021).

Certain bioactive components of saffron are known to have antitumor actions because they inhibit cell development.

Intriguingly, these substances do not impact healthy cells (Bolhassani et al., 2014). Hepatocarcinoma HepG2 cells exhibit cytotoxicity in response to crocin, a bioactive compound of saffron. Crocin and crocetin decreased the growth and invasion of colorectal cancer cells as well as the size of tumors and HL-60 xenografts in nude mice. Additionally, the colorectal cancer cell lines HCT-116, SW-480, and HT-29 are significantly inhibited in their ability to proliferate by these compounds (Noureini & Wink, 2012; Sun et al., 2013; Amerizadeh et al., 2018; Zhuang et al., 2018; Xing et al., 2021). Because it inhibits cell proliferation by generating cell cycle arrest through p53-dependent or p53-independent P21-mediated pathways, crocetin has special anticancer properties (C.-Y. Li et al., 2012). It inhibits growth factor signaling pathways, inhibits nucleic acid synthesis, stimulates the immune system, causes apoptosis, and affects the formation of cancer cells (Gutheil et al., 2012).

3.5 Black Pepper

Black pepper (*Piper nigrum L.*), sometimes known as "pepper," is a perennial woody aromatic climber that can reach heights of 50–60 cm (Bui et al., 2017). The word "pepper" derives from the Sanskrit word pippali, which means berry (Kumar et al., 2011). Because of its enormous trading share on the international market, black pepper is regarded as the "king of spices" (Srinivasan, 2007). Black pepper can be used as a spice, preservative, pesticide, and in herbal medicine, among other things (Wang et al., 2017).

Most of the time, *Piper nigrum* (*P. nigrum*) is grown in hot and humid places. The South Indian Peninsula's Western Ghats are where black pepper is primarily grown. It spread to additional South and Southeast Asian nations (Takooree et al., 2019a). Currently, Vietnam produces the most black pepper in the world, with the majority of it being farmed in the southern part of the nation (Hao et al., 2012). The top four countries in the world for pepper production are Vietnam, Indonesia, India, and Brazil (Takooree et al., 2019b). The cultivation of pepper in countries such as Indonesia and Vietnam has substantially impacted India's production, resulting in a significant decline over time (Hussain et al., 2017).

The primary usage of *P. nigrum* is as a component in food. It is largely used in Western cuisine as a flavor enhancer and preservation (Ravindran & Kallupurackal, 2012). *P. nigrum* is well-known for its use in traditional medicine to cure a variety of ailments as well as its culinary applications. Current cell, animal, and human studies indicate that piperine has immunomodulatory, anti-inflammatory, antioxidant, and anticarcinogenic properties (Ravindran & Kallupurackal, 2012). The main alkaloid components of black pepper, piperine, and piperidine have antitumor effects on a number of cancers (Zheng et al., 2016b; Mitra et al., 2022).

These substances possess the capacity to initiate various molecular mechanisms, subsequently leading to cancer cell apoptosis. The recent discovery of the anticancer effect of piperidine and piperine has shed light on their underlying mechanism. This mechanism entails activating signaling pathways such as NF-κB and PI3K/Akt, which play crucial roles in cancer progression. Notably, this activation triggers the caspase-dependent pathway, ultimately leading to cell death (Rather & Bhagat, 2018; Zadorozhna et al., 2019). The application of piperine resulted in breast cancer cells reduced cell proliferation and elevated apoptosis by activating caspase-3 and cleaving PARP. Piperine's interference with the ERK1/2 and p38 MAPK signaling pathways was found to suppress EGF-induced MMP-9 synthesis and subsequent migration. Piperine administration increased the paclitaxel responsiveness of breast cancer cells that overexpress the human epidermal growth factor receptor (HER 2) in a 2013 study by Do et al. Si et al. (2018) found that the dosage and duration of exposure affect piperine's ability to inhibit the proliferation of human ovarian cancer A2780 cells. However, this effect is not observed in healthy human surface epithelial (OSE) cells. Previous studies have demonstrated that the interleukin-6 (IL-6) cytokine can promote the invasion of gastric cancer cells by activating the c-Src/RhoA/ROCK signaling pathway. Conversely, piperine has exhibited its efficacy in inhibiting gastric cancer through various trials (Lin et al., 2007). The study conducted by Xia et al. (2015) revealed that piperine has the capability to inhibit the expression of IL-6, thereby impeding the invasive potential of gastric cancer cells (TMK-1) concerning their ability to infiltrate neighboring cells.

3.6   Red Chili Pepper

The red chili pepper, or *Capsicum annuum*, of the genus Capsicum, is an herb or small shrub that may grow to a height of 0.3–1.2 meters (1–4 feet), and it is family "Solanaceae" member. It is one of the world's most popular spices. The ancestors of the C. annuum species are believed to have originated in northern South America, according to genetic and archaeological data (Surh et al., 1998; Britannica, 2020). Currently, the top red pepper-producing countries are China, Mexico, Turkey, Africa, India, and Peru (https://uses.plantnetproject.org/e/index.php?title=Capsicum_annuum_(PROTA)&oldid=328098). Chili peppers are used in food but also play a part in various illnesses, including obesity, gastrointestinal and cardiovascular disorders, malignancies, neurogenic bladder, and dermatological issues (Sharma et al., 2013).

The active ingredient in chili peppers, capsaicin ($C_{18}H_{27}NO_3$, 8-methyl-N-vanillyl-6-nonenamide, is an alkaloid (capsaicinoid). This capsaicinoid is responsible for the spice's pungency and is also an irritant that induces a burning sensation in whatever tissue it comes into contact with (Srinivasan, 2016). For its capacity to prevent chemo, capsaicin has received much research. Capsaicin has anti-growth properties against many cancer cell lines (Liu et al., 2012). According to research findings, capsaicin has an inhibitory effect on the multiplication of breast cancer cells, as demonstrated by tests conducted by Cao et al. in 2019. Chou et al. (2009) found that after a 24-hour exposure to capsaicin, MCF-7 cells demonstrated a dose-dependent activation of apoptosis in an *in vitro* setting. This apoptotic response was observed to occur through a caspase-independent mechanism. In an alternative investigation, the application of capsaicin decreased *in vitro* proliferation and inhibited the migratory capabilities of various cell lines, namely, MDA-MB231, MCF-7, SKBR-3, T47D, and BT-474. According to Thoennissen et al. (2010), the application of capsaicin demonstrated significant inhibition of preneoplastic breast lesions by 80% in an *in vivo* setting.

Additionally, the treatment of capsaicin reduced the size of mice's breast tumors by 50% without causing any obvious negative effects. By limiting the breakdown of IκBα and subsequently obstructing the translocation of p65 into the nucleus, capsaicin successfully suppresses the activation of NF-κB in human promyelocytic leukemia HL-60 cells, especially when TPA stimulation is present (Han et al., 2002). It should be mentioned that there is debate concerning capsaicin's connection to cancer. According to several researches, capsaicin alone is mutagenic, encourages the growth of tumors, and may raise cancer risk in people (Li et al., 2017).

3.7 Oregano

The term "oregano" is used to describe a wide range of plants that all have a similar flavor and aroma. Oregano is a name that refers to at least 60 species and 17 genera that are members of numerous plant families (Gutiérrez-Grijalva et al., 2017). The Greek words "oros" (meaning mountain) and "ganos" (meaning joy), which describe the area where the plant is cultivated, are the source of the name Origanum (Gómez & Ramírez, 2007). Additionally, it is grown in Greece, the Dominican Republic, Turkey, Italy, Mexico, and Italy. It is present throughout the temperate Himalayas of India, from Kashmir to Sikkim (Oregano | Spices Board, n.d.).

Typically, the genus exhibits characteristics of a perennial herb or subshrub, possessing creeping roots, erect woody stems, and leaves ranging from sub-sessile to petiolate, displaying a hairy texture (Salvo et al., 2019). Although stem lengths might vary, most species have stems between 30 and 60 cm long (Sharifi-Rad et al., 2021). Different cultures actively employ Origanum plants in daily life. The Origanum plant, often known as "oregano" or "pizza spice," has been used as a spice for centuries and was once very common in Southern European nations, including Italy, Greece, France, and Spain, as well as Mexico (Sharifi-Rad et al., 2021). Despite its use in food, this spice has a long history of use in herbal medicine worldwide. Origanum plants have a wide range of biological actions, including hepatoprotective, antidiabetic, and anticancer characteristics (Teixeira et al., 2013).

The main bioactive compound in oregano, specifically in the essential oils derived from *Origanum vulgare*, is carvacrol (CV; C10H14O). Carvacrol is a liquid phenolic monoterpenoid characterized by its chemical structure as 2 methyl-5-(1-methyl ethyl) phenol. It is responsible for the various biological effects of oregano, including its anticancer, antioxidant, and anti-microbial properties (Sharifi-Rad, 2018a). Multiple studies have provided evidence indicating that CV exhibits significant genotoxic, cytotoxic, and proapoptotic properties on cancer cells, with the intensity of these effects dependent on the dosage administered. According to the studies, it has been observed to influence cell invasion by downregulating matrix metalloproteases 2 and 9 the expression. Multiple studies have documented the impact of cardiovascular exercise on breast cancer (Arunasree, 2010; Yin et al., 2012; Fan et al., 2015). The p53 gene regulates apoptosis, through its interaction with the Bcl2 family. It accomplishes this by directly activating the transcription of the Bax gene through the promoter of the Bax, thereby increasing its expression. Simultaneously, it reduces the expression of the Bcl2 gene. According to a study, the administration of CV, a chemotherapeutic agent, to MCF7 cells, a breast cancer cell line known for its sensitivity to chemotherapy, resulted in the reduction of the Bcl2 gene expression and a dose-dependent Bax gene upregulation (Al-Fatlawi et al., 2014). CV caused G0/G1 arrest of cell cycle and reactive oxygen species-mediated death in prostate cancer cells from humans (Khan et al., 2017).

Numerous studies have shown that CV nano-emulsion is effective at killing A549 lung cancer cells. These studies have collectively determined that the primary mechanism through which CV nano-emulsion induces the production of reactive oxygen species (ROS) within the mitochondria of A549 cells is by initiating diverse cellular processes that ultimately activate the mitochondria-mediated intrinsic apoptotic pathway (Ren et al., 2015; Elmore, 2007). Colorectal cancer, commonly called colon cancer, is a malignant neoplasm originating in the colon or rectum. A separate study on the disease observed that treating HCT116 and LoVo cells with CV resulted in a dose-dependent decrease in proliferation, invasion, and migration (Sharifi-Rad, 2018b).

3.8   Rosemary

The Mediterranean region is the primary source of therapeutic rosemary (*Rosmarinus officinalis*). It is a perennial herb of the Lamiaceae family that is evergreen. It can grow to a height of 2 meters and has green leaves with a distinctive scent (De Oliveira et al., 2019; Kammath et al., 2021). It is grown in California, the US, and Europe. Additionally, it is grown in China, Algeria, India, the Middle East, Romania, Morocco, Russia, Tunisia, Serbia, and Turkey. The cultivation of rosemary is ideal for a temperate climate (Rosemary | Spices Board, n.d.). *R. Officinalis* is a plant that can be used as a decorative, medicinal, cooking spice, and natural food preservative (De Oliveira et al., 2019). Besides other, anti-inflammatory and anticancer properties are also present (Begum et al., 2013; Ojeda-Sana et al., 2013; Ribeiro-Santos et al., 2015).

The primary polyphenols found in rosemary extract (RE) are the diterpenes rosmarinic acid (RA) and carnosic acid (CA) (Cuvelier et al., 1994). Recent research has indicated that rosemary extract and its polyphenols CA and RA have anticancer effects. Several *in vitro* experiments using colon cancer cell lines have shown that RE has anticancer properties. The formation of colonies in CaCo-2 (Colorectal adenocarcinoma) colon cancer cells was significantly reduced after exposure to RE at a specified dosage (Slameňová et al., 2002). Other studies point to the ability of RE to, at certain dosages, inhibit pancreatic and breast cancer cell survival and proliferation and cause apoptosis (Tsiani et al., 2016). Another study found that rosemary ethanol extracts significantly decreased prostate cancer cell (LNCaP) viability concentration-dependently (Bourhia et al., 2019).

3.9   Cardamom

Elettaria cardamomum, commonly referred to as the "Queen of Spices," belongs to the Zingiberaceae family. This aromatic spice is characterized by its sweet fragrance and is recognized for its thick, evergreen stems that can reach heights of 2–4 meters. Following saffron and vanilla on the list of most costly spices is cardamom. The plant produces green or real cardamom, segmented scented pods or capsules with 15–20 seeds. (Krishnan et al., 2005; Ryes et al., 2006).

The *Elettaria cardamomum* plant originated on India's Malabar coast and is the type of cardamom that Guatemala cultivates and is the world's top producer. India is the world's second-largest producer of cardamom. It is widely grown in India, particularly in the South Indian hills. Cardamom is also produced in Tanzania, Papua New Guinea, and Sri Lanka. The primary markets for cardamom include the Middle East, South Asia, Southeast Asia, and Europe. The largest import market for cardamom is Saudi Arabia (The World Market for Cardamom, n.d.). The entire cardamom pod contains tough black seeds used in specific recipes. The spice's essential oil, which has traces of mint and lemon and gives the spice its flavor and aroma, is present in these seeds. The seeds are pounded using a mortar and pestle before being added to South Asian dishes like curries and chai. In addition, cardamom is a staple of Middle Eastern cooking. It is also used in pastries, particularly in Scandinavian nations, where it is a coffee and tea flavoring. It is also a component of the Indian spice mixture, garam masala.

It has also been used for centuries as a natural remedy, particularly for the common cold. Additionally, cardamom has been used to treat digestive issues, lung congestion, pulmonary tuberculosis, and infections of the teeth, gums, and throat (Das et al., 2012a). Cardamom's bioactive components have been researched for its chemo-preventive, anti-inflammatory, and anticancer activities (Bhattacharjee et al., 2007; Das et al., 2012b).

Terpenes and phenolic compounds, which have potent antioxidant capabilities, are the major bioactive components of cardamom. They contain the following primary bioactive substances: α-terpinyl acetate, 1,8-cineole, sabinene, α-pinene, nerolidol, g-terpinene limonene, α-terpineol, β-pinene, methyl linoleate, and n-hexadecanoic acid, which are some of the compounds found in this mixture. The main bioactive ingredients in cardamom are 1,8-cineole and α-terpinyl acetate (Ahmad et al., 2022).

Leukemia (Moteki et al., 2002), skin (Sampath et al., 2018), oral (Cha et al., 2010), colon (Murata et al., 2013), breast (Efferth et al., 2011), liver (Rodenak-Kladniew et al., 2020), and ovarian cancer (Wang et al., 2012) are all confirmed to be susceptible to 1,8-cineole's anticancer properties. The activation of the tumor suppressor protein p53 signaling pathway is the main underlying factor contributing to the observed anticancer effects. This pathway initiates apoptosis, a programmed cell death process, specifically targeting cancer cells. According to Sampath et al. (2018), the upregulation of p53 protein expression by 1,8-cineole has demonstrated efficacy in inducing apoptosis and G2/M phase arrest, specifically in skin cancer cells, with minimal impact observed on normal keratinocytes. Furthermore, it should be noted that 1,8-cineole induces mitochondrial stress and facilitates apoptosis in human oral epidermoid carcinoma cells via the caspase-dependent and MAPK-mediated pathways (Cha et al., 2010). Additionally, 1,8-cineole can cause apoptosis in human colorectal cancer via activating p38 MAPK and Akt, leading to caspase-3 cleavage (Murata et al., 2013).

3.10 Turmeric

Turmeric, scientifically referred to as *Curcuma longa* and colloquially known as "*Curcuma domestica*," is a member of the family Zingiberaceae, commonly known as the ginger family. The plant is a perennial herbaceous species characterized by its rhizomatous growth habit. It is naturally found in the tropical regions of South Asia (Prasad & Aggarwal, 2011; Unlu et al., 2016). Turmeric is cultivated extensively in tropical areas and is recognized by several names in various countries and cultures. Turmeric is generally referred to as "haldi" in North India, "manjal" in the South, and "Kurkum" in Arabic (Prasad & Aggarwal, 2011).

India is the primary producer of turmeric crop in the world as well as the primary consumer of it. India consumes about 80% of the total crop produced. The greatest production and most significant trading hub for turmeric in the world is Erode, a city in the state of Tamil Nadu in Southern India, which is also popular by other names like "Yellow City," "Turmeric City," and "Textile City" (Prasad & Aggarwal, 2011). It is a commonly used spice in traditional dishes in India, China, Bangladesh, Malaysia, Jamaica, Pakistan, El Salvador, Indonesia, and Haiti (Krishnaswamy, 2006). It is a common ingredient in Eastern delicacies like fresh turmeric pickles and is used in savory and sweet recipes (Prasad & Aggarwal, 2011).

Turmeric consumption in Asian countries has been reported to be 200–1000 mg/day (Thimmayamma et al., 1983; Polasa et al., 1991) or 160–440 g/person/year range (Krishnaswamy, 1996). Although turmeric contains over 300 active ingredients, curcumin is the primary biochemically active component extracted from its root (Aggarwal et al., 2006; Lüer et al., 2014). Curcumin has been used for over 2,500 years in Asia, especially in traditional Indian medicine (Ayurveda) (Gupta et al., 2013). Various studies have been done on curcumin, a polyphenol-structured compound, to see how it affects various enzymes, cytokines, kinases, transcription factors, growth factors, and receptors (Kocaadam & Şanlier, 2017). It has been found to have anti-microbial (Zhu et al., 2015), anti-inflammatory (Zhang et al., 2015), antioxidant (Kavakli et al., 2011; Meng et al., 2013), immunomodulatory (Jantan et al., 2012), renoprotective (Trujillo et al., 2013), hepatoprotective (Kiso et al., 1983), and hypoglycemic (Fujiwara et al., 2008) properties. The anti-inflammatory properties of curcumin have been demonstrated in various research, and as inflammation is one of the risk factors for cancer development; therefore, it could be used for cancer prevention and therapy (Devassy et al., 2015; Unlu et al., 2016; Kumar et al., 2017).

Numerous modes of action for curcumin's anticancer activities have been identified as a result of extensive research into this substance. Curcumin shields biomembranes by scavenging reactive free radicals and halting peroxidative deterioration (Aggarwal et al., 2007). Inflammation is a major factor in the majority of modern disease processes, including tumor growth and metastasis (Mantovani et al., 2008). Nuclear factor-κB (NFκB), inducible nitric oxide synthase (iNOS), lipoxygenase (LOX), and cyclooxygenase-2 (COX-2) are all inhibited by curcumin, which reduces inflammation (Aggarwal et al., 2007; Bachmeier et al., 2008). Angiogenesis is a critical factor in the growth of tumors and the development of metastases. The tumor can be fed and allowed to spread to other parts of the body thanks to the blood supply. Curcumin has been demonstrated to have direct angiogenesis inhibitory actions by limiting endothelial cell motility and invasion. By blocking COX-2, vascular endothelial growth factor, and NF-κB, curcumin has been found to indirectly decrease angiogenesis (Hutchins-Wolfbrandt & Mistry, 2011).

3.11   Garlic

Garlic (*Allium sativum L.*) is a member of the family Alliaceae that has been used for over 5,000 years as a flavoring agent, condiment, and medicine (Adaki et al., 2014). Garlic is believed to have originated in Central Asia and subsequently spread to China, the Near East, and the Mediterranean region before eventually arriving in Southern and Central Europe, Mexico, and Northern Africa (Egypt) (Singh & Singh, 2008). Certain evidence suggests that garlic has been used for thousands of years for culinary and therapeutic purposes. Sanskrit literature indicates that it was used for medicinal purposes around 5,000 years ago. Greeks, Romans, Babylonians, Chinese, and Egyptians used garlic as a remedy (Londhe et al., 2011).

Garlic is currently being grown worldwide, with China, South Korea, India, Thailand, Spain, and Egypt being major producers. The FDA estimates yearly global production at 2,315,000 metric tons. Gilroy, California, a major garlic producer in the United States, is well-known for its garlic festival (Nagourney, 1998). Garlic consumption is the highest in China, India, and Korea. Spain and Turkey have Europe's greatest per capita consumption (about 1.5 kg per year). The average annual garlic intake in the United States is 1 kg, a considerable decrease from 1.5 kg in 1990 (Wiczkowski, 2018).

Garlic is composed of various bioactive constituents, such as saponins, organosulfur compounds, phenolic compounds, and polysaccharides (Bradley et al., 2016; Diretto et al., 2017; Szychowski et al., 2018; Wang et al., 2018). Garlic's main active components include organosulfur compounds such as diallyl disulfide (DADS), diallyl sulfide (DAS), S-allyl-cysteine (SAC), diallyl thiosulfonate (allicin), E/Z-ajoene, diallyl trisulfide (DATS), and S-allyl-cysteine sulfoxide (alliin) (Shang et al., 2019).

The chemicals being studied for their biological activity have shown extraordinary biological effects, such as anti-inflammatory, antioxidant, and anticancer capabilities. According to Shang et al.'s study from 2019, which was based on Nicastro et al.'s study from 2015, it has been discovered that garlic and its sulfur compounds have the power to reduce the activation of carcinogens, potentially reducing the susceptibility to cancer. According to the research done by Bagul et al. (2015), the growth of several human cancer cell lines, including prostate (PC-3), liver (HepG2), breast (MCF-7), and colon (Caco2) cancer cells, was inhibited by crude garlic extract. Human leukemic cells can be made to undergo apoptosis, a form of programmed cell death when exposed to ajoene, a key chemical component of garlic. Additionally, it has demonstrated therapeutic efficacy in the treatment of acute myeloid leukemia, a form of cancer that affects the myeloid line of blood cells (Bhagat & Chaturvedi, 2016).

3.12   Ginger

Ginger, scientifically known as *Zingiber officinale*, is widely utilized as a culinary spice, condiment, and herbal remedy globally (Moghaddasi & Kashani, 2012). Ginger, a widely used spice, is derived from the subterranean stems or rhizomes of the herbaceous tropical perennial plant known as *Zingiber officinale* (Rosc.), which belongs to the Zingiberaceae family (Vasala, 2012). According to Purseglove et al. (1981) and Burkill (1966), ginger is widely believed to have origins in Southeast Asia, particularly in India. In the first century CE period, ginger was introduced to the Mediterranean region by traders from India. During the 13th century CE, ginger was introduced to East Africa by the Arabs. At the same time, the Portuguese facilitated its introduction to West Africa and the Pacific islands, primarily for commercial cultivation (Kizhakkayil & Sasikumar, 2011).

Ginger cultivation is widespread globally, with significant production occurring in India, China, Nepal, Indonesia, Nigeria,

Thailand, Japan, Bangladesh, and the Philippines. According to Vasala (2012), India and China are recognized as the primary contributors to the global market. Ginger is commonly employed as a culinary additive, with an estimated average daily intake of fresh ginger root ranging from 8 to 10 grams in India (Moghaddasi & Kashani, 2012). Ginger, in its diverse manifestations, is employed in culinary applications to enhance flavor, provide antioxidant properties, exhibit antibacterial attributes, and serve as a deodorizing agent. Throughout history, various medical systems, including those of China, India, Tibet, and the Arab world, have acknowledged the therapeutic properties of ginger (Altman & Marcussen, 2001). The Chinese have used ginger for at least 2500 years as a digestive aid, anti-nausea medication, and treatment for blood disorders and rheumatism, as well as for baldness, toothaches, snakebites, and respiratory conditions (Duke & Ayensu, 1985). In Ayurveda, the traditional medicine of India, ginger is frequently used to treat arthritis, decrease cholesterol, and avoid excessive blood clotting (heart disease). In Malaysia and Indonesia, new mothers are fed ginger soup for 30 days following delivery in order to keep them warm and help them sweat away impurities. In Arabian medicine, ginger is regarded as an aphrodisiac (Qureshi et al., 1989). According to certain Africans (Duke & Ayensu, 1985), eating ginger regularly will deter mosquitoes. Ginger had made its way to Europe by the time of the Greek and Roman eras. By Greek and Roman times, ginger had spread westward to Europe. The Greeks ate ginger wrapped in bread after meals as a digestive aid (Moghaddasi & Kashani, 2012).

Bioactive compounds like phenolic and terpene molecules are abundant in ginger. In ginger, gingerols, paradols, and shogaols are the main phenolic components. Additionally, ginger is known to contain a wide variety of terpene compounds, including -curcumene, -bisabolene, zingiberene, -farnesene, and -sesquiphellandrene, which are recognized as the main ingredients in ginger essential oils (Mao et al., 2019).

Various studies have demonstrated the anti-inflammatory properties (Hudson et al., 2006), anticancer effects (Shukla & Singh, 2007), antioxidant activity (Jeyakumar et al., 1999), anti-angiogenic effects (Huang et al., 2000), and anti-atherosclerotic properties (Coppola & Novo, 2007) of phenolic compounds such as shogoal, paradol, and gingerol. The compounds mentioned above can impede the expression of gene products regulated by NF-κB, including IL-8 (Nonn et al., 2007), VEGF (Kim et al., 2005), and ovarian cancer cells (Rhode et al., 2007). These gene products play a crucial role in cellular proliferation and angiogenesis. Multiple laboratory studies conducted on different experimental models have identified several pathways that could potentially contribute to the chemo-preventive effects of ginger and its constituents. The compound known as 6-gingerol can impede the viability of gastric cancer cells, thus restricting the dissemination of cancer within the body (Surh et al., 1999; Shukla & Singh, 2007). Ginger oil has been found to prevent skin cancer in mice, and gingerols have been shown to kill ovarian cancer cells in a study at the University of Michigan (Moghaddasi & Kashani, 2012).

3.13   Cinnamon

Cinnamon, scientifically known as *Cinnamomum cassia*, is a perennial tree under the botanical family Lauraceae (Bhagat & Chaturvedi, 2016). Cinnamon is a spice and aromatic crop that has been used since ancient times and has a wide range of applications in flavoring, fragrance, and medicine (Ribeiro-Santos et al., 2017). Cinnamon, a plant species known as *Cinnamomum verum*, originates from Sri Lanka. This country holds a prominent position in the production and exportation of cinnamon bark oil and leaf oil. Thomas and Kuruvilla (2012) stated that Sri Lanka cultivates cinnamon on approximately 24,000 hectares of land. Based on the findings of the Food and Agriculture Organization of the United Nations, it is evident that Indonesia emerged as the foremost contributor to cinnamon production, with a recorded output of 83,176.79 tons, during the period spanning from 2000 to 2014. China followed suit with a production volume of 53,176.79 tons, while Sri Lanka, Vietnam, and Madagascar produced 13,938.21 tons, 13,894.43 tons, and 1797.36 tons of cinnamon, respectively (Ribeiro-Santos et al., 2017). Mexico, West

Germany, the United States, the United Kingdom, Saudi Arabia, Taiwan, Singapore, Hong Kong, and France are widely recognized as the principal importers of spice (Thomas & Kuruvilla, 2012).

Cinnamon is used in a variety of ways around the world. It is used to flavor pastries and beverages in North America. Cinnamon is used in sweet and savory foods in European and Middle Eastern cuisines, such as pastries and bread. Cinnamon is used in curries, rice dishes, and chai blends in South Asian cooking, particularly in India and Sri Lanka. Cinnamon is used in meat-based dishes and sweets in Southeast Asian cuisines such as Indonesian and Thai. It is also used in Latin America's mole sauces, hot chocolate, and Caribbean jerk chicken. (Different Types of Cinnamon Explained - WebstaurantStore, n.d.).

In addition to its usage as a spice and flavoring, cinnamon has long been utilized in traditional Chinese, Indian, Persian, and Unani medicine. Flatulence, amenorrhea, diarrhea, toothaches, fever, leukorrhea, common cold, and headaches are just a few of the illnesses it addresses (Bandara et al., 2012; R. Deng, 2012). Cinnamon's antibacterial, antiviral, antifungal, antioxidant, anticancer, antihypertensive, antilipemic, antidiabetic, gastroprotective, and immunomodulatory effects have shown promise in a number of research investigations (Shen et al., 2012; Beejmohun et al., 2014; Hajimonfarednejad et al., 2018; Zare et al., 2019).

The bark of this plant contains various compounds such as essential oils (cinnamic aldehyde and cinnamyl aldehyde), eugenol, tannin, terpinene, carvacrol, safrole, linalool, benzyl benzoate, and coumarin. Additionally, it also contains mucus and glucose (Tanaka, 2008). These compounds exhibit various properties, including anti-inflammatory, antioxidant, and antitumor activities (Schoene et al., 2005; Youn et al., 2008; Kwon et al., 2010). Cinnamon exhibits antioxidant properties and can potentially mitigate lipid peroxidation, a process implicated in cancer development. Research indicates that the effectiveness of cinnamon extracts in combating cancer is associated with their ability to regulate angiogenesis and AP-1 in CD8+ T cells. In the murine melanoma model, the activities of NFB and AP1 target genes, including Bcl-2 and Bcl-xL, were inhibited by cinnamon extract. According to the study conducted by Kwon et al. (2010), the results of this study provide compelling evidence that the anti-tumoral effects of the cinnamon extract are mediated through multiple signaling pathways (Bhagat & Chaturvedi, 2016).

3.14 Coriander

Coriander, scientifically known as *Coriandrum sativum L.*, is a spice from a plant belonging to the Umbelliferae (Apiaceae) family (Singletary, 2016). The herb is utilized for culinary purposes as a flavoring agent in various regions, including Asia, the Middle East, and Central and South America (Sharma & Sharma, 2012). *Coriandrum sativum L.*, commonly referred to as cilantro, Chinese parsley, Mexican parsley, Arab parsley, Dhania, and Yuen sai, is indigenous to southern Asia and North Africa (Sachan et al., 2018).

Both Greek and Roman cultures used it as a spice; the Romans used it to preserve meats and flavor bread. Coriander was also introduced to Britain by the Romans and was often used in English cuisine. Coriander leaves are also used in the culinary traditions of Latin America, India, and China. The plant is thought to have been known in India since the Vedic Period, but it was primarily used for its fresh leaves at the time (Sharma & Sharma, 2012). India is the world's largest producer of coriander, with an estimated area of $4.0–6.1 \times 105$ ha and an annual production of $3.0–4.0 \times 105$ tons. Coriander is commercially grown in many countries, including Morocco, Myanmar, Romania, Italy, Bulgaria, France, Spain, Turkey, the Netherlands, Pakistan, Argentina, Mexico, Canada, Australia, and, to a lesser extent, the United Kingdom and the United States. India is also the world's biggest coriander seed exporter (Sharma & Sharma, 2012). Coriander has been extensively utilized as a culinary ingredient and in traditional medicinal practices across diverse civilizations (Sahib et al., 2013). Traditionally, this substance has been employed for treating infections affecting the digestive, respiratory, and urinary systems while exhibiting stimulatory properties (Gilani et al., 2007).

Table 3.1 Spices, major bioactive compounds and their chemical structure with anti-cancer properties.

S. No.	Spice	Major bioactive compound	Chemical structure*	Anti-cancer properties	References
1.	Clove (*Syzygium aromaticum L.*)	Eugenol (EUG) or 4-allyl-2-methoxyphenol ($C_{10}H_{12}O_2$)		Inhibit breast cancer related oncogene, like NF-κB and cyclin D1.	(Zari et al., 2021b) (Nisar et al., 2021)
				Prevent the proliferation of MCF-7 cells.	(Anuj & Sanjay, 2010)
				Suppress E2F1 and its downstream antiapoptotic target in breast cancer.	(Al-Sharif et al., 2013)
2.	Black cumin (*Nigella sativa*)	Thymoquinone (TQ) or 2-isopropyl-5-methyl-1,4-benzoquinone		Act as an Akt suppressor.	(Randhawa & Al-Ghamdi, 2002)
				Anti-proliferative impact on human myeloblastic leukemia HL-60 cells.	(Schneider-Stock et al., 2014);
				Induce cell death by apoptosis in MCF-7/Topo breast carcinoma and in KB-V1/Vb1 cervical carcinoma.	(Franke & Cantley, 1997); (El-Mahdy et al., 2005)
					(Effenberger et al., 2010)

(Continued)

Table 3.1 (*Continued*)

S. No.	Spice	Major bioactive compound	Chemical structure*	Anti-cancer properties	References
3.	Saffron (*Crocus sativus*)	Picrocrocin[1] ($C_{16}H_{26}O_7$), Crocin[2] ($C_{44}H_{64}O_{24}$), Crocetin[3] ($C_{20}H_{24}O_{40}$), and Safranal[4] ($C_{10}H_{14}O$)		Causes cytotoxicity in Hepatocarcin-oma HepG2 cells.	(Ashktorab et al., 2019);
				Anti-proliferative effects on the colorectal cancer cell lines.	(Noureini & Wink, 2012);
				Slows down cell division by causing cell cycle arrest through p53-dependent or p53-independent P21-mediated pathways.	(Amerizadeh et al (Zari et al., 2018) (C.-Y. Li et al., 2012)

S. No.	Spice	Major bioactive compound	Chemical structure*	Anti-cancer properties	References
4.	Black pepper (*Piper nigrum L.*)	Piperine[1] and Piperidine[2]		Reduced proliferation and promoted apoptosis in breast cancer cells via triggering caspase-3 and PARP cleavage.	[Zheng et al., 2016]; [Do et al., 2013];
				Inhibits the proliferation of human ovarian cancer A2780 cells.	[Si et al., 2018]; [Xia et al., 2015]
				Inhibit IL-6 expression, thereby reduce the ability of gastric cancer cell (TMK-1) to penetrate other cells.	
5.	Red chili pepper (*Capsicum annuum*)	Capsaicin		Antiproliferative effect on breast cancer cells via a caspase-independent mechanism.	[Srinivasan, 2016]; [Cao et al., 2019];
				Inhibits TPA-stimulated activation of NF-κB in human promyelocytic leukemia HL-60 cells.	[Chou et al., 2009] [Han et al., 2002]

(*Continued*)

Table 3.1 (*Continued*)

S. No.	Spice	Major bioactive compound	Chemical structure*	Anti-cancer properties	References
6.	Oregano (*Origanum vulgare*)	Carvacrol		Cell cycle arrest at G0/G1 and reactive oxygen species-mediated death in prostate cancer cells from humans.	(Sharifi-Rad, 2018a); (F. Khan et al., 2017);
				Showed reduced proliferation, invasion, and migration in Colon cancer HCT116 and LoVo cells.	(Sharifi-Rad, 2018b)
7.	Rosemary (*Rosmarinus officinalis*)	Carnosic Acid[1] and Rosmarinic Acid[2]		Reduced colony formation in CaCo-2 (Colorectal adenocarcinoma) colon cancer cells.	(Cuvelier et al., 1994);
				Decreased prostate cancer cells (LNCaP) viability.	(Slameňová et al., 2002);
				Inhibit cell survival and proliferation and cause apoptosis in pancreatic and breast cancer.	(Bourhia et al., 2019) (Tsiani et al., 2016)

S. No.	Spice	Major bioactive compound	Chemical structure*	Anti-cancer properties	References
8.	Cardamom (*Elettaria cardamomum*)	Eucalyptol (1,8-cineole)[1] and α-terpinyl acetate[2]		Causes apoptosis and G2/M phase arrest in skin cancer cells by upregulating the expression of the p53 protein. Causes apoptosis in human colorectal cancer via activating p38 MAPK and Akt. Promoted apoptosis in human oral epidermoid carcinoma cells through the caspase-dependent pathway and the MAPK-mediated pathway.	(Ahmad et al., 2022); (Sampath et al., 2018); (Murata et al., 2013); (Cha et al., 2010)
9.	Turmeric (*Curcuma longa*)	Curcumin		Anti-inflammatory role by inhibiting cyclooxygenase-2 (COX-2), lipoxygenase (LOX), inducible nitric oxide synthase (iNOS), and nuclear factor-κB (NFκB).	(Aggarwal et al., 2006);

(Continued)

Table 3.1 (*Continued*)

S. No.	Spice	Major bioactive compound	Chemical structure*	Anti-cancer properties	References
				Inhibit angiogenesis directly by reducing endothelial cell migration and invasion & indirectly by inhibiting vascular endothelial growth factor (VEGF), COX-2, and NFκB.	(Aggarwal et al., 2007); (Bachmeier et al., 2008) [Hutchins-Wolfbrandt & Mistry, 2011]
10.	Garlic (*Allium sativum L.*)	Allicin		Anti-proliferative effects on human cancer cell lines such as liver (HepG2), colon (Caco2), prostate (PC-3) and breast (MCF-7) cancer cells. Suppress proliferation and cause apoptosis in human leukaemic cells.	(Salehi et al., 2019); (Bagul et al., 2015); (Bhagat & Chaturvedi, 2016)
11.	Ginger (*Zingiber officinale*)	Gingerol		Inhibit NF-κB-regulated gene products such as IL-8, and VEGF. Inhibit the viability of gastric cancer cells.	(Mao et al., 2019); (Nonn et al., 2007); (Kim et al., 2005);

S. No.	Spice	Major bioactive compound	Chemical structure*	Anti-cancer properties	References
				Inhibit the growth of human colorectal cancer cells.	(Shukla & Singh, 2007); (Bode, 2003)
12.	Cinnamon (*Cinnamomum cassia*)	Cinnamaldehyde		Anti-tumoral actions, mediated by numerous action pathways.	(Banerjee & Banerjee, 2023);
				Inhibited the activities of NFB and AP1 target genes such as Bcl-2 and Bcl-xL in a murine melanoma model.	(Bhagat & Chaturvedi, 2016); (Kwon et al., 2010)
13.	Coriander (*Coriandrum sativum L.*)	Linalool		Anticancer properties in sarcoma-180 (S-180) solid tumour cells through the development of oxidative stress.	(Gu et al., 2010); (Jana et al., 2014);
				Suppress cell growth in breast cancer.	(Laribi et al., 2015);
				Shows reverse doxorubicin resistance in human breast cancer cells.	(Ravizza et al., 2008)

* All structures are takes from the *http://www.chemspider.com/*

Coriander extracts and phytochemicals have been known to have a variety of biological activities, including antioxidant, anticancer, and anti-inflammatory properties (Laribi et al., 2015). These therapeutic qualities are primarily mediated by the coriander extracts' strong antioxidant properties and its primary component, linalool. Essential oils, lipids, polyphenols, and other types of bioactive substances have also been obtained from *C. sativum* (Prachayasittikul et al., 2018).

Linalool has demonstrated anticancer properties in various cancer cell lines, such as leukemia (Gu et al., 2010), lymphoma (Chiang et al., 2003), breast, liver (Paik et al., 2005; Usta et al., 2009), melanoma, and renal cancer cell lines (Loizzo et al., 2008). According to Jana et al. (2014), evidence indicates that linalool possesses anticancer properties in sarcoma-180 (S-180) solid tumor cells. The data suggest that the mechanism underlying its anticancer activity involves the induction of oxidative stress. According to Ravizza et al. (2008), linalool can counteract doxorubicin resistance in human breast cancer cells. This naturally occurring chemical significantly inhibits cellular proliferation, potentially enhancing the therapeutic efficacy of anthracyclines in managing breast cancer (Laribi et al., 2015). Table 3.1 summarizes the spices, their major bioactive compounds, their chemical structure, and their various anticancer properties.

3.15   Conclusion

Spices are used worldwide for their culinary and medicinal properties. Spices' widespread popularity reflects their flexible role in improving the sensory experience of food while also providing a variety of health benefits, making them essential components of cuisines and lifestyles all over the world. The comprehensive exploration of anti-cancerous properties of various spices showed potent role of spices as alternative therapies for prevention and treatment of cancer. The bioactive compounds found in various spices such as eugenol, thymoquinone, crocetin, piperidine, curcumin, gingerol, and others exerts various pharmacological effects including anti-proliferative, anti-inflammatory, anti-apoptotic and immunomodulatory effects emphasizing their role in not only flavoured delightful complements to cuisine, but also intriguing sources of medicinal substances with anti-cancer properties. As most of the available anti-cancer therapies are having side effects hence an alternative therapy with lesser side effects is much needed at the time. The bioactive compound from these spices offers a promising alternative, which is a hidden gem for future research and development. The health benefits offered by various spices speaks of the fact that the mother nature itself offers cure to every disease.

References

Adaki, S., Adaki, R., Shah, K., & Karagir, A. (2014). Garlic: review of literature. *Indian Journal of Cancer*, *51*(4), 577–581. https://doi.org/10.4103/0019-509X.175383.

Aggarwal, B. B., Bhatt, I. D., Ichikawa, H., Ahn, K. S., Sethi, G., Sandur, S. K., Natarajan, C., Seeram, N., & Shishodia, S. (2006). *10 Curcumin—biological and medicinal properties*.

Aggarwal, B. B., Surh, Y.-J., & Shishodia, S. (2007). *The molecular targets and therapeutic uses of curcumin in health and disease* (Vol. 595). Springer Science & Business Media.

Ahmad, N., Tian, W., Zengliu, S., Zou, Y., Farooq, S., Huang, Q., & Xiao, J. (2022). Recent advances in the extraction, chemical composition, therapeutic potential, and delivery of cardamom phytochemicals. *Frontiers in Nutrition*, *9*, 1024820.

Ahrazem, O., Rubio-Moraga, A., Nebauer, S. G., Molina, R. V., & Gomez-Gomez, L. (2015). Saffron: its phytochemistry, developmental processes, and biotechnological prospects. *Journal of Agricultural and Food Chemistry*, *63*(40), 8751–8764.

Al-Fatlawi, A. A., Al-Fatlawi, A. A., Irshad, M., Zafaryab, M., Alam Rizvi, M. M., & Ahmad, A. (2014). Rice bran phytic acid induced apoptosis through regulation of Bcl-2/Bax and p53 genes in HepG2 human hepatocellular carcinoma cells. *Asian Pacific Journal of Cancer Prevention*, *15*(8), 3731–3736.

Al-Jishi, S. A. A. (2000). A study of Nigella sativa on blood hemostatic functions. King Faisal University.

Al-Sharif, I., Remmal, A., & Aboussekhra, A. (2013). Eugenol triggers apoptosis in breast cancer cells through E2F1/survivin down-regulation. *BMC Cancer*, *13*, 1–10.

Altman, R., & Marcussen, K. C. (2001). Effects of a ginger extract on knee pain in patients with osteoarthritis. *Arthritis & Rheumatism*, *44*(11), 2531–2538.

Amara, S., Ivy, M. T., Myles, E. L., & Tiriveedhi, V. (2016). Sodium channel γENaC mediates IL-17 synergized high salt induced inflammatory stress in breast cancer cells. *Cellular Immunology*, *302*, 1–10. https://doi.org/10.1016/J.CELLIMM.2015.12.007.

Amerizadeh, F., Rezaei, N., Rahmani, F., Hassanian, S. M., Moradi-Marjaneh, R., Fiuji, H., Boroumand, N., Nosrati-Tirkani, A., Ghayour-Mobarhan, M., & Ferns, G. A. (2018). Crocin synergistically enhances the antiproliferative activity of 5-flurouracil through Wnt/PI3K pathway in a mouse model of colitis-associated colorectal cancer. *Journal of Cellular Biochemistry*, *119*(12), 10250–10261.

Anuj, G., & Sanjay, S. (2010). Eugenol: a potential phytochemical with multifaceted therapeutic activities. *Pharmacologyonline*, *2*, 108–120.

Arunasree, K. M. (2010). Anti-proliferative effects of carvacrol on a human metastatic breast cancer cell line, MDA-MB 231. *Phytomedicine*, *17*(8–9), 581–588.

Ashktorab, H., Soleimani, A., Singh, G., Amin, A., Tabtabaei, S., Latella, G., Stein, U., Akhondzadeh, S., Solanki, N., & Gondré-Lewis, M. C. (2019). Saffron: the golden spice with therapeutic properties on digestive diseases. *Nutrients*, *11*(5), 943.

Bachmeier, B. E., Mohrenz, I. V, Mirisola, V., Schleicher, E., Romeo, F., Höhneke, C., Jochum, M., Nerlich, A. G., & Pfeffer, U. (2008). Curcumin downregulates the inflammatory cytokines CXCL1 and-2 in breast cancer cells via NFκB. *Carcinogenesis*, *29*(4), 779–789.

Bagul, M., Kakumanu, S., & Wilson, T. A. (2015). Crude garlic extract inhibits cell proliferation and induces cell cycle arrest and apoptosis of cancer cells *in vitro*. *Journal of Medicinal Food*, *18*(7), 731–737.

Bandara, T., Uluwaduge, I., & Jansz, E. R. (2012). Bioactivity of cinnamon with special emphasis on diabetes mellitus: a review. *International Journal of Food Sciences and Nutrition*, *63*(3), 380–386.

Banerjee, S., & Banerjee, S. (2023). Anticancer potential and molecular mechanisms of cinnamaldehyde and its congeners present in the cinnamon plant. *Physiologia*, *3*(2), 173–207.

Bathaie, S. Z., & Mousavi, S. Z. (2010). New applications and mechanisms of action of saffron and its important ingredients. *Critical Reviews in Food Science and Nutrition*, *50*(8), 761–786.

Beejmohun, V., Peytavy-Izard, M., Mignon, C., Muscente-Paque, D., Deplanque, X., Ripoll, C., & Chapal, N. (2014). Acute effect of Ceylon cinnamon extract on postprandial glycemia: alpha-amylase inhibition, starch tolerance test in rats, and randomized crossover clinical trial in healthy volunteers. *BMC Complementary and Alternative Medicine*, *14*, 1–11.

Begum, A., Sandhya, S., Vinod, K. R., Reddy, S., & Banji, D. (2013). An in-depth review on the medicinal flora Rosmarinus officinalis (Lamiaceae). *Acta ScientiarumPolonorumTechnologia Alimentaria*, *12*(1), 61–74.

Bensimon, J., Biard, D., Paget, V., Goislard, M., Morel-Altmeyer, S., Konge, J., Chevillard, S., & Lebeau, J. (2016). Forced extinction of CD24 stem-like breast cancer marker alone promotes radiation resistance through the control of oxidative stress. *Molecular Carcinogenesis*, *55*(3), 245–254. https://doi.org/10.1002/MC.22273.

Bhagat, N., & Chaturvedi, A. (2016). Spices as an alternative therapy for cancer treatment. *Systematic Reviews in Pharmacy*, *7*, 46–56. https://doi.org/10.5530/srp.2016.7.7.

Bhandari, P. R. (2015). Crocus sativus L.(saffron) for cancer chemo-prevention: a mini review. *Journal of Traditional and Complementary Medicine*, *5*(2), 81–87.

Bhattacharjee, S., Rana, T., & Sengupta, A. (2007). Inhibition of lipid peroxidation and enhancement of GST activity by cardamom and cinnamon during chemically induced colon carcinogenesis in Swiss albino mice. *Asian Pac J Cancer Prev*, *8*(4), 578–582.

Bode, A. (2003). *Ginger is an effective inhibitor of HCT116 human colorectal carcinoma in vivo.*

Bolhassani, A., Khavari, A., & Bathaie, S. Z. (2014). Saffron and natural carotenoids: Biochemical activities and anti-tumor effects. *Biochimica et Biophysica Acta (Bba)-Reviews on Cancer*, *1845*(1), 20–30.

Bononi, M., Tateo, F., Scaglia, B., & Quaglia, G. (2020). δ13C data of the total water-soluble fraction and triacylglycerols as related indexes for differentiating the geographical origin of saffron (Crocus sativus L.). *Food Chemistry*, *315*, 126292.

Bourhia, M., Laasri, F. E., Aourik, H., Boukhris, A., Ullah, R., Bari, A., Ali, S. S., El Mzibri, M., Benbacer, L., & Gmouh, S. (2019). Antioxidant and antiproliferative activities of bioactive compounds contained in Rosmarinus officinalis used in the Mediterranean diet. *Evidence-Based Complementary and Alternative Medicine*, *2019*.

Bradley, J. M., Organ, C. L., & Lefer, D. J. (2016). Garlic-derived organic polysulfides and myocardial protection. *The Journal of Nutrition, 146*(2), 403S–409S.

Broadhead, G. K., Chang, A., Grigg, J., & McCluskey, P. (2016). Efficacy and safety of saffron supplementation: current clinical findings. *Critical Reviews in Food Science and Nutrition, 56*(16), 2767–2776.

Bui, T. T., Piao, C. H., Song, C. H., Shin, H. S., Shon, D.-H., & Chai, O. H. (2017). Piper nigrum extract ameliorated allergic inflammation through inhibiting Th2/Th17 responses and mast cells activation. *Cellular Immunology, 322*, 64–73.

Burkill, I. H. (1966). A dictionary of the economic products of the Malay Peninsula. *A Dictionary of the Economic Products of the Malay Peninsula.* (2nd edition).

Butt, M. S., Naz, A., Sultan, M. T., & Qayyum, M. M. N. (2013). Anti-oncogenic perspectives of spices/herbs: a comprehensive review. *EXCLI Journal, 12*, 1043. /pmc/articles/PMC4827078/.

Cao, S.-Y., Li, Y., Meng, X., Zhao, C.-N., Li, S., Gan, R.-Y., & Li, H.-B. (2019). Dietary natural products and lung cancer: effects and mechanisms of action. *Journal of Functional Foods, 52*, 316–331.

Cha, J.-D., Kim, Y.-H., & Kim, J.-Y. (2010). Essential oil and 1, 8-cineole from Artemisia lavandulaefolia induces apoptosis in KB cells via mitochondrial stress and caspase activation. *Food Science and Biotechnology, 19*, 185–191.

Chang, H. S., Tang, J. Y., Yen, C. Y., Huang, H. W., Wu, C. Y., Chung, Y. A., Wang, H. R., Chen, I. S., Huang, M. Y., & Chang, H. W. (2016). Antiproliferation of Cryptocarya concinna-derived cryptocaryone against oral cancer cells involving apoptosis, oxidative stress, and DNA damage. *BMC Complementary and Alternative Medicine, 16*(1). https://doi.org/10.1186/S12906-016-1073-5.

Chiang, L.-C., Chiang, W., Chang, M.-Y., Ng, L.-T., & Lin, C.-C. (2003). Antileukemic activity of selected natural products in Taiwan. *The American Journal of Chinese Medicine, 31*(01), 37–46.

Chou, C.-C., Wu, Y.-C., Wang, Y.-F., Chou, M.-J., Kuo, S.-J., & Chen, D.-R. (2009). Capsaicin-induced apoptosis in human breast cancer MCF-7 cells through caspase-independent pathway. *Oncology Reports, 21*(3), 665–671.

Coppola, G., & Novo, S. (2007). Statins and peripheral arterial disease: effects on claudication, disease progression, and prevention of cardiovascular events. *Archives of Medical Research, 38*(5), 479–488.

Cuvelier, M. E., Berset, C., & Richard, H. (1994). Antioxidant constituents in sage (Salvia officinalis). *Journal of Agricultural and Food Chemistry*, *42*(3), 665–669.

Darriet, A. (2007). Herbs, spices, and essential oils. *Handbook of Food Products Manufacturing; Hui, YH (Ed.), John Wiley & Sons: Hoboken, NJ, USA*, 205–220.

Das, I., Acharya, A., Berry, D. L., Sen, S., Williams, E., Permaul, E., Sengupta, A., Bhattacharya, S., & Saha, T. (2012a). Antioxidative effects of the spice cardamom against non-melanoma skin cancer by modulating nuclear factor erythroid-2-related factor 2 and NF-κB signalling pathways. *British Journal of Nutrition*, *108*(6), 984–997.

Das, I., Acharya, A., Berry, D. L., Sen, S., Williams, E., Permaul, E., Sengupta, A., Bhattacharya, S., & Saha, T. (2012b). Antioxidative effects of the spice cardamom against non-melanoma skin cancer by modulating nuclear factor erythroid-2-related factor 2 and NF-κB signalling pathways. *British Journal of Nutrition*, *108*(6), 984–997.

De Oliveira, J. R., Camargo, S. E. A., & De Oliveira, L. D. (2019). Rosmarinus officinalis L.(rosemary) as therapeutic and prophylactic agent. *Journal of Biomedical Science*, *26*(1), 1–22.

Deng, G.-F., Xu, X.-R., Guo, Y.-J., Xia, E.-Q., Li, S., Wu, S., Chen, F., Ling, W.-H., & Li, H.-B. (2012). Determination of antioxidant property and their lipophilic and hydrophilic phenolic contents in cereal grains. *Journal of Functional Foods*, *4*(4), 906–914.

Deng, R. (2012). A review of the hypoglycemic effects of five commonly used herbal food supplements. *Recent Patents on Food, Nutrition & Agriculture*, *4*(1), 50–60.

Dessie, A. B., Abate, T. M., Adane, B. T., Tesfa, T., & Getu, S. (2020). Estimation of technical efficiency of black cumin (Nigella sativa L.) farming in northwest Ethiopia: a stochastic frontier approach. *Journal of Economic Structures*, *9*(1), 1–14.

Devassy, J. G., Nwachukwu, I. D., & Jones, P. J. H. (2015). Curcumin and cancer: barriers to obtaining a health claim. *Nutrition Reviews*, *73*(3), 155–165.

Different Types of Cinnamon Explained - WebstaurantStore. (n.d.). Retrieved July 4, 2023, from https://www.webstaurantstore.com/blog/3782/cinnamon-types.html.

Diretto, G., Rubio-Moraga, A., Argandoña, J., Castillo, P., Gómez-Gómez, L., &Ahrazem, O. (2017). Tissue-specific accumulation of sulfur compounds and saponins in different parts of garlic cloves from purple and white ecotypes. *Molecules*, *22*(8), 1359.

Do, M. T., Kim, H. G., Choi, J. H., Khanal, T., Park, B. H., Tran, T. P., Jeong, T. C., & Jeong, H. G. (2013). Antitumor efficacy of piperine in the treatment of human HER2-overexpressing breast cancer cells. *Food Chemistry, 141*(3), 2591–2599.

Dornenburg, A., & Page, K. (2003). The new American chef: cooking with the best flavors and techniques from around the world. *(No Title).*

Duke, J. A., & Ayensu, E. S. (1985). *Medicinal plants of China. Medicinal plants of the world.* Reference Publications, Algonac, MI, Inc, *1*, 362.

Effenberger, K., Breyer, S., & Schobert, R. (2010). Terpene conjugates of the Nigella sativa seed-oil constituent thymoquinone with enhanced efficacy in cancer cells. *Chemistry & Biodiversity, 7*(1), 129–139.

Efferth, T., Herrmann, F., Tahrani, A., & Wink, M. (2011). Cytotoxic activity of secondary metabolites derived from Artemisia annua L. towards cancer cells in comparison to its designated active constituent artemisinin. *Phytomedicine, 18*(11), 959–969.

El-Kadi, A., & Kandil, O. (1986). Effect of Nigella sativa (the black seed) on immunity. *Proceeding of the 4th International Conference on Islamic Medicine, Kuwait. Bull Islamic Med, 4*, 344–348.

El-Mahdy, M. A., Zhu, Q., Wang, Q., Wani, G., & Wani, A. A. (2005). Thymoquinone induces apoptosis through activation of caspase-8 and mitochondrial events in p53-null myeloblastic leukemia HL-60 cells. *International Journal of Cancer, 117*(3), 409–417.

Elmore, S. (2007). Apoptosis: a review of programmed cell death. *Toxicologic Pathology, 35*(4), 495–516.

Fonnegra Gómez, R., & Jiménez Ramírez, S. L. (2007). Plantas medicinales aprobadas en Colombia. Universidad de Antioquia.

Franke, T. F., & Cantley, L. C. (1997). A Bad kinase makes good. *Nature, 390*(6656), 116–117.

Fridlender, M., Kapulnik, Y., & Koltai, H. (2015). Plant derived substances with anti-cancer activity: from folklore to practice. *Frontiers in Plant Science, 6*(OCTOBER). https://doi.org/10.3389/FPLS.2015.00799.

Fu, L., Xu, B.-T., Xu, X.-R., Gan, R.-Y., Zhang, Y., Xia, E.-Q., & Li, H.-B. (2011). Antioxidant capacities and total phenolic contents of 62 fruits. *Food Chemistry, 129*(2), 345–350.

Fujiwara, H., Hosokawa, M., Zhou, X., Fujimoto, S., Fukuda, K., Toyoda, K., Nishi, Y., Fujita, Y., Yamada, K., & Yamada, Y. (2008). Curcumin inhibits glucose production in isolated mice hepatocytes. *Diabetes Research and Clinical Practice, 80*(2), 185–191.

G Gutheil, W., Reed, G., Ray, A., Anant, S., & Dhar, A. (2012). Crocetin: an agent derived from saffron for prevention and therapy for cancer. *Current Pharmaceutical Biotechnology*, *13*(1), 173–179.

Gemma, A., Takenaka, K., Hosoya, Y., Matuda, K., Seike, M., Kurimoto, F., Ono, Y., Uematsu, K., Takeda, Y., & Hibino, S. (2001). Altered expression of several genes in highly metastatic subpopulations of a human pulmonary adenocarcinoma cell line. *European Journal of Cancer*, *37*(12), 1554–1561.

Ghosh, S. S., Gehr, T. W. B., & Ghosh, S. (2014). Curcumin and chronic kidney disease (CKD): major mode of action through stimulating endogenous intestinal alkaline phosphatase. *Molecules (Basel, Switzerland)*, *19*(12), 20139–20156. https://doi.org/10.3390/MOLECULES191220139.

Giacosa, A., Morazzoni, P., Bombardelli, E., Riva, A., Bianchi Porro, G., & Rondanelli, M. (2015). Can nausea and vomiting be treated with ginger extract. *Eur Rev Med Pharmacol Sci*, *19*(7), 1291–1296.

Gilani, A. H., Bashir, S., & Khan, A. (2007). Pharmacological basis for the use of Borago officinalis in gastrointestinal, respiratory and cardiovascular disorders. *Journal of Ethnopharmacology*, *114*(3), 393–399.

Gismondi, A., Serio, M., Canuti, L., & Canini, A. (2012). Biochemical, antioxidant and antineoplastic properties of Italian saffron (Crocus sativus L.). *American Journal of Plant Sciences*, *3*(11), 1573.

Gu, Y., Ting, Z., Qiu, X., Zhang, X., Gan, X., Fang, Y., Xu, X., & Xu, R. (2010). Linalool preferentially induces robust apoptosis of a variety of leukemia cells via upregulating p53 and cyclin-dependent kinase inhibitors. *Toxicology*, *268*(1–2), 19–24.

Guo, Y. J., Deng, G. F., Xu, X. R., Wu, S., Li, S., Xia, E. Q., Li, F., Chen, F., Ling, W. H., & Li, H. Bin. (2012). Antioxidant capacities, phenolic compounds and polysaccharide contents of 49 edible macro-fungi. *Food & Function*, *3*(11), 1195–1205. https://doi.org/10.1039/C2FO30110E.

Gupta, S. C., Sung, B., Kim, J. H., Prasad, S., Li, S., & Aggarwal, B. B. (2013). Multitargeting by turmeric, the golden spice: from kitchen to clinic. *Molecular Nutrition & Food Research*, *57*(9), 1510–1528.

Gutiérrez-Grijalva, E. P., Picos-Salas, M. A., Leyva-López, N., Criollo-Mendoza, M. S., Vazquez-Olivo, G., & Heredia, J. B. (2017). Flavonoids and phenolic acids from oregano: occurrence, biological activity and health benefits. *Plants, 7* (1): 2.

Hajimonfarednejad, M., Nimrouzi, M., Heydari, M., Zarshenas, M. M., Raee, M. J., & Jahromi, B. N. (2018). Insulin resistance improvement by cinnamon powder in polycystic ovary syndrome: a randomized double-blind placebo controlled clinical trial. *Phytotherapy Research, 32*(2), 276–283.

Han, S.-S., Keum, Y.-S., Chun, K.-S., & Surh, Y.-J. (2002). Suppression of phorbol ester-induced NF-κB activation by capsaicin in cultured human promyelocytic leukemia cells. *Archives of Pharmacal Research, 25*, 475–479.

HAO, C., Rui, F. A. N., Ribeiro, M. C., TAN, L., WU, H., YANG, J., ZHENG, W., & Huan, Y. (2012). Modeling the potential geographic distribution of black pepper (Piper nigrum) in Asia using GIS tools. *Journal of Integrative Agriculture, 11*(4), 593–599.

Hegde, P. S., Karanikas, V., & Evers, S. (2016). The where, the when, and the how of immune monitoring for cancer immunotherapies in the era of checkpoint inhibition. *Clinical Cancer Research: An Official Journal of the American Association for Cancer Research, 22*(8), 1865–1874. https://doi.org/10.1158/1078-0432.CCR-15-1507

UNIDO and FAO (2005). Herbs, spices and essential oils post-harvest operations in developing countries.

Herbst, S. T. (2001). The new food lover's companion: comprehensive definitions of nearly 6000 food, drink, and culinary terms. *(No Title)*.

Huang, S., DeGuzman, A., Bucana, C. D., & Fidler, I. J. (2000). Nuclear factor-κB activity correlates with growth, angiogenesis, and metastasis of human melanoma cells in nude mice. *Clinical Cancer Research, 6*(6), 2573–2581.

Hudson, E. A., Fox, L. H., Luckett, J. C. A., & Manson, M. M. (2006). Ex vivo cancer chemoprevention research possibilities. *Environmental Toxicology and Pharmacology, 21*(2), 204–214.

Hussain, M. D. S., Hegde, L., Sharatbabu, A. G., Hegde, N. K., Shantappa, T., Gurumurthy, S. B., Manju, M. J., & Shivakumar, K. M. (2017). Evaluation of local black pepper (Piper nigrum L.) genotypes for yield and quality under arecanut based cropping system. *Int J Pure ApplBiosci, 5*, 1396–1400.

Hutchins-Wolfbrandt, A., & Mistry, A. M. (2011). Dietary turmeric potentially reduces the risk of cancer. *Asian Pac J Cancer Prev, 12*(12), 3169–3173.

IJpma, I., Renken, R. J., ter Horst, G. J., & Reyners, A. K. L. (2015). Metallic taste in cancer patients treated with chemotherapy. *Cancer*

Treatment Reviews, *41*(2), 179–186. https://doi.org/10.1016/J. CTRV.2014.11.006.

ISO 676:1995(en), Spices and condiments —Botanical nomenclature. (n.d.). Retrieved June 24, 2023, from https://www.iso.org/obp/ ui/#iso:std:iso:676:ed-2:v1:en.

Jana, S., Patra, K., Sarkar, S., Jana, J., Mukherjee, G., Bhattacharjee, S., & Mandal, D. P. (2014). Antitumorigenic potential of linalool is accompanied by modulation of oxidative stress: an *in vivo* study in sarcoma-180 solid tumor model. *Nutrition and Cancer*, *66*(5), 835–848.

Jantan, I., Bukhari, S. N. A., Lajis, N. H., Abas, F., Wai, L. K., & Jasamai, M. (2012). Effects of diarylpentanoid analogues of curcumin on chemiluminescence and chemotactic activities of phagocytes. *Journal of Pharmacy and Pharmacology*, *64*(3), 404–412.

Jessica Elizabeth, D. L. T., Gassara, F., Kouassi, A. P., Brar, S. K., & Belkacemi, K. (2017). Spice use in food: properties and benefits. *Critical Reviews in Food Science and Nutrition*, *57*(6), 1078–1088. https://doi.org/10.1080/10408398.2013.858235.

Jeyakumar, S. M., Nalini, N., & Menon, V. P. (1999). Antioxidant activity of ginger (Zingiber officinale Rosc) in rats fed a high fat diet. *Medical Science Research*, *27*(5), 341–344.

Kafi, M. (2006). *Saffron (Crocus Sativus): Production and Processing*, Science Publishers.

Kamatou, G. P., Vermaak, I., & Viljoen, A. M. (2012). Eugenol—from the remote Maluku Islands to the international market place: a review of a remarkable and versatile molecule. *Molecules*, *17*(6), 6953–6981.

Kammath, A. J., Nair, B., P, S., & Nath, L. R. (2021). Curry versus cancer: potential of some selected culinary spices against cancer with *in vitro, in vivo*, and human trials evidences. *Journal of Food Biochemistry*, *45*(3), e13285.

Kaseb, A. O., Chinnakannu, K., Chen, D., Sivanandam, A., Tejwani, S., Menon, M., Dou, Q. P., & Reddy, G. P.-V. (2007). Androgen receptor–and E2F-1–targeted thymoquinone therapy for hormone-refractory prostate cancer. *Cancer Research*, *67*(16), 7782–7788.

Kavakli, H. S., Koca, C., & Alici, O. (2011). Antioxidant effects of curcumin in spinal cord injury in rats. *Ulus TravmaAcilCerrahiDerg*, *17*(1), 14–18.

Khan, A., Chen, H. C., Tania, M., & Zhang, D. Z. (2011). Anticancer activities of Nigella sativa (black cumin). *African Journal of Traditional, Complementary and Alternative Medicines*, *8*(5S).

Khan, F., Khan, I., Farooqui, A., & Ansari, I. A. (2017). Carvacrol induces reactive oxygen species (ROS)-mediated apoptosis along with cell cycle arrest at G0/G1 in human prostate cancer cells. *Nutrition and Cancer, 69*(7), 1075–1087.

Kim, E.-C., Min, J.-K., Kim, T.-Y., Lee, S.-J., Yang, H.-O., Han, S., Kim, Y.-M., & Kwon, Y.-G. (2005). [6]-Gingerol, a pungent ingredient of ginger, inhibits angiogenesis *in vitro* and *in vivo. Biochemical and Biophysical Research Communications, 335*(2), 300–308.

Kiso, Y., Suzuki, Y., Watanabe, N., Oshima, Y., & Hikino, H. (1983). Antihepatotoxic principles of Curcuma longa rhizomes. *Planta Medica, 49*(11), 185–187.

Kizhakkayil, J., & Sasikumar, B. (2011). Diversity, characterization and utilization of ginger: a review. *Plant Genetic Resources, 9*(3), 464–477. https://doi.org/DOI: 10.1017/S1479262111000670.

Kocaadam, B., & Şanlier, N. (2017). Curcumin, an active component of turmeric (Curcuma longa), and its effects on health. *Critical Reviews in Food Science and Nutrition, 57*(13), 2889–2895.

Krishnan, S., Bhosale, R., & Singhal, R. S. (2005). Microencapsulation of cardamom oleoresin: evaluation of blends of gum Arabic, maltodextrin and a modified starch as wall materials. *Carbohydrate Polymers, 61*(1), 95–102.

Krishnaswamy, K. (1996). Indian functional foods: role in prevention of cancer. *Nutrition Reviews, 54*(11 Pt 2). https://doi.org/10.1111/J.1753-4887.1996.TB03832.X.

Krishnaswamy, K. (2006). *Turmeric: The Salt of the Orient is the Spice of Life*, Allied Publishers.

Kumar, A., Sharma, B., Sharma, U., Parashar, G., Parashar, N. C., Rani, I., Ramniwas, S., Kaur, S., Haque, S., & Tuli, H. S. (2023). Apoptotic and antimetastatic effect of cucurbitacins in cancer: recent trends and advancement. *Naunyn-Schmiedeberg's Archives of Pharmacology, 396*(9), 1867–1878. https://doi.org/10.1007/s00210-023-02471-z

Kumar, S., Kamboj, J., & Sharma, S. (2011). Overview for various aspects of the health benefits of Piper longum linn. fruit. *Journal of Acupuncture and Meridian Studies, 4*(2), 134–140.

Kumar, U., Sharma, U., & Rathi, G. (2017). Reversal of hypermethylation and reactivation of glutathione S-transferase pi 1 gene by curcumin in breast cancer cell line. *Tumour Biology: The Journal of the International Society for Oncodevelopmental Biology and Medicine, 39*(2), 1010428317692258. https://doi.org/10.1177/1010428317692258.

Kunnumakkara, A., Bicer, C., Dey, S., Danda, D., Sung, B., & Aggarwal, B. (2009). Traditional uses of spices: an overview. *Molecular Targets and Therapeutic Uses of Spices*. https://doi.org/10.1142/9789812837912_0001.

Kwon, H.-K., Hwang, J.-S., So, J.-S., Lee, C.-G., Sahoo, A., Ryu, J.-H., Jeon, W. K., Ko, B. S., Im, C.-R., & Lee, S. H. (2010). Cinnamon extract induces tumor cell death through inhibition of NFκB and AP1. *BMC Cancer*, *10*, 1–10.

Laribi, B., Kouki, K., M'Hamdi, M., & Bettaieb, T. (2015). Coriander (*Coriandrum sativum L.*) and its bioactive constituents. *Fitoterapia*, *103*, 9–26.

Li, C.-Y., Huang, W.-F., Wang, Q.-L., Wang, F., Cai, E., Hu, B., Du, J.-C., Wang, J., Chen, R., & Cai, X.-J. (2012). Crocetin induces cytotoxicity in colon cancer cells via p53-independent mechanisms. *Asian Pacific Journal of Cancer Prevention*, *13*(8), 3757–3761.

Li, F., Li, S., Li, H. Bin, Deng, G. F., Ling, W. H., & Xu, X. R. (2013). Antiproliferative activities of tea and herbal infusions. *Food & Function*, *4*(4), 530–538. https://doi.org/10.1039/C2FO30252G.

Li, F., Li, S., Li, H.-B., Deng, G.-F., Ling, W.-H., Wu, S., Xu, X.-R., & Chen, F. (2013). Antiproliferative activity of peels, pulps and seeds of 61 fruits. *Journal of Functional Foods*, *5*(3), 1298–1309.

Li, S., Li, S.-K., Gan, R.-Y., Song, F.-L., Kuang, L., & Li, H.-B. (2013). Antioxidant capacities and total phenolic contents of infusions from 223 medicinal plants. *Industrial Crops and Products*, *51*, 289–298.

Li, Y., Li, S., Meng, X., Gan, R.-Y., Zhang, J.-J., & Li, H.-B. (2017). Dietary natural products for prevention and treatment of breast cancer. *Nutrients*, *9*(7), 728.

Lin, M., Lin, B., Chang, C., Chu, C., Su, H., Chen, S., Jeng, Y., & Kuo, M. (2007). IL-6 induces AGS gastric cancer cell invasion via activation of the c-Src/RhoA/ROCK signaling pathway. *International Journal of Cancer*, *120*(12), 2600–2608.

Liu, N.-C., Hsieh, P.-F., Hsieh, M.-K., Zeng, Z.-M., Cheng, H.-L., Liao, J.-W., & Chueh, P. J. (2012). Capsaicin-mediated tNOX (ENOX2) up-regulation enhances cell proliferation and migration *in vitro* and *in vivo*. *Journal of Agricultural and Food Chemistry*, *60*(10), 2758–2765.

Loizzo, M. R., Tundis, R., Menichini, F., Saab, A. M., Statti, G. A., & Menichini, F. (2008). Antiproliferative effects of essential oils and their major constituents in human renal adenocarcinoma and amelanotic melanoma cells. *Cell Proliferation*, *41*(6), 1002–1012.

Londhe, V., Gavasane, A., Nipate, S., D.D, B., & P.D, C. (2011). Role of garlic (Allium sativum) in various diseases: an overview. *Journal of Pharmaceutical Research and Opinion, 1*, 129–134.

Lüer, S. C., Goette, J., Troller, R., & Aebi, C. (2014). Synthetic versus natural curcumin: bioequivalence in an *in vitro* oral mucositis model. *BMC Complementary and Alternative Medicine, 14*(1), 1–7.

Maghsoodi, V., Kazemi, A., & Akhondi, E. (2012). Effect of different drying methods on saffron (Crocus sativus L) quality. *Iranian Journal of Chemistry and Chemical Engineering*.

Maisonneuve, P., Shivappa, N., Hébert, J. R., Bellomi, M., Rampinelli, C., Bertolotti, R., Spaggiari, L., Palli, D., Veronesi, G., & Gnagnarella, P. (2016). Dietary inflammatory index and risk of lung cancer and other respiratory conditions among heavy smokers in the COSMOS screening study. *European Journal of Nutrition, 55*(3), 1069–1079. https://doi.org/10.1007/S00394-015-0920-3.

Majdalawieh, A. F., & Fayyad, M. W. (2015). Immunomodulatory and anti-inflammatory action of Nigella sativa and thymoquinone: a comprehensive review. *International Immunopharmacology, 28*(1), 295–304. https://doi.org/10.1016/J.INTIMP.2015.06.023.

Mantovani, A., Allavena, P., Sica, A., & Balkwill, F. (2008). Cancer-related inflammation. *Nature, 454*(7203), 436–444.

Mao, Q.-Q., Xu, X.-Y., Cao, S.-Y., Gan, R.-Y., Corke, H., Beta, T., & Li, H.-B. (2019). Bioactive compounds and bioactivities of ginger (Zingiber officinale Roscoe). *Foods, 8*(6), 185.

Meng, B., Li, J., & Cao, H. (2013). Antioxidant and anti-inflammatory activities of curcumin on diabetes mellitus and its complications. *Current Pharmaceutical Design, 19*(11), 2101–2113.

Mitra, S., Anand, U., Jha, N. K., Shekhawat, M. S., Saha, S. C., Nongdam, P., Rengasamy, K. R. R., Proćków, J., & Dey, A. (2022). Anticancer applications and pharmacological properties of piperidine and piperine: a comprehensive review on molecular mechanisms and therapeutic perspectives. *Frontiers in Pharmacology, 12*, 772418.

Moghaddasi, M. S., & Kashani, H. H. (2012). Ginger (Zingiber officinale): a review. *Journal of Medicinal Plants Research, 6*(26), 4255–4258.

Moteki, H., Hibasami, H., Yamada, Y., Katsuzaki, H., Imai, K., & Komiya, T. (2002). Specific induction of apoptosis by 1, 8-cineole in two human leukemia cell lines, but not a in human stomach cancer cell line. *Oncology Reports, 9*(4), 757–760.

Murata, S., Shiragami, R., Kosugi, C., Tezuka, T., Yamazaki, M., Hirano, A., Yoshimura, Y., Suzuki, M., Shuto, K., & Ohkohchi, N. (2013). Antitumor effect of 1, 8-cineole against colon cancer. *Oncology Reports*, *30*(6), 2647–2652.

Nabavi, S. F., Di Lorenzo, A., Izadi, M., Sobarzo-Sánchez, E., Daglia, M., & Nabavi, S. M. (2015). Antibacterial effects of cinnamon: from farm to food, cosmetic and pharmaceutical industries. *Nutrients*, *7*(9), 7729. https://doi.org/10.3390/NU7095359.

Nagi, M. N., & Almakki, H. A. (2009). Thymoquinone supplementation induces quinone reductase and glutathione transferase in mice liver: possible role in protection against chemical carcinogenesis and toxicity. *Phytotherapy Research: An International Journal Devoted to Pharmacological and Toxicological Evaluation of Natural Product Derivatives*, *23*(9), 1295–1298.

Nagourney, R. A. (1998). Garlic: medicinal food or nutritious medicine? *Journal of Medicinal Food*, *1*(1), 13–28.

Neveu, V., Perez-Jiménez, J., Vos, F., Crespy, V., Chaffaut, L., & Mennen, L. (2010a). An online comprehensive database on polyphenol contents in foods. *Database (Oxford), Phenol-Explorer*.

Neveu, V., Perez-Jiménez, J., Vos, F., Crespy, V., Chaffaut, L., & Mennen, L. (2010b). An online comprehensive database on polyphenol contents in foods. *Database (Oxford), Phenol-Explorer*.

Nicastro, H. L., Ross, S. A., & Milner, J. A. (2015). Garlic and onions: their cancer prevention properties garlic and onions: their cancer prevention properties. *Cancer Prevention Research*, *8*(3), 181–189.

Nilius, B., & Appendino, G. (2013). Spices: the savory and beneficial science of pungency. *Reviews of Physiology, Biochemistry and Pharmacology*, *164*, 1–76. https://doi.org/10.1007/112_2013_11/COVER.

Nisar, M. F., Khadim, M., Rafiq, M., Chen, J., Yang, Y., & Wan, C. C. (2021). Pharmacological properties and health benefits of eugenol: a comprehensive review. *Oxidative Medicine and Cellular Longevity*, *2021*.

Nonn, L., Duong, D., & Peehl, D. M. (2007). Chemopreventive anti-inflammatory activities of curcumin and other phytochemicals mediated by MAP kinase phosphatase-5 in prostate cells. *Carcinogenesis*, *28*(6), 1188–1196.

Noureini, S. K., & Wink, M. (2012). Antiproliferative effects of crocin in HepG2 cells by telomerase inhibition and hTERT down-regulation. *Asian Pacific Journal of Cancer Prevention*, *13*(5), 2305–2309.

Nova, R., Hoemardani, A. S. D., & Louisa, M. (2021). Potential of herbal medicines in cancer therapy. *The Indonesian Journal of Cancer Control, 1*(1), 32–42.

Ojeda-Sana, A. M., van Baren, C. M., Elechosa, M. A., Juárez, M. A., & Moreno, S. (2013). New insights into antibacterial and antioxidant activities of rosemary essential oils and their main components. *Food Control, 31*(1), 189–195.

Oliveira, R. A., Oliveira, F. F., & Sacramento, C. K. (2007). Essential oils: prospects for agribusiness spices in Bahia. *Bahia Agric, 8*(1), 46–48.

Oregano|Spices Board. (n.d.). Retrieved July 16, 2023, from http://www.indianspices.com/spice-catalog/oregano.html.

Paik, S.-Y., Koh, K.-H., Beak, S.-M., Paek, S.-H., & Kim, J.-A. (2005). The essential oils from Zanthoxylum schinifolium pericarp induce apoptosis of HepG2 human hepatoma cells through increased production of reactive oxygen species. *Biological and Pharmaceutical Bulletin, 28*(5), 802–807.

Park, J. M., Lee, H. J., Yoo, J. H., Ko, W. J., Cho, J. Y., & Hahm, K. B. (2015). Overview of gastrointestinal cancer prevention in Asia. *Best Practice & Research. Clinical Gastroenterology, 29*(6), 855–867. https://doi.org/10.1016/J.BPG.2015.09.008.

Parthasarathy, V. A., Chempakam, B., & Zachariah, T. J. (2008). *Chemistry of Spices*, Cabi.

Polasa, K., Sesikaran, B., Krishna, T. P., & Krishnaswamy, K. (1991). Turmeric (Curcuma longa)-induced reduction in urinary mutagens. *Food and Chemical Toxicology: An International Journal Published for the British Industrial Biological Research Association, 29*(10), 699–706. https://doi.org/10.1016/0278-6915(91)90128-T.

Prachayasittikul, V., Prachayasittikul, S., Ruchirawat, S., & Prachayasittikul, V. (2018). Coriander (Coriandrum sativum): a promising functional food toward the well-being. *Food Research International, 105*, 305–323.

Prasad, S., & Aggarwal, B. B. (2011). Turmeric, the golden spice. *Herbal Medicine: Biomolecular and Clinical Aspects,* Second Edition, 263–288. https://www.ncbi.nlm.nih.gov/books/NBK92752/.

Purseglove, J. W., Brown, E. G., Green, C. L., & Robbins, S. R. J. (1981). *Spices, Vol. 2,* Longman Group Ltd.

Qureshi, S., Shah, A. H., Tariq, M., & Ageel, A. M. (1989). Studies on herbal aphrodisiacs used in Arab system of medicine. *The American Journal of Chinese Medicine, 17*(01n02), 57–63.

Rahaiee, S., Moini, S., Hashemi, M., & Shojaosadati, S. A. (2015). Evaluation of antioxidant activities of bioactive compounds and various extracts obtained from saffron (Crocus sativus L.): a review. *Journal of Food Science and Technology*, *52*, 1881–1888.

Randhawa, M. A., & Al-Ghamdi, M. S. (2002). A review of the pharmaco-therapeutic effects of Nigella sativa. *Pakistan J Med Res*, *41*(2), 77–83.

Randhawa, M. A., & Alghamdi, M. S. (2011). Anticancer activity of Nigella sativa (black seed)—a review. *The American Journal of Chinese Medicine*, *39*(06), 1075–1091.

Rather, R. A., & Bhagat, M. (2018). Cancer chemoprevention and piperine: molecular mechanisms and therapeutic opportunities. *Frontiers in Cell and Developmental Biology*, *6*, 10.

Ravindran, P. N., & Kallupurackal, J. A. (2012). Black pepper. In *Handbook of Herbs and Spices* (pp. 86–115), Elsevier.

Ravizza, R., Gariboldi, M. B., Molteni, R., & Monti, E. (2008). Linalool, a plant-derived monoterpene alcohol, reverses doxorubicin resistance in human breast adenocarcinoma cells. *Oncology Reports*, *20*(3), 625–630.

Ren, J., Xu, Y., Huang, Q., Yang, J., Yang, M., Hu, K., & Wei, K. (2015). Chabamide induces cell cycle arrest and apoptosis by the Akt/MAPK pathway and inhibition of P-glycoprotein in K562/ADR cells. *Anti-Cancer Drugs*, *26*(5), 498–507.

Rhode, J., Fogoros, S., Zick, S., Wahl, H., Griffith, K. A., Huang, J., & Liu, J. R. (2007). Ginger inhibits cell growth and modulates angiogenic factors in ovarian cancer cells. *BMC Complementary and Alternative Medicine*, *7*, 1–9.

Ribeiro-Santos, R., Andrade, M., Madella, D., Martinazzo, A. P., Moura, L. de A. G., de Melo, N. R., & Sanches-Silva, A. (2017). Revisiting an ancient spice with medicinal purposes: cinnamon. *Trends in Food Science & Technology*, *62*, 154–169.

Ribeiro-Santos, R., Carvalho-Costa, D., Cavaleiro, C., Costa, H. S., Albuquerque, T. G., Castilho, M. C., Ramos, F., Melo, N. R., & Sanches-Silva, A. (2015). A novel insight on an ancient aromatic plant: the rosemary (Rosmarinus officinalis L.). *Trends in Food Science & Technology*, *45*(2), 355–368.

Rodenak-Kladniew, B., Castro, A., Stärkel, P., Galle, M., & Crespo, R. (2020). 1, 8-Cineole promotes G0/G1 cell cycle arrest and oxidative stress-induced senescence in HepG2 cells and sensitizes cells to anti-senescence drugs. *Life Sciences*, *243*, 117271.

Rosemary | Spices Board. (n.d.). Retrieved July 16, 2023, from http://www. indianspices.com/spice-catalog/rosemary.html.

Rubió, L., Motilva, M. J., & Romero, M. P. (2013). Recent advances in biologically active compounds in herbs and spices: a review of the most effective antioxidant and anti-inflammatory active principles. *Critical Reviews in Food Science and Nutrition, 53*(9), 943–953. https://doi.org/10.1080/10408398.2011.574802.

Ryes, T., Luukkanen, O., & Quiroz, R. (2006). Small cardamom-precious for people, harmful for mountainforests: possibilities for sustainable cultivation in the East Usambaras, Tanzania. *Mt Res Dev, 26*, 131–137.

Sachan, A. K., Kumar, S., Kumari, K., & Singh, D. (2018). Medicinal uses of spices used in our traditional culture: worldwide. *Journal of Medicinal Plants Studies, 6*(3), 116–122.

Sahib, N. G., Anwar, F., Gilani, A., Hamid, A. A., Saari, N., & Alkharfy, K. M. (2013). Coriander (*Coriandrum sativum L.*): a potential source of high-value components for functional foods and nutraceuticals – a review. *Phytotherapy Research, 27*(10), 1439–1456.

Salehi, B., Zucca, P., Orhan, I. E., Azzini, E., Adetunji, C. O., Mohammed, S. A., Banerjee, S. K., Sharopov, F., Rigano, D., & Sharifi-Rad, J. (2019). Allicin and health: a comprehensive review. *Trends in Food Science & Technology, 86*, 502–516.

Salvo, A., La Torre, G. L., Rotondo, A., Cicero, N., Gargano, R., Mangano, V., Casale, K. E., & Dugo, G. (2019). Multiple analytical approaches for the organic and inorganic characterization of Origanum vulgare L. samples. *Natural Product Research, 33*(19), 2815–2822.

Sampath, S., Subramani, S., Janardhanam, S., Subramani, P., Yuvaraj, A., & Chellan, R. (2018). Bioactive compound 1,8-Cineole selectively induces G2/M arrest in A431 cells through the upregulation of the p53 signaling pathway and molecular docking studies. *Phytomedicine, 46*, 57–68.

Schneider-Stock, R., Fakhoury, I. H., Zaki, A. M., El-Baba, C. O., & Gali-Muhtasib, H. U. (2014). Thymoquinone: fifty years of success in the battle against cancer models. *Drug Discovery Today, 19*(1), 18–30.

Schoene, N. W., Kelly, M. A., Polansky, M. M., & Anderson, R. A. (2005). Water-soluble polymeric polyphenols from cinnamon inhibit proliferation and alter cell cycle distribution patterns of hematologic tumor cell lines. *Cancer Letters, 230*(1), 134–140.

Shahi, T., Assadpour, E., & Jafari, S. M. (2016). Main chemical compounds and pharmacological activities of stigmas and tepals of 'red gold': saffron. *Trends in Food Science & Technology, 58*, 69–78.

Shang, A., Cao, S. Y., Xu, X. Y., Gan, R. Y., Tang, G. Y., Corke, H., Mavumengwana, V., & Li, H. Bin. (2019). Bioactive compounds and biological functions of garlic (Allium sativum L.). *Foods*, *8*(7). https://doi.org/10.3390/FOODS8070246.

Sharifi-Rad, M. (2018a). *CARVACROL and human health: A comprehensive review, || Phyther. Res.*

Sharifi-Rad, M. (2018b). *CARVACROL and human health: A comprehensive review, || Phyther. Res.*

Sharifi-Rad, M., Berkay Yýlmaz, Y., Antika, G., Salehi, B., Tumer, T. B., Kulandaisamy Venil, C., Das, G., Patra, J. K., Karazhan, N., & Akram, M. (2021). Phytochemical constituents, biological activities, and health-promoting effects of the genus Origanum. *Phytotherapy Research*, *35*(1), 95–121.

Sharma, M. M., & Sharma, R. K. (2012). Coriander. In *Handbook of Herbs and Spices* (pp. 216–249), Elsevier.

Sharma, S. K., Vij, A. S., & Sharma, M. (2013). Mechanisms and clinical uses of capsaicin. *European Journal of Pharmacology*, *720*(1–3), 55–62.

Shen, Y., Jia, L.-N., Honma, N., Hosono, T., Ariga, T., & Seki, T. (2012). Beneficial effects of cinnamon on the metabolic syndrome, inflammation, and pain, and mechanisms underlying these effects–a review. *Journal of Traditional and Complementary Medicine*, *2*(1), 27–32.

Shukla, Y., & Singh, M. (2007). Cancer preventive properties of ginger: a brief review. *Food and Chemical Toxicology*, *45*(5), 683–690.

Si, L., Yang, R., Lin, R., & Yang, S. (2018). Piperine functions as a tumor suppressor for human ovarian tumor growth via activation of JNK/p38 MAPK-mediated intrinsic apoptotic pathway. *Bioscience Reports*, *38*(3), BSR20180503.

Singh Tuli, H., Kumar, A., Ramniwas, S., Coudhary, R., Aggarwal, D., Kumar, M., Sharma, U., Chaturvedi Parashar, N., Haque, S., & Sak, K. (2022). Ferulic acid: a natural phenol that inhibits neoplastic events through modulation of oncogenic signaling. *Molecules*, *27*(21), 7653.

Singh Tuli, H., Kumar, A., Ramniwas, S., Coudhary, R., Aggarwal, D., Kumar, M., Sharma, U., Chaturvedi Parashar, N., Haque, S., & Sak, K. (2022b). Ferulic acid: a natural phenol that inhibits neoplastic events through modulation of oncogenic signaling. *Molecules* (Basel, Switzerland), 27(21), 7653. https://doi.org/10.3390/molecules27217653.

Singh, V. K., & Singh, D. K. (2008). Pharmacological effects of garlic (Allium sativum L.). *Annual Review of Biomedical Sciences*, *10*.

Singletary, K. (2016). Coriander: overview of potential health benefits. *Nutrition Today*, *51*(3). https://journals.lww.com/nutritiontodayonline/Fulltext/2016/05000/Coriander_Overview_of_Potential_Health_Benefits.8.aspx.

Slameňová, D., Kubošková, K., Horváthová, E., & Robichová, S. (2002). Rosemary-stimulated reduction of DNA strand breaks and FPG-sensitive sites in mammalian cells treated with H_2O_2 or visible light-excited Methylene Blue. *Cancer Letters*, *177*(2), 145–153.

Srinivasan, K. (2007). Black pepper and its pungent principle-piperine: a review of diverse physiological effects. *Critical Reviews in Food Science and Nutrition*, *47*(8), 735–748.

Srinivasan, K. (2014). Antioxidant potential of spices and their active constituents. *Critical Reviews in Food Science and Nutrition*, *54*(3), 352–372. https://doi.org/10.1080/10408398.2011.585525.

Srinivasan, K. (2016). Biological activities of red pepper (Capsicum annuum) and its pungent principle capsaicin: a review. *Critical Reviews in Food Science and Nutrition*, *56*(9), 1488–1500.

Sung, H., Ferlay, J., Siegel, R. L., Laversanne, M., Soerjomataram, I., Jemal, A., & Bray, F. (2021). Global Cancer Statistics 2020: GLOBOCAN estimates of incidence and mortality worldwide for 36 cancers in 185 countries. *CA: a cancer journal for clinicians*, *71*(3), 209–249. https://doi.org/10.3322/caac.21660.

Surh, Y.-J., Lee, E., & Lee, J. M. (1998). Chemoprotective properties of some pungent ingredients present in red pepper and ginger. *Mutation Research/Fundamental and Molecular Mechanisms of Mutagenesis*, *402*(1–2), 259–267.

Surh, Y.-J., Park, K.-K., Chun, K.-S., Lee, L. J., Lee, E., & Lee, S. S. (1999). Anti-tumor-promoting activities of selected pungent phenolic substances present in ginger. *Journal of Environmental Pathology, Toxicology and Oncology: Official Organ of the International Society for Environmental Toxicology and Cancer*, *18*(2), 131–139.

Szychowski, K. A., Rybczynska-Tkaczyk, K., Gawel-Beben, K., Swieca, M., Karas, M., Jakuczyk, A., Matysiak, M., Binduga, U. E., & Gminski, J. (2018). Characterization of active compounds of different garlic (Allium sativum L.) cultivars. *Polish Journal of Food and Nutrition Sciences*, *68*(1).

Takooree, H., Aumeeruddy, M. Z., Rengasamy, K. R. R., Venugopala, K. N., Jeewon, R., Zengin, G., & Mahomoodally, M. F. (2019a). A systematic review on black pepper (Piper nigrum L.): from folk uses to pharmacological applications. *Critical Reviews in Food Science and Nutrition, 59*(sup1), S210–S243.

Takooree, H., Aumeeruddy, M. Z., Rengasamy, K. R. R., Venugopala, K. N., Jeewon, R., Zengin, G., & Mahomoodally, M. F. (2019b). A systematic review on black pepper (Piper nigrum L.): from folk uses to pharmacological applications. *Critical Reviews in Food Science and Nutrition, 59*(sup1), S210–S243.

Tanaka, T. (2008). Chemical studies on plant polyphenols and formation of black tea polyphenols. *YakugakuZasshi: Journal of the Pharmaceutical Society of Japan, 128*(8), 1119–1131.

Teixeira, B., Marques, A., Ramos, C., Neng, N. R., Nogueira, J. M. F., Saraiva, J. A., & Nunes, M. L. (2013). Chemical composition and antibacterial and antioxidant properties of commercial essential oils. *Industrial Crops and Products, 43*, 587–595.

The World Market for Cardamom. (n.d.). Retrieved July 16, 2023, from https://www.yumpu.com/en/document/read/20609955/the-world-market-for-cardamom.

Thimmayamma, B. V. S., Rau, P., & Radhaiah, G. (1983). Use of spices and condiments in the dietaries of urban and rural families. *The Indian Journal of Nutrition and Dietetics*, 153–162.

Thoennissen, N. H., O'kelly, J., Lu, D., Iwanski, G. B., La, D. T., Abbassi, S., Leiter, A., Karlan, B., Mehta, R., & Koeffler, H. P. (2010). Capsaicin causes cell-cycle arrest and apoptosis in ER-positive and-negative breast cancer cells by modulating the EGFR/HER-2 pathway. *Oncogene, 29*(2), 285–296.

Thomas, J., & Kuruvilla, K. M. (2012). Cinnamon. In *Handbook of Herbs and Spices* (pp. 182–196), Elsevier.

Tong, Y., Zhu, X., Yan, Y., Liu, R., Gong, F., Zhang, L., Hu, J., Fang, L., Wang, R., & Wang, P. (2015). The influence of different drying methods on constituents and antioxidant activity of saffron from China. *International Journal of Analytical Chemistry, 2015*.

Trujillo, J., Chirino, Y. I., Molina-Jijón, E., Andérica-Romero, A. C., Tapia, E., & Pedraza-Chaverrí, J. (2013). Renoprotective effect of the antioxidant curcumin: recent findings. *Redox Biology, 1*(1), 448–456.

Tsiani, E., Moore, J., & Yousef, M. (2016). Anticancer effects of rosemary (rosmarinus officinalis l.) extract and rosemary extract polyphenols.

Ubillos, L., Freire, T., Berriel, E., Chiribao, M. L., Chiale, C., Festari, M. F., Medeiros, A., Mazal, D., Rondán, M., Bollati-Fogolín, M., Rabinovich, G. A., Robello, C., & Osinaga, E. (2016). Trypanosoma cruzi extracts elicit protective immune response against chemically induced colon and mammary cancers. *International Journal of Cancer*, *138*(7), 1719–1731. https://doi.org/10.1002/IJC.29910.

Ulanowska, M., & Olas, B. (2021). Biological Properties and prospects for the application of eugenol—A review. *International Journal of Molecular Sciences*, *22*(7), 3671.

Unlu, A., Nayir, E., Kalenderoglu, M. D., Kirca, O., & Ozdogan, M. (2016). Curcumin (Turmeric) and cancer. *J Buon*, *21*(5), 1050–1060.

Usta, J., Kreydiyyeh, S., Knio, K., Barnabe, P., Bou-Moughlabay, Y., & Dagher, S. (2009). Linalool decreases HepG2 viability by inhibiting mitochondrial complexes I and II, increasing reactive oxygen species and decreasing ATP and GSH levels. *Chemico-Biological Interactions*, *180*(1), 39–46.

Vasala, P. A. (2012). 18 - Ginger. In K. V Peter (Ed.), *Handbook of Herbs and Spices* (Second Edition) (pp. 319–335). Woodhead Publishing. https://doi.org/https://doi.org/10.1533/9780857095671.319.

Vidhya, N., & Devaraj, S. N. (2011). Induction of apoptosis by eugenol in human breast cancer cells.

Wang, B., Zhang, Y., Huang, J., Dong, L., Li, T., & Fu, X. (2017). Anti-inflammatory activity and chemical composition of dichloromethane extract from Piper nigrum and P. longum on permanent focal cerebral ischemia injury in rats. *RevistaBrasileira de Farmacognosia*, *27*, 369–374.

Wang, W., Li, N., Luo, M., Zu, Y., & Efferth, T. (2012). Antibacterial activity and anticancer activity of Rosmarinus officinalis L. essential oil compared to that of its main components. *Molecules*, *17*(3), 2704–2713.

Wang, Y., Guan, M., Zhao, X., & Li, X. (2018). Effects of garlic polysaccharide on alcoholic liver fibrosis and intestinal microflora in mice. *Pharmaceutical Biology*, *56*(1), 325–332.

Wiczkowski, W. (2018). Garlic and onion: production, biochemistry, and processing. *Handbook of Vegetables and Vegetable Processing*, 661–682.

Willard, P. (2002). *Secrets of Saffron: The Vagabond Life of the World's Most Seductive Spice*, Beacon Press.

Xia, Y., Khoi, P. N., Yoon, H. J., Lian, S., Joo, Y. E., Chay, K. O., Kim, K. K., & Jung, Y. Do. (2015). Piperine inhibits IL-1β-induced IL-6 expression by suppressing p38 MAPK and STAT3 activation in gastric cancer cells. *Molecular and Cellular Biochemistry*, *398*, 147–156.

Xing, B., Li, S., Yang, J., Lin, D., Feng, Y., Lu, J., & Shao, Q. (2021). Phytochemistry, pharmacology, and potential clinical applications of saffron: a review. *Journal of Ethnopharmacology*, *281*, 114555.

Yi, J.-L., Shi, S., Shen, Y.-L., Wang, L., Chen, H.-Y., Zhu, J., & Ding, Y. (2015). Myricetin and methyl eugenol combination enhances the anticancer activity, cell cycle arrest and apoptosis induction of cis-platin against HeLa cervical cancer cell lines. *International Journal of Clinical and Experimental Pathology*, *8*(2), 1116.

Youn, H. S., Lee, J. K., Choi, Y. J., Saitoh, S. I., Miyake, K., Hwang, D. H., & Lee, J. Y. (2008). Cinnamaldehyde suppresses toll-like receptor 4 activation mediated through the inhibition of receptor oligomerization. *Biochemical Pharmacology*, *75*(2), 494–502.

Zare, R., Nadjarzadeh, A., Zarshenas, M. M., Shams, M., & Heydari, M. (2019). Efficacy of cinnamon in patients with type II diabetes mellitus: a randomized controlled clinical trial. *Clinical Nutrition*, *38*(2), 549–556.

Zari, A. T., Zari, T. A., & Hakeem, K. R. (2021a). Anticancer properties of eugenol: a review. *Molecules (Basel, Switzerland)*, *26*(23). https://doi.org/10.3390/MOLECULES26237407.

Zari, A. T., Zari, T. A., & Hakeem, K. R. (2021b). Anticancer properties of eugenol: a review. *Molecules*, *26*(23), 7407.

Zhang, N., Li, H., Jia, J., & He, M. (2015). Anti-inflammatory effect of curcumin on mast cell-mediated allergic responses in ovalbumin-induced allergic rhinitis mouse. *Cellular Immunology*, *298*(1–2), 88–95.

Zheng, J., Zhou, Y., Li, Y., Xu, D.-P., Li, S., & Li, H.-B. (2016a). Spices for prevention and treatment of cancers. *Nutrients*, *8*(8), 495. https://doi.org/10.3390/nu8080495.

Zheng, J., Zhou, Y., Li, Y., Xu, D.-P., Li, S., & Li, H.-B. (2016b). Spices for prevention and treatment of cancers. *Nutrients*, *8*(8), 495.

Zhou, Y., Li, Y., Zhou, T., Zheng, J., Li, S., & Li, H. Bin. (2016). Dietary natural products for prevention and treatment of liver cancer. *Nutrients*, *8*(3). https://doi.org/10.3390/NU8030156.

Zhu, L., Ding, X., Zhang, D., Ch, Y., Wang, J., Ndegwa, E., & Zhu, G. (2015). Curcumin inhibits bovine herpesvirus type 1 entry into MDBK cells. *Acta Virologica*, *59*(3), 221–227.

Zhuang, X., Dong, A., Wang, R., & Shi, A. (2018). Crocetin treatment inhibits proliferation of colon cancer cells through down-regulation of genes involved in the inflammation. *Saudi Journal of Biological Sciences*, *25*(8), 1767–1771.

Zick, S. M., Turgeon, D. K., Ren, J., Ruffin, M. T., Wright, B. D., Sen, A., Djuric, Z., & Brenner, D. E. (2015). Pilot clinical study of the effects of ginger root extract on eicosanoids in colonic mucosa of subjects at increased risk for colorectal cancer. *Molecular Carcinogenesis*, 54(9), 908–915. https://doi.org/10.1002/MC.22163.

Chapter 4

Apoptosis and Autophagy Induction Mechanisms of Spices in Cancer

Attuluri Vamsi Kumar,[a] Vivek Kumar Garg,[a] and Saahil Kumar Sharma[b]

[a]*Department of Medical Lab Technology,*
University Institute of Allied Health Sciences, Chandigarh University,
Mohali, Punjab, India
[b]*Department of Clinical Research, Desh Bhagat University, Mandi Gobindgarh,*
Fatehgarh Sahib, Punjab, India

garg.vivek85@gmail.com

4.1 Introduction

Cancer encompasses a wide variety of diseases marked by the unchecked growth of irregular cells, culminating in the development of tumors with the potential to metastasize (Gupta, Patchva, et al., 2013). Both genetic and environmental elements have roles in its onset, with mutations in certain genes being particularly influential (Stratton et al., 2009). In 2020, cancer was responsible for nearly 10 million deaths, with 19.3 million new diagnoses (Sung et al., 2021). Notably, the impact of cancer varies across regions and populations due to differences in risk exposure and healthcare accessibility (Bray et al., 2018). Primary

Anticancer Spices: Dietary Input to Health
Edited by Hardeep Singh Tuli
Copyright © 2025 Jenny Stanford Publishing Pte. Ltd.
ISBN 978-981-5129-28-1 (Hardcover), 978-1-003-53466-2 (eBook)
www.jennystanford.com

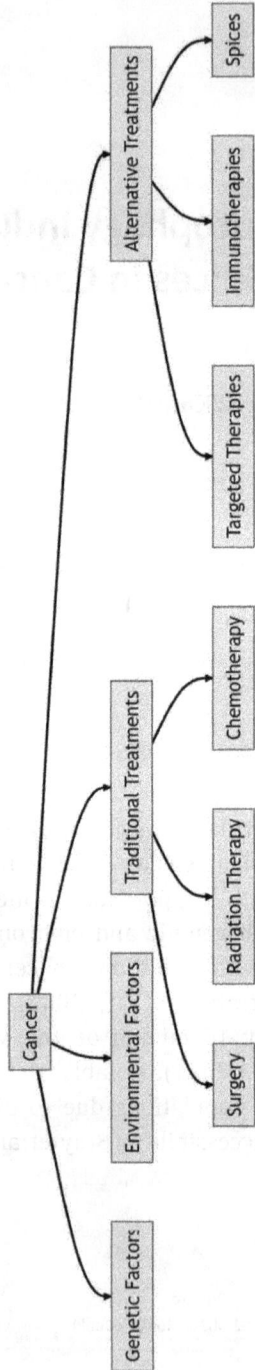

Figure 4.1 Overview of cancer: causes, traditional treatments, and alternative approaches.

cancer treatments like surgery, radiation, and chemotherapy can lead to significant side effects such as pain, tiredness, and heightened infection susceptibility (Miller et al., 2019). Moreover, treatments like chemotherapy and radiation can inadvertently harm healthy cells, causing more health issues (Baskar et al., 2014). Thus, there is a growing urgency to explore more efficient and less detrimental treatment alternatives. Current research is delving into targeted and immune-based therapies, which either focus on cancer cells or activate the body's own defense against them (Scott et al., 2012). Furthermore, natural substances found in spices are being investigated for their anticancer properties, which may work by triggering specific cellular death processes (Xiao et al., 2014). This article aims to delve deeper into these mechanisms and assess the potential of spices in cancer treatment (Fig. 4.1).

4.2   Apoptosis and Autophagy

Apoptosis, or programmed cell death, is a crucial process in development, immunity, and tissue homeostasis (Elmore, 2007). It is characterized by cell shrinkage, chromatin condensation, and DNA fragmentation, leading to cell death. At the molecular level, apoptosis is controlled by various proteins, including the Bcl-2 family proteins, the caspase family, and the tumor necrosis factor (TNF) family (Hengartner, 2000). Dysregulation of apoptosis can lead to cancer, as cells evade apoptosis and proliferate uncontrollably (Kimmelman & White, 2017).

Autophagy is a cellular degradation pathway that delivers cytoplasmic constituents to the lysosome for degradation (Mizushima & Komatsu, 2011a). It helps cells survive under stress conditions such as nutrient starvation. Autophagy can also act as a tumor suppressor by maintaining cellular homeostasis and preventing the accumulation of damaged proteins and organelles (Kimmelman & White, 2017). Yet, in established tumors, autophagy can promote cancer cell survival by providing nutrients and removing toxic substances (Kimmelman & White, 2017). In cancer, both apoptosis and autophagy can be dysregulated.

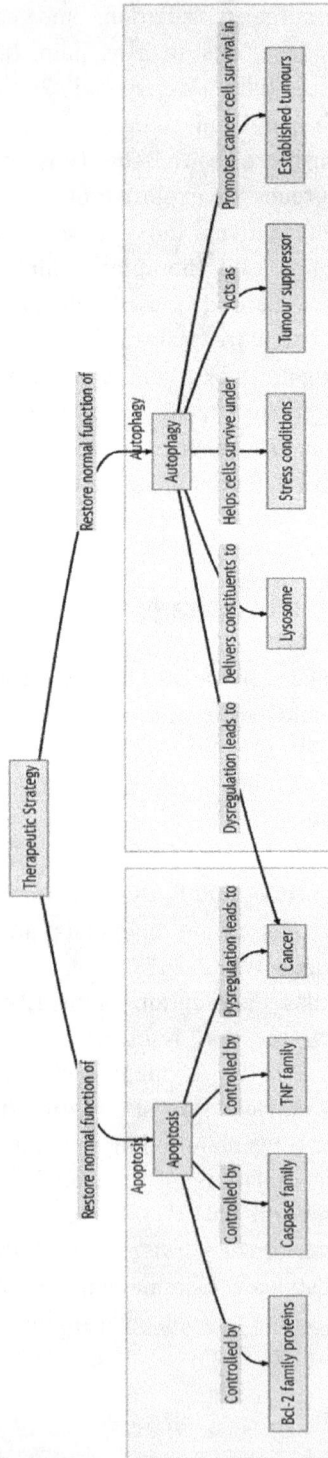

Figure 4.2 The interplay of apoptosis and autophagy in cellular functioning.

For instance, overexpression of anti-apoptotic proteins or downregulation of pro-apoptotic proteins can help cancer cells evade apoptosis (Adams & Cory, 2007). Meanwhile, the role of autophagy in cancer is complex and context-dependent, with both pro-tumorigenic and anti-tumorigenic roles described (Levine & Kroemer, 2008). Restoring the normal function of apoptosis and autophagy has shown promise as a therapeutic strategy in cancer (Fig. 4.2). Agents that can induce apoptosis or autophagy in cancer cells, such as those derived from spices, have the potential to slow tumor growth and overcome resistance to conventional treatments (Adams & Cory, 2007).

4.3 Spices and Their Bioactive Components

Historically, spices have been valued for their potential health-enhancing properties, largely attributed to their abundance of active biological compounds (Gupta, Sung, et al., 2013). These bioactive ingredients can exhibit antioxidant, anti-inflammatory, and anticancer capabilities (Tapsell et al., 2006). A notable example is curcumin, found in turmeric, acclaimed for its anticancer effects. Studies have revealed curcumin's ability to deter various tumor cell growth, initiate cell death, and prevent both angiogenesis and metastasis (Ravindran et al., 2009). The compound's effectiveness is believed to arise from its influence on diverse cellular signaling routes like NF-kB, Akt, MAPK, p53, and more (Prakobwong et al., 2011). Similarly, capsaicin, present in chili peppers, possesses anticancer attributes. Specifically, capsaicin has shown the capacity to trigger cell death and halt the cell cycle in certain cancer cells, and to suppress the activity of NF-kB (Chapa-Oliver & Mejía-Teniente, 2016). A variety of other spices contain bioactive components showcasing anticancer potentials, such as thymoquinone in black seed, piperine in black pepper, zingerone in ginger, and eugenol in cloves (Baliga et al., 2011). While each compound operates through distinct pathways, many prompt cell death processes in cancerous cells, marking them as intriguing subjects for continued study.

4.3.1 Spices and Cancer

Many *in vitro* studies have demonstrated the potential anticancer effects of spices (Fig. 4.3). For example, curcumin has been shown to inhibit the growth of various cancer cell lines and induce apoptosis (Ravindran et al., 2009). Similarly, capsaicin has been shown to induce cell death in several cancer cell types, including colon, breast, and pancreatic cancer cells (Garufi et al., 2016). Studies using animal models have also supported the anticancer effects of spices. In mice, curcumin was found to inhibit tumor growth and metastasis in breast cancer (Aggarwal & Harikumar, 2009). Likewise, capsaicin was shown to inhibit the growth of lung cancer xenografts in mice (Mori et al., 2006). While the evidence from *in vitro* and animal studies is promising, human studies are less conclusive. A few clinical trials have suggested the potential benefits of spices in cancer patients, but these studies were often small, lacked control groups, or had other methodological issues (Gupta, Sung, et al., 2013). More high-quality human studies are needed to confirm the anticancer effects of spices. While the current evidence for the anticancer effects of spices is promising, there are several limitations to the current research. These include the use of high doses in *in vitro* studies that may not be achievable in humans, the potential for adverse effects at high doses, and the lack of standardized dosing regimens. Future research should focus on overcoming these limitations and further exploring the mechanisms of action of spices in cancer (Baliga et al., 2011).

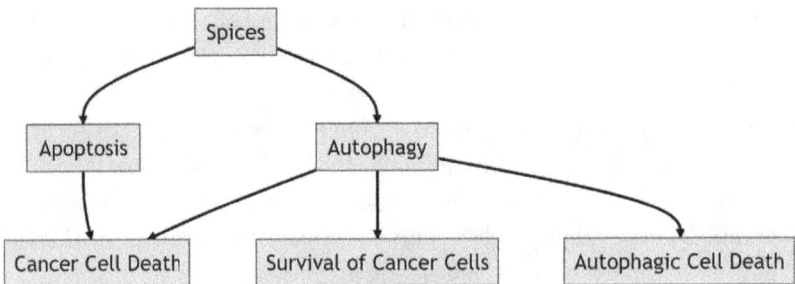

Figure 4.3 Anticancer mechanisms of spices: apoptosis and autophagy.

Spice-derived compounds' capacity to initiate apoptosis in cancer cells is a heavily researched aspect of their anticancer properties. Apoptosis refers to the programmed demise of cells, a process that often goes awry in cancer cells, resulting in unchecked cell growth (Elmore, 2007). These compounds from spices can instigate this programmed death in cancerous cells through diverse mechanisms, potentially leading to tumor shrinkage. Among these, curcumin stands out for its powerful apoptotic properties. It instigates apoptosis by influencing various routes, including those connected to p53, Bcl-2 family proteins, and caspases. Studies show that curcumin decreases levels of anti-apoptotic proteins like Bcl-2 and Bcl-xL and augments levels of pro-apoptotic proteins such as Bax and Bak (Ravindran et al., 2009). Similarly, capsaicin prompts apoptosis across several cancer cell varieties. It stimulates the external death pathway by boosting death receptor expression and their binding molecules, subsequently leading to caspase triggering and apoptosis. Additionally, capsaicin impairs mitochondrial operations, resulting in cytochrome c release and the initiation of the inherent apoptotic route (Brown et al., 2022). Other spice-based compounds, such as thymoquinone, piperine, zingerone, and eugenol, also display the ability to initiate apoptosis across different cancer cells (Baliga et al., 2011). These compounds, akin to curcumin and capsaicin, engage numerous cellular communication routes to activate apoptosis in cancer cells.

Spice-derived compounds are not only capable of inducing apoptosis, but they can also trigger autophagy, a cellular process involving the degradation and recycling of cellular components (Mizushima & Komatsu, 2011). While the role of autophagy in cancer is complex and can vary depending on the context, it generally acts as a tumor suppressor mechanism in the early stages of cancer but may support the survival of established tumors under certain conditions (Kimmelman & White, 2017). Curcumin has been shown to induce autophagy in several cancer cell lines. This involves the activation of AMP-activated protein kinase (AMPK), which inhibits the mTOR pathway and triggers autophagy. Additionally, curcumin can increase the expression of autophagy-related genes such as Beclin-1 and LC3 (Li et al., 2013). Like curcumin, capsaicin can also stimulate autophagy in cancer cells. It has been reported to induce autophagy via the JNK1 pathway, leading to the inhibition of the Akt/mTOR pathway (Park et al., 2014). Moreover, capsaicin-induced autophagy may contribute to the death of cancer cells, further underlining its anticancer potential. Other bioactive compounds from spices, such as piperine, thymoquinone, and eugenol, have also been reported to induce autophagy in various cancer cell models (Kundu & Surh, 2012). These findings suggest a potential therapeutic use of spices for cancer treatment through the modulation of autophagy. Inducing autophagy in cancer cells can have both beneficial and detrimental effects. On the one hand, autophagy can lead to cell death and potentially halt tumor progression. On the other hand, autophagy can provide nutrients to cancer cells and enhance their survival under stressful conditions, such as during chemotherapy (Kimmelman & White, 2017). Thus, the context-specific role of autophagy in cancer should be considered when evaluating the therapeutic potential of spice compounds (Fig. 4.4).

Apoptosis and autophagy are two pivotal cellular functions that intricately interact, especially in the realm of cancer. At times, autophagy can serve as a survival mechanism, aiding cancer cells to fend off apoptosis when faced with metabolic challenges. However, in specific scenarios, heightened autophagy can result in a type of cell death that's separate from apoptosis, known as autophagic cell death (Maiuri et al., 2007). In situations like nutrient scarcity or low oxygen levels, which are frequent in tumors, autophagy might promote cancer cell resilience. This is achieved by breaking down and recycling cellular parts, which furnish the resources and energy required for cancer cells to avoid apoptosis and keep multiplying (Degenhardt et al., 2006). On the flip side, uncontrolled or excessive autophagy can culminate in cell death, termed type II or autophagic cell death, marked by significant degradation of cellular elements (Galluzzi et al., 2014; Tasdemir et al., 2008). The relationship between apoptosis and autophagy is crucial for cancer treatments. Compounds that can influence these processes, like those sourced from spices, might offer more efficient and less harmful substitutes to conventional chemotherapy. Nonetheless, a profound grasp of how apoptosis and autophagy interact, contingent on specific contexts, is essential for crafting such treatments (Galluzzi et al., 2015, 2017).

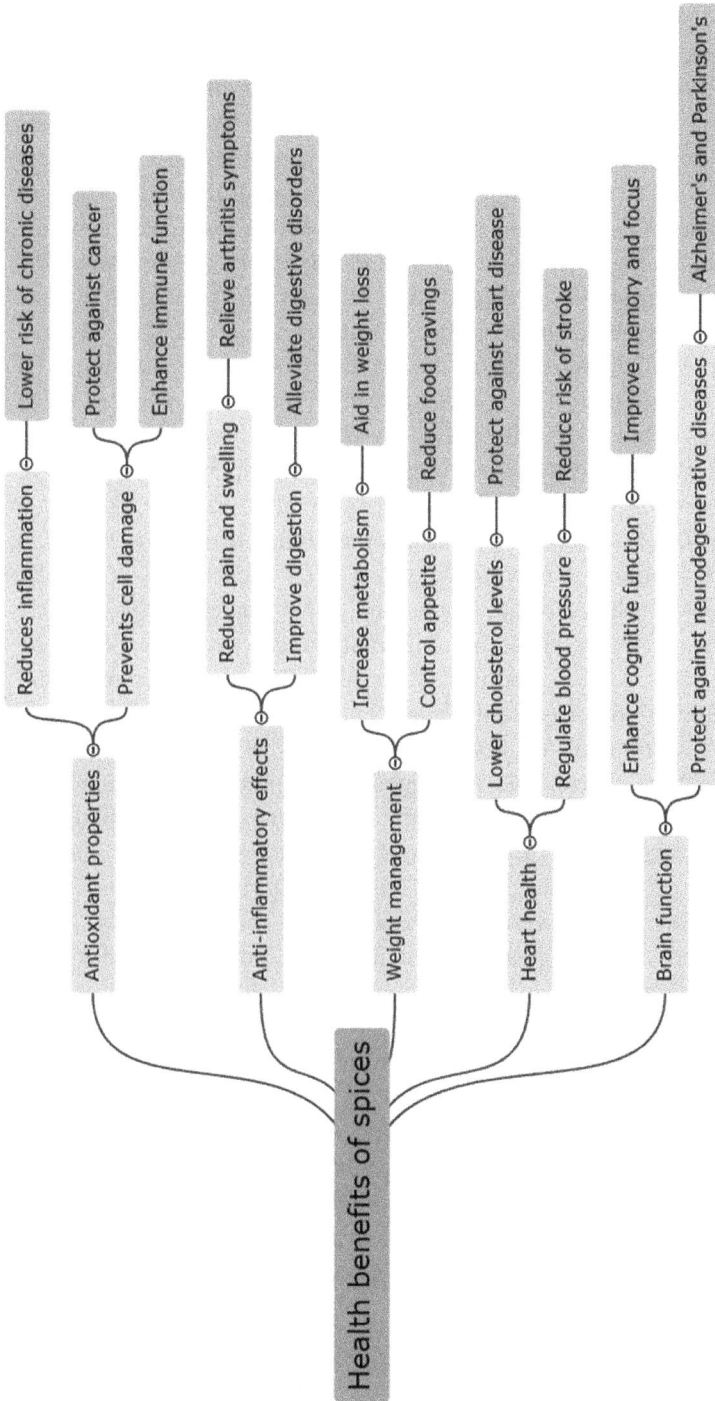

Figure 4.4 Health benefits of spices.

Despite the wealth of preclinical data showing the anticancer potential of spices, there remains a gap in our understanding of the molecular mechanisms underlying their effects, particularly in the context of the complex interplay between apoptosis and autophagy. These two cellular processes are intricately linked, with the balance between them potentially determining the fate of a cancer cell (Maiuri et al., 2007). Moreover, a better understanding of these processes could pave the way for novel therapeutic strategies that harness the power of dietary compounds to combat cancer. To date, numerous studies have demonstrated the capacity of various spices to induce apoptosis and/or autophagy in different cancer models. However, these studies often focus on one or the other of these processes, and a comprehensive understanding of the interplay between them in the context of spice-induced cell death is lacking (Kundu & Surh, 2012). Furthermore, while the ability of certain spices to affect apoptosis and autophagy has been reported, a systematic review of the various spices and their corresponding effects on these processes across different cancer types is yet to be undertaken. Given the increasing global burden of cancer and the limitations of current treatments, including their toxicity and the development of resistance, there is a pressing need for alternative therapeutic strategies. With the growing interest in dietary interventions and the use of natural compounds for cancer prevention and treatment, this topic is timely and of broad relevance (Liu, 2003). Moreover, this review will provide a comprehensive resource for researchers in the field, summarizing the state of knowledge and pointing to potential avenues for future research.

This review aims to provide a comprehensive overview of the evidence relating to the anticancer effects of spices, with a particular focus on their ability to modulate the processes of apoptosis and autophagy. We will first discuss the biological relevance of apoptosis and autophagy and their interplay in cancer. We will then introduce various spices and their bioactive compounds that have demonstrated anticancer potential, delving into their reported effects on apoptosis and autophagy (Fig. 4.5). Subsequent sections will categorize and elaborate on how different types of cancers respond to these spices and the specific apoptosis and autophagy mechanisms that these spices are reported to affect. We will also examine the experimental evidence from both *in vivo* and *in vitro* studies, as well as data from human clinical trials, where available.

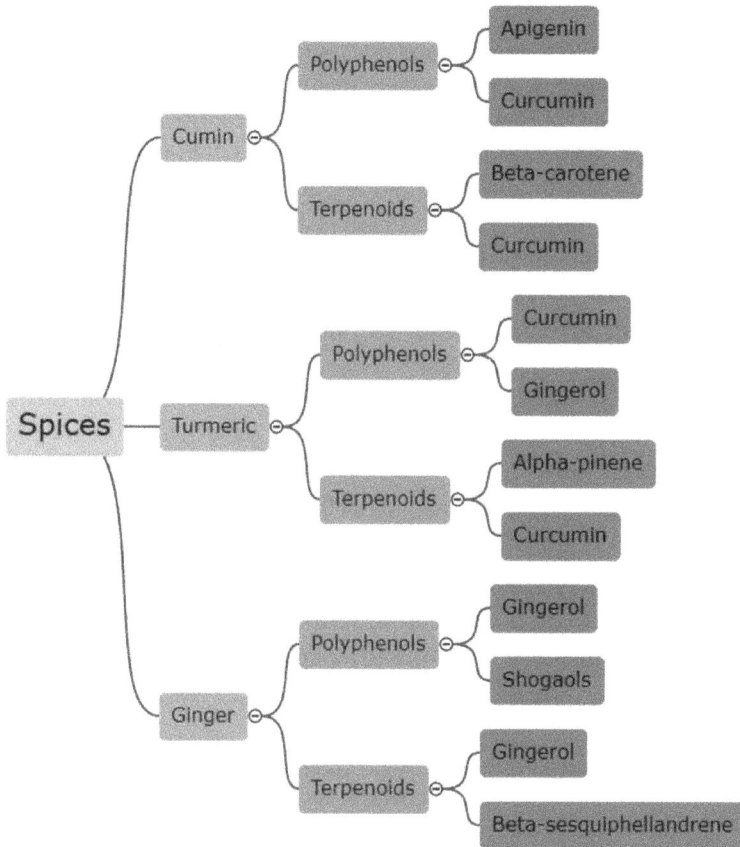

Figure 4.5 Bioactive compounds in spices.

Lastly, we will address the challenges that researchers and clinicians face when attempting to translate these findings into viable therapeutic strategies. We will also highlight gaps in the current body of knowledge that future research needs to address and offer perspectives on future directions for the field.

This review aims to serve as a resource for both researchers in the field of nutrition and oncology and healthcare providers interested in the potential use of dietary interventions in cancer prevention and treatment.

4.3.2 Classification of Spices

Spices have been used since ancient times for culinary and medicinal purposes. Their use in traditional medicine has been recognized for millennia, particularly in countries with rich histories in herbal medicine, such as India, China, and Egypt (Aggarwal & Kunnumakkara, 2009). Recent scientific advances have allowed for the identification and isolation of several bioactive compounds from these spices, many of which show promise in the prevention and treatment of cancer. While spices are typically grouped based on their culinary uses or plant families, this review will focus on classifying them based on their demonstrated anticancer properties (Table 4.1). We will focus on spices that have shown the ability to induce apoptosis and/or autophagy in cancer cells. These include, but are not limited to, turmeric, pepper, garlic, ginger, and cinnamon.

Table 4.1 Bioactive components in spices and their anticancer properties

Spice	Bioactive component	Anticancer effects
Turmeric	Curcumin	Induces apoptosis in cancer cells through various pathways
Pepper	Piperine	Triggers apoptosis possibly by altering the expression of apoptosis-related proteins
Garlic	Allicin	Induces apoptosis possibly through effects on mitochondrial function and caspase activation
Ginger	Gingerol	Has anti-inflammatory and anti-carcinogenic properties; may affect the expression of apoptosis-related proteins
Cinnamon	Cinnamaldehyde	May inhibit the proliferation of cancer cells and induce apoptosis through effects on cell cycle regulation and apoptosis-related pathways

Turmeric (Curcumin): Curcumin, the main bioactive compound in turmeric, has been widely studied for its anticancer effects. Curcumin has been shown to trigger apoptosis in a variety of cancer cell lines, potentially through its effects on Bcl-2 and caspase family proteins, among other pathways (Aggarwal et al., 2003).

Pepper (Piperine): Piperine, the compound that gives black pepper its pungency, has also shown promise as a cancer therapeutic. Studies have suggested that piperine can induce apoptosis in cancer cells, possibly by increasing the expression of pro-apoptotic proteins and decreasing the expression of anti-apoptotic proteins (Greenshields et al., 2015).

Garlic (Allicin): Garlic contains a number of bioactive compounds, including allicin, which has demonstrated anticancer properties. Allicin has been shown to induce apoptosis in cancer cells, possibly through its effects on mitochondrial function and the activation of caspases (Zhang et al., 2019).

Ginger (Gingerols): Gingerols, the bioactive compounds in ginger, have been shown to have anti-inflammatory and anti-carcinogenic properties. They may induce apoptosis in cancer cells, possibly by affecting the expression of apoptosis-related proteins (Lee & Surh, 1998).

Cinnamon (Cinnamaldehyde): Cinnamaldehyde, the compound that gives cinnamon its flavor and aroma, has been shown to have anticancer effects. Studies suggest that cinnamaldehyde may inhibit the proliferation of cancer cells and induce apoptosis, possibly through its effects on cell cycle regulation and the activation of apoptosis-related pathways (Koppikar et al., 2010).

4.3.3   Spices and Specific Cancer Types

Dietary factors, including spices, play a significant role in cancer prevention and treatment, and an increasing body of evidence supports their potential therapeutic benefits (Table 4.2). Epidemiological studies have demonstrated a correlation between spice consumption and reduced cancer incidence, with specific spices exhibiting chemo-preventive and chemotherapeutic properties against various types of cancer (Aggarwal & Shishodia, 2006; Liu et al., 2014).

Table 4.2 Effects of specific spices on different cancer types

Spice	Bioactive component	Cancer type	Effect on cancer cells	Mechanisms of action	Evidence level (*in vitro, in vivo*, clinical trials)	References
Turmeric	Curcumin	Breast cancer	Induces apoptosis and autophagy	Activates caspase pathways, inhibits NF-κB signaling	*In vitro, in vivo*	(Aggarwal & Shishodia, 2006; Liu et al., 2014)
Ginger	Gingerol	Prostate cancer	Induces apoptosis and inhibits proliferation	Inhibits MAPK and PI3K/Akt signaling pathways	*In vitro, in vivo*	(Banerjee et al., 2010; Pommier et al., 2010)
Garlic	Allicin	Colorectal cancer	Induces apoptosis, inhibits cell cycle	Activates p53, increases ROS production	*In vitro, in vivo*, limited clinical trials	(Butt et al., 2009; Ravindran et al., 2009)
Black pepper	Piperine	Lung cancer	Induces apoptosis and autophagy	Inhibits STAT3, Akt/ mTOR signaling	*In vitro, in vivo*	(Kaefer & Milner, 2008; Prasad et al., 2014)
Cinnamon	Cinnamaldehyde	Pancreatic cancer	Induces apoptosis, inhibits metastasis	Inhibits NF-κB, MMP-2/9 expression	*In vitro, in vivo*	(Sarkar et al., 2010; Srinivasan, 2014)

Breast Cancer: Several spices such as turmeric and ginger have demonstrated effects on breast cancer cells. The bioactive components of these spices, notably curcumin in turmeric and gingerol in ginger, have been shown to induce apoptosis and autophagy in breast cancer cells, thereby inhibiting their growth and proliferation (Banerjee et al., 2010; Pommier et al., 2010).

Prostate Cancer: Bioactive components of spices, like curcumin from turmeric and piperine from black pepper, have shown significant anticancer effects against prostate cancer. These compounds can induce apoptosis and autophagy in prostate cancer cells, halting their progression (Butt et al., 2009; Ravindran et al., 2009).

Colorectal Cancer: Spices such as turmeric and garlic have been associated with reduced risk and improved treatment outcomes for colorectal cancer. The bioactive compounds within these spices induce apoptosis and autophagy in colorectal cancer cells, thereby inhibiting their growth (Kaefer & Milner, 2008; Prasad et al., 2014).

Lung Cancer: Certain spices and their bioactive components have demonstrated inhibitory effects on lung cancer cells, with emphasis on apoptosis and autophagy. For instance, capsaicin from chili peppers has shown the potential to induce apoptosis in lung cancer cells (Srinivasan, 2014).

Pancreatic Cancer: Various spices have been observed to impact pancreatic cancer cells, with mechanisms involving apoptosis and autophagy. Curcumin, a bioactive component of turmeric, has shown promise in inducing apoptosis and autophagy in pancreatic cancer cells (Sarkar et al., 2010).

Despite the promising potential of spices as anticancer agents, several challenges exist. These include the lack of extensive human trials, variability in spice composition, issues with the bioavailability of the bioactive compounds, and potential adverse effects (Baer-Dubowska et al., 1998). The use of spices as anticancer agents opens a promising avenue for cancer prevention and treatment. Their bioactive compounds induce apoptosis and autophagy in various types of cancer, thus halting their progression. However, more extensive human trials are required to conclusively establish their therapeutic potential and overcome the current challenges.

4.4   Mechanism of Inducing Apoptosis

Apoptosis plays a vital role in maintaining homeostasis and preventing the development of cancer by eliminating cells that are damaged, infected, or no longer needed (Elmore, 2007). It is primarily regulated by two major pathways: the intrinsic (mitochondrial) pathway and the extrinsic (death receptor) pathway. The BCL-2 family proteins are pivotal regulators of the intrinsic apoptosis pathway. This family includes both pro-apoptotic members (such as BAX, BAK, and BAD) and anti-apoptotic members (such as BCL-2 and BCL-XL). A delicate balance between pro- and anti-apoptotic proteins is essential for cell survival and death; an imbalance can lead to diseases such as cancer (Adams & Cory, 2007). Notably, certain bioactive components from spices, such as curcumin and capsaicin, have been shown to modulate the BCL-2 family proteins to promote apoptosis in cancer cells (Bimonte et al., 2013). Caspases, cysteine-dependent aspartate-directed proteases, are the executioners of apoptosis. They are categorized as initiator caspases (like caspases 8 and 9) that kick start the apoptosis process, and executioner caspases (like caspases 3, 6, and 7) that carry out the demolition phase, leading to cell death (Julien and Wells, 2017). Intriguingly, several bioactive compounds from spices, including curcumin, capsaicin, and piperine, have been reported to trigger caspase-dependent apoptosis in various types of cancer cells (Bimonte et al., 2013; Greenshields et al., 2015; Prasad & Aggarwal, 2011). The tumor necrosis factor-related apoptosis-inducing ligand (TRAIL) pathway plays a crucial role in immune surveillance against tumor cells. TRAIL binds to death receptors (DR4 and DR5) to form the death-inducing signaling complex (DISC), leading to caspase activation and apoptosis (Ashkenazi, 2008). Emerging studies have suggested that certain spices, like garlic and ginger, can upregulate TRAIL expression or enhance the sensitivity of cancer cells to TRAIL-induced apoptosis (Zhang et al., 2010).

Curcumin, the active compound of turmeric, has been reported to induce apoptosis in various types of cancer cells by altering the expression of Bcl-2 family proteins, activating caspases, and enhancing TRAIL-induced apoptosis (Anand et al., 2008; Ravindran et al., 2009). Piperine, an active compound in black pepper, has been found to induce apoptosis in breast cancer cells by inhibiting the PI3K/Akt/mTOR pathway, a signaling pathway often hyperactivated in cancer (Greenshields et al., 2015). Allicin, a compound in garlic, can induce apoptosis in gastric cancer cells by upregulating TRAIL and activating caspases (Kwon et al., 2010). Gingerols in ginger can trigger apoptosis in colon cancer cells through modulation of the Bcl-2 family proteins and activation of caspases (Rhode et al., 2007). Cinnamaldehyde, a bioactive compound in cinnamon, has been found to induce apoptosis in leukemia cells by disrupting the mitochondrial membrane potential and triggering caspase activation (Zhang et al., 2010).

Table 4.3 Spice-specific mechanisms of apoptosis induction in cancer cells

Spice	Bioactive compound	Mechanism of action	References
Turmeric	Curcumin	Alters the expression of Bcl-2 family proteins, activates caspases, enhances TRAIL-induced apoptosis	(Anand et al., 2008; Ravindran et al., 2009)
Pepper	Piperine	Inhibits the PI3K/Akt/mTOR pathway	(Greenshields et al., 2015)
Garlic	Allicin	Upregulates TRAIL, activates caspases	(Zhang et al., 2010)
Ginger	Gingerols	Modulates the Bcl-2 family proteins, activates caspases	(Rhode et al., 2007)
Cinnamon	Cinnamaldehyde	Disrupts the mitochondrial membrane potential, triggers caspase activation	(Kwon et al., 2010)

There is emerging evidence that combining different bioactive compounds from spices can produce a synergistic effect, leading to enhanced induction of apoptosis. For example, co-treatment with curcumin and piperine has been found to increase the apoptotic effect in various cancer cells (Kakarala et al., 2010). Despite the promising anticancer properties of spices, significant challenges remain, such as the need for more human trials, the bioavailability of bioactive compounds, and difficulties in standardizing doses. Nanotechnology-based delivery systems and structural modifications of bioactive compounds are potential solutions that could increase the bioavailability and therapeutic efficacy of these compounds (Shanmugam et al., 2015). Understanding the mechanisms through which spices induce apoptosis in cancer cells could pave the way for novel cancer therapies (Table 4.3). Given their relative safety, spices and their bioactive compounds hold great potential as part of a natural, less-toxic approach to cancer prevention and treatment.

4.5   Mechanism of Inducing Autophagy

Autophagy, a self-degradative process crucial for maintaining cellular homeostasis, has been the subject of burgeoning interest in cancer research due to its dual role as both a potential tumor suppressor and a survival mechanism for established tumors (Amaravadi et al., 2016). Autophagy can be categorized into macroautophagy, microautophagy, and chaperone-mediated autophagy, each characterized by different processes and functions (Mizushima et al., 2008). The autophagy pathway, intricately coordinated by various proteins and complexes, encompasses several stages: induction, nucleation, elongation, fusion, and degradation (Dikic & Elazar, 2018). The ULK1 complex initiates autophagy, followed by the nucleation phase led by the PI3K complex. Autophagy-related (ATG) proteins then facilitate membrane elongation, leading to the formation of autophagosomes. These autophagosomes eventually fuse with lysosomes, where enclosed materials are degraded by lysosomal enzymes (Levine & Klionsky, 2017). Autophagy is modulated by several key pathways, including the nutrient-sensing mTOR pathway and energy-sensing AMPK pathway. The tumor suppressor protein p53 also plays a crucial role in coordinating autophagic responses (Kunnumakkara et al., 2017; Maiuri et al., 2009).

These regulatory mechanisms respond to diverse cellular stresses, precisely modulating the degree of autophagy to ensure cellular homeostasis. Spices, including turmeric, pepper, garlic, ginger, and cinnamon, have long been recognized for their medicinal properties. Recent studies suggest that their bioactive compounds can modulate autophagic responses in cancer cells (Kunnumakkara et al., 2017). For instance, curcumin in turmeric can inhibit mTOR signaling, thus activating autophagy (Xiao et al., 2014). Similarly, allicin from garlic can induce autophagy in human hepatocellular carcinoma cells through the AMPK pathway (Xiao et al., 2014). These findings underline the potential of spices as modulators of autophagy in cancer treatment. The relationship between autophagy and cancer is complex. While autophagy may suppress tumorigenesis by removing damaged proteins and organelles, it can also promote cancer cell survival under stress conditions. However, excessively activated autophagy can induce a form of cell death, known as autophagic or type II cell death (Galluzzi et al., 2015). There is emerging evidence that combinations of spices or their bioactive components can synergistically enhance autophagy, leading to more potent anticancer effects (Cao et al., 2015; Mulcahy Levy & Thorburn, 2020). Despite promising preclinical findings, translating autophagy modulation into cancer therapy faces several challenges. The complexity of autophagy regulation, difficulty in accurately monitoring autophagy in humans, and the scarcity of clinical trials testing the efficacy of autophagy modulators are some current limitations (Mulcahy Levy & Thorburn, 2020). Future studies should focus on addressing these challenges and explore potential solutions, such as combining autophagy-modulating spices with conventional therapies. Therefore, spices and their bioactive compounds hold promising potential as autophagy modulators in cancer therapy. However, a more comprehensive understanding of the complex regulation and role of autophagy in cancer is necessary. As we continue to unravel the mechanisms underlying the effects of spices on autophagy, it is hoped that novel and more effective strategies for cancer therapy will emerge (Table 4.4).

Table 4.4 Spice-specific mechanisms of autophagy induction in cancer cells

Spice	Bioactive compound	Autophagy-related targets or pathways	Evidence source
Turmeric	Curcumin	mTOR, AMPK, Beclin-1, LC3-II	(Aoki et al., 2007)
Pepper	Piperine	mTOR, p70S6K, ULK1	(Yaffe et al., 2015)
Garlic	Allicin	Beclin-1, LC3-II, p62	(Chen et al., 2020)
Ginger	Gingerols	AMPK, mTOR, ULK1	(Jeong et al., 2009)
Cinnamon	Cinnamaldehyde	AMPK, PI3K/Akt/mTOR	(Koppikar et al., 2010)

4.6 Crosstalk Between Apoptosis and Autophagy

The existence of intertwined pathways between apoptosis and autophagy, two critical cellular responses to stress, has been the subject of intensive investigation. Both these processes are essential for maintaining cellular homeostasis; however, they play different roles. Apoptosis is a form of programmed cell death, while autophagy, primarily a survival mechanism, may lead to cell death under certain circumstances (Maiuri, 2007). Apoptosis and autophagy are not isolated events, rather, they share a complex interplay that ultimately dictates cell fate. While autophagy is generally cytoprotective, it can facilitate cell death under certain conditions. Conversely, apoptosis functions as a programmed cell death pathway. Depending on the cellular context and stimuli, these processes can cooperate, compete, or substitute for each other to decide the cell's fate (Berghe et al., 2014). The common molecular machinery and signaling pathways underpin the intricate crosstalk between apoptosis and autophagy. The anti-apoptotic BCL-2 protein, for instance, inhibits apoptosis while also controlling autophagy through its binding to Beclin-1 (Pattingre et al., 2005). The p53 tumor suppressor, depending on its location, can both promote apoptosis and inhibit autophagy (Tasdemir et al., 2008). Additionally, the mTOR complex, a central regulator of cell growth, can inhibit autophagy and influence apoptosis (Mo et al., 2010). Certain caspases, essential to apoptosis, can cleave autophagy-related proteins and thereby inhibit autophagy (Wirawan et al., 2010).

Research suggests that bioactive components from certain spices can modulate the interplay between apoptosis and autophagy. For instance, curcumin, found in turmeric, is known to induce both autophagy and apoptosis in cancer cells. The delicate balance between these two processes, modulated by curcumin, may be a critical factor in determining cell fate (Mo et al., 2010). The nuanced interplay between apoptosis and autophagy has considerable implications for cancer therapy. By modulating this crosstalk, the response of cancer cells to therapy could be influenced. For example, the application of spices known to enhance apoptosis or autophagy could offer a new therapeutic avenue (White, 2012). Despite these promising findings, challenges remain. Manipulating the balance between apoptosis and autophagy with precision remains difficult. Furthermore, there is a pressing need for clinical evidence to substantiate the potential of these spice-derived compounds in cancer treatment. Future research should aim to identify new modulators of apoptosis-autophagy crosstalk and explore combination strategies for cancer therapy (Kimmelman & White, 2017). In summary, the crosstalk between apoptosis and autophagy, albeit complex, offers intriguing possibilities for cancer therapy (Table 4.5). Exploiting this relationship using bioactive compounds from spices opens up novel therapeutic opportunities. However, a comprehensive understanding and successful application of this strategy necessitate further research in this promising field.

4.7   *In vivo* and *in vitro* Studies

Both cell culture (*in vitro*) and animal model (*in vivo*) studies have been instrumental in shedding light on the anticancer properties of spices (Table 4.6). These distinct study methods yield mutually informative perspectives on the therapeutic potential of spice-derived bioactive ingredients. While *in vitro* studies give intricate insights into the molecular and cellular

Table 4.5 Modulation of apoptosis–autophagy crosstalk by spice-derived compounds

Spice	Bioactive compound	Effect on apoptosis	Effect on autophagy	Mechanism of action	References
Turmeric	Curcumin	Induces	Induces	Inhibits BCL-2, activates caspases and autophagy-related proteins	(Prakobwong et al., 2011)
Pepper	Piperine	Induces	Induces	Inhibits BCL-2, induces Beclin-1, regulates mTOR and p53	(Huang et al., 2013)
Garlic	Allicin	Induces	Induces	Induces reactive oxygen species (ROS generation, caspase activation, and Beclin-1 expression	(Liu et al., 2010)
Ginger	Gingerol	Induces	Induces	Inhibits BCL-2, activates caspases, induces LC3-II expression	(Prasad & Tyagi, 2015)
Cinnamon	Cinnamaldehyde	Induces	Induces	Inhibits NF-κB and Akt/mTOR signaling, induces ROS generation	(Liu et al., 2010)

Table 4.6 Key *in vitro* and *in vivo* studies on anticancer effects of spices

Study type	Spice	Bioactive compound	Cancer type	Key findings	Reference
In vitro	Grapes & berries, black pepper	Resveratrol, piperine	Prostate cancer	Enhanced bioavailability and efficacy of resveratrol in killing prostate cancer cells	[Johnson et al., 2011]
In vitro	Turmeric, cruciferous vegetables	Curcumin, phenethyl isothiocyanate	Prostate cancer	Synergistic inhibition of growth of human PC-3 prostate cancer cells	[Khor et al., 2006]
In vivo	Black pepper	Piperine	Breast cancer	Inhibition of tumor growth and metastasis	[Wang et al., 2012]
In vivo	Turmeric	Curcumin	Prostate cancer	Inhibition of proliferation of prostate cancer cells, induction of apoptosis, and inhibition of angiogenesis	[Dorai et al., 2001]

activities of these substances, *in vivo* studies portray a comprehensive picture of their impact on the intricate systems of living beings (Levine & Klionsky, 2017). Various *in vitro* research has unveiled the anticancer capabilities of numerous spices. For instance, a study by Johnson et al. showed that when resveratrol, present in grapes and berries, is paired with piperine from black pepper, it greatly improves resveratrol's absorption and potency against prostate cancer cells (Johnson, 2011). Another research by Khor et al. determined that merging curcumin, sourced from turmeric, with phenethyl isothiocyanate from cruciferous veggies, collaboratively halted the expansion of human PC-3 prostate cancer cells (Khor et al., 2006).

Despite these promising results, *in vitro* studies come with their own set of limitations. For one, the experimental conditions of cell culture studies do not fully replicate the complexity of biological systems within a living organism. Additionally, differences in the bioavailability and metabolism of spice compounds between *in vitro* conditions and the human body may influence their anticancer effects.

Animal model-based (*in vivo*) studies offer a closer-to-reality evaluation of spices' anticancer capabilities. For example, a study by Wang et al. found that piperine reduced tumor growth and spread in a mouse breast cancer model (Lai et al., 2012). In another research, Dorai et al. discovered that curcumin not only curtailed the growth of prostate cancer cells in mice but also triggered apoptosis and restricted angiogenesis (Dorai et al., 2001). However, similar to *in vitro* research, *in vivo* investigations carry their set of constraints. Even though animal models present a context more akin to real-life situations compared to cell cultures, they do not flawlessly emulate human cancer due to biological disparities between different species.

While both *in vitro* and *in vivo* studies have advanced our understanding of the anticancer effects of spices, discrepancies between their findings can sometimes arise due to the different experimental conditions and biological complexities (Knight, 2008). Such discrepancies highlight the need for more integrated research approaches, including more sophisticated *in vitro* models like organoids or micro-physiological systems, and better *in vivo* models that can more accurately mimic human cancer.

One major challenge for both *in vitro* and *in vivo* studies is the variability in the composition of spices, which can influence the bioavailability and metabolism of their bioactive compounds. More standardized protocols for preparing and administering spice extracts or compounds may help address this issue. Furthermore, more advanced *in vitro* models like organoids and micro-physiological systems could provide more realistic cellular environments for testing the anticancer effects of spices (Ronaldson-Bouchard & Vunjak-Novakovic, 2018). In summary, both *in vitro* and *in vivo* studies play integral roles in exploring the anticancer potential of spices. They provide complementary insights into the mechanisms and efficacy of spice compounds, thereby paving the way for their potential use in cancer therapy. Nevertheless, more research is required to overcome the current challenges and further our understanding of this promising field (Mould-Quevedo et al., 2009).

4.8   Clinical Trials

Several clinical trials have assessed the anticancer effects of various spices, particularly turmeric (curcumin), pepper (piperine), and ginger (6-gingerol) (Table 4.7). A randomized, double-blind, placebo-controlled trial involving 44 patients with lesions (precancerous lesions) showed that oral curcumin effectively reduced the lesions' size and number by 40% within 30 days (Cruz–Correa et al., 2006). This indicated that curcumin could potentially prevent cancer at its earliest stages. In another study involving 114 patients, the combination of curcumin and piperine significantly decreased oxidative stress markers and enhanced the antioxidant status in oral submucous fibrosis patients (Sharma et al., 2021). Furthermore, a phase II trial of ginger showed significant improvement in chemotherapy-induced nausea symptoms in cancer patients (Ryan et al., 2012). While these trials provide promising results, they also have limitations. Many of the trials had small sample sizes and short durations, limiting the generalizability of their results. Also, the bioavailability of these bioactive compounds is a significant concern due to their poor absorption and rapid metabolism (Anand et al., 2007).

Table 4.7 Summary of key clinical trials investigating the anticancer properties of spice-derived compounds

Spice/compound	Clinical trial phase	Cancer type	Study design	Number of participants	Key findings	References
Curcumin	Completed	Pre-cancerous lesions	Randomized, double-blind, placebo-controlled	44	Reduced lesions' size and number by 40%	(Cruz–Correa et al., 2006)
Curcumin and Piperine	Completed	Oral submucous fibrosis	Randomized, double-blind, placebo-controlled	114	Decreased oxidative stress markers and enhanced antioxidant status	(Sharma et al., 2021)
Ginger (6-gingerol)	Completed	Chemotherapy-induced nausea	Double-blind, randomized, placebo-controlled	576	Significant improvement in chemotherapy-induced nausea	(Ryan et al., 2012)
Curcumin	Ongoing (phase II)	Colon cancer	Randomized, double-blind, placebo-controlled	Not available	Not available	(Center, n.d.)
Piperine	Ongoing	Non-specified	Non-specified	Not available	Not available	

Numerous clinical trials are currently underway to further investigate the anticancer effects of spices. For example, a phase II trial is investigating the effects of curcumin on colon cancer, while another trial is studying the effects of piperine on bioavailability and the immune system in cancer patients (Center, n.d.). These trials could provide vital evidence regarding the therapeutic efficacy and safety of these spices in treating different types of cancers.

Despite the promising anticancer potential of spices, several challenges remain. The bioavailability of these compounds remains a significant concern. Furthermore, patient compliance and potential side effects also pose significant challenges. Future research should focus on improving the bioavailability of these compounds, possibly through novel delivery systems. There is also a need for larger and more rigorous trials and a deeper investigation into the effects of combinations of different spices. Clinical trials and human studies play a crucial role in translating preclinical findings into potential therapeutic applications. The current evidence suggests a promising potential for spices in cancer therapy, although further research is required to overcome the existing challenges and validate these effects.

4.9 Challenges and Future Directions

Indeed, translating preclinical findings into effective clinical applications has always been a major challenge in biomedical research, and the use of spices as anticancer agents is no exception (Pammolli et al., 2011).

Bioavailability of bioactive compounds is one of the first hurdles to tackle. These compounds' absorption and subsequent availability to exert their pharmacological effects is influenced by several factors including method of administration, individual differences in metabolism, and interaction with other dietary components (Singh & Lillard Jr, 2009). Future research needs to address these issues, possibly with innovative drug delivery systems or using adjunct substances that can enhance absorption and bioavailability. Another challenge is potential side effects.

While generally recognized as safe, certain spices when consumed in large doses may exert toxicity or elicit allergic reactions. For instance, excessive intake of curcumin has been associated with gastrointestinal discomfort, and in rare cases, hypersensitivity reactions (Reeta & Kalia, 2022). Furthermore, potential interactions of these bioactive compounds with conventional chemotherapy need to be thoroughly investigated to avoid undesirable consequences (Hermann & von Richter, 2012).

The standardization of doses poses yet another significant challenge. The concentration of bioactive compounds varies widely among different varieties of spices and is also greatly influenced by cooking and processing methods. Thus, developing accurate, reliable, and reproducible methods for measurement and standardization is a critical need for this field (Johnson, 2011). The design of clinical trials to evaluate the safety and efficacy of spices as anticancer agents presents unique challenges. These include the need for appropriate control treatments, recruitment of a sufficiently large and diverse sample of participants, and ethical considerations inherent in using a non-conventional treatment (Sironi et al., 2017). The commercialization of these natural compounds and regulatory issues are additional hurdles. For instance, patenting natural substances is often difficult, and ensuring consistency in product quality can be a major challenge (Yamagata, 2019). Regulatory bodies require rigorous safety and efficacy data for approval of any substance as a therapeutic agent (Wang et al., 2013).

Moving forward, research should focus on improving the bioavailability of bioactive compounds, investigating the detailed mechanisms of their anticancer actions, conducting more rigorous clinical trials, and addressing standardization issues. Besides, innovative approaches to overcome the commercial and regulatory challenges are also required. In conclusion, although numerous challenges persist in the journey of spices from the kitchen to the clinic as anticancer agents, the potential benefits they offer make it a venture worth pursuing (Table 4.8). Overcoming these challenges could open new avenues for cancer therapy and bring hope to millions of patients worldwide.

Table 4.8 Key challenges and future directions in utilizing spices for cancer prevention and treatment

Challenge	Description	Possible future directions	Reference
Bioavailability	Variability in the absorption of bioactive compounds from spices due to factors such as the method of consumption, food matrix, and individual metabolism.	Research into methods to improve the bioavailability of bioactive compounds, such as new formulations or delivery methods.	(Di Meo et al., 2019)
Side effects	Potential adverse effects of bioactive compounds in spices, including direct toxic effects, allergic reactions, or interactions with other substances.	Further investigation into the risk profile of these compounds, as well as research into methods to minimize side effects.	(Jurenka, et al., 2009)
Standardization of doses	Difficulty standardizing the doses of bioactive compounds from spices due to variations in spice varieties and the effect of cooking or processing.	Development of methods to standardize the concentration of bioactive compounds in spices.	(Shobha et al., 1998)
Clinical trial design	Challenges related to the selection of control treatments, the need for large sample sizes, and ethical considerations when designing clinical trials for spices as anticancer agents.	Development of guidelines for designing rigorous and ethically sound clinical trials in this field.	(Kotecha et al., 2021)
Regulatory and commercial	Regulatory requirements for safety and efficacy testing, and challenges related to patenting natural substances or achieving consistency in product quality.	Advocacy for clear regulatory guidelines for natural anticancer agents, and exploration of commercial strategies that ensure product quality.	(Jones et al., 2016)

4.10   Conclusion

In this review, we have delved into the profound promise of spices as anticancer agents, primarily focusing on their role in inducing apoptosis and autophagy. This relationship presents an opportunity for therapeutic intervention in the fight against cancer, a leading cause of death worldwide (Bray et al., 2018). The bioactive compounds present in various spices such as curcumin, piperine, capsaicin, and many others, have shown anticancer effects in different cancer types (Bray et al., 2018; Shanmugam et al., 2016). Their mechanism of action involves disrupting cell homeostasis, leading to programmed cell death and autophagy, therefore inhibiting cancer progression (Hanahan & Weinberg, 2011; Kroemer et al., 2010). The interplay between apoptosis and autophagy is complex and still under intensive investigation, but emerging data have shed light on their coordinated action in regulating cell death and survival (Gong et al., 2013; Levy et al., 2017).

Preclinical *in vitro* and *in vivo* studies have contributed significantly to our understanding of the anticancer properties of spices (Aggarwal et al., 2009; Toden et al., 2015). However, there remain discrepancies between these studies, underlining the need for further investigations and more sophisticated study models. Clinical trials and human studies have attempted to translate preclinical findings into the clinical realm, with some promising results (Ryan et al., 2013). Yet, limitations exist, including issues of bioavailability, dosing standardization, and potential side effects, which need to be addressed in future studies (Kotecha et al., 2016).

Given these challenges, future research directions should focus on improving the bioavailability of bioactive compounds, clarifying their mechanisms of action, conducting rigorous clinical trials, and developing standardization methods (Hejazi et al., 2016). In conclusion, the potential of spices as anticancer agents presents a fascinating field of research. Despite the complexity and challenges, spices and their bioactive components hold promising potential as a new frontier in cancer therapy. However, more rigorous, comprehensive, and well-designed studies are required to fully comprehend and exploit the potential of these natural compounds in the fight against cancer. The take-home message from this review is clear: spices, commonplace in our diets, could be key players in the field of oncology. Their journey from the kitchen shelf to the medicine cabinet, while fraught with challenges, represents a promising and exciting direction for cancer research.

References

Adams, J. M., & Cory, S. (2007). The Bcl-2 apoptotic switch in cancer development and therapy. *Oncogene, 26*(9), 1324–1337. https://doi.org/10.1038/sj.onc.1210220.

Aggarwal, B. B., & Harikumar, K. B. (2009). Potential therapeutic effects of curcumin, the anti-inflammatory agent, against neurodegenerative, cardiovascular, pulmonary, metabolic, autoimmune and neoplastic diseases. *The International Journal of Biochemistry & Cell Biology, 41*(1), 40–59.

Aggarwal, B. B., Kumar, A., & Bharti, A. C. (2003). Anticancer potential of curcumin: preclinical and clinical studies. *Anticancer Research, 23*(1/A), 363–398.

Aggarwal, B. B., & Kunnumakkara, A. B. (2009). *Molecular targets and therapeutic uses of spices: modern uses for ancient medicine.* World Scientific.

Aggarwal, B. B., & Shishodia, S. (2006). Guggulsterone inhibits NF-kappa and lkappaBalpha kinase activation, suppresses expression of anti-apoptotic gene products, and enhances apoptosis. *Biochem Pharmacol, 71*, 1397–1421.

Aggarwal, B. B., Van Kuiken, M. E., Iyer, L. H., Harikumar, K. B., & Sung, B. (2009). Molecular targets of nutraceuticals derived from dietary spices: potential role in suppression of inflammation and tumorigenesis. *Experimental Biology and Medicine, 234*(8), 825–849.

Amaravadi, R., Kimmelman, A. C., & White, E. (2016). Recent insights into the function of autophagy in cancer. *Genes & Development, 30*(17), 1913–1930.

Anand, P., Kunnumakkara, A. B., Newman, R. A., & Aggarwal, B. B. (2007). Bioavailability of curcumin: problems and promises. *Molecular Pharmaceutics, 4*(6), 807–818.

Anand, P., Sundaram, C., Jhurani, S., Kunnumakkara, A. B., & Aggarwal, B. B. (2008). Curcumin and cancer: an "old-age" disease with an "age-old" solution. *Cancer Letters, 267*(1), 133–164.

Aoki, H., Takada, Y., Kondo, S., Sawaya, R., Aggarwal, B. B., & Kondo, Y. (2007). Evidence that curcumin suppresses the growth of malignant gliomas *in vitro* and *in vivo* through induction of autophagy: role of Akt and extracellular signal-regulated kinase signaling pathways. *Molecular Pharmacology, 72*(1), 29–39.

Ashkenazi, A. (2008). Targeting the extrinsic apoptosis pathway in cancer. *Cytokine & Growth Factor Reviews, 19*(3–4), 325–331.

Baer-Dubowska, W., Szaefer, H., & Krajka-Kuzniak, V. (1998). Inhibition of murine hepatic cytochrome P450 activities by natural and synthetic phenolic compounds. *Xenobiotica, 28*(8), 735–743.

Baliga, M. S., Haniadka, R., Pereira, M. M., D'Souza, J. J., Pallaty, P. L., Bhat, H. P., & Popuri, S. (2011). Update on the chemopreventive effects of ginger and its phytochemicals. *Critical Reviews in Food Science and Nutrition, 51*(6), 499–523.

Banerjee, S., Padhye, S., Azmi, A., Wang, Z., Philip, P. A., Kucuk, O., Sarkar, F. H., & Mohammad, R. M. (2010). Review on molecular and therapeutic potential of thymoquinone in cancer. *Nutrition and Cancer, 62*(7), 938–946.

Baskar, R., Dai, J., Wenlong, N., Yeo, R., & Yeoh, K. W. (2014). Biological response of cancer cells to radiation treatment. *Frontiers in Molecular Biosciences, 1*(NOV). https://doi.org/10.3389/FMOLB.2014.00024.

Berghe, T. Vanden, Linkermann, A., Jouan-Lanhouet, S., Walczak, H., & Vandenabeele, P. (2014). Regulated necrosis: the expanding network of non-apoptotic cell death pathways. *Nature Reviews Molecular Cell Biology, 15*(2), 135–147.

Bimonte, S., Barbieri, A., Palma, G., Luciano, A., Rea, D., & Arra, C. (2013). Curcumin inhibits tumor growth and angiogenesis in an orthotopic mouse model of human pancreatic cancer. *BioMed Research International, 2013*.

Bray, F., Ferlay, J., Soerjomataram, I., Siegel, R. L., Torre, L. A., & Jemal, A. (2018). Global cancer statistics 2018: GLOBOCAN estimates of incidence and mortality worldwide for 36 cancers in 185 countries. *CA: A Cancer Journal for Clinicians, 68*(6), 394–424.

Brown, K. C., Modi, K. J., Light, R. S., Cox, A. J., Long, T. E., Gadepalli, R. S., Rimoldi, J. M., Miles, S. L., Rankin, G., Valentovic, M., Denning, K. L., Tirona, M. T., Finch, P. T., Hess, J. A., & Dasgupta, P. (2022). Anticancer Activity of Region B Capsaicin Analogs. *Journal of Medicinal Chemistry*. https://doi.org/10.1021/acs.jmedchem.2c01594

Butt, M. S., Sultan, M. T., Butt, M. S., & Iqbal, J. (2009). Garlic: nature's protection against physiological threats. *Critical Reviews in Food Science and Nutrition, 49*(6), 538–551.

Cao, A.-L., Tang, Q.-F., Zhou, W.-C., Qiu, Y.-Y., Hu, S.-J., & Yin, P.-H. (2015). Ras/ERK signaling pathway is involved in curcumin-induced cell cycle arrest and apoptosis in human gastric carcinoma AGS cells. *Journal of Asian Natural Products Research, 17*(1), 56–63.

Center, S. (n.d.). ClinicalTrials. gov [Internet] Bethesda (MD): National Library of Medicine (US); 2000–. *Vaccine Therapy With or Without Imiquimod in Treating Patients With Grade, 3.*

Chapa-Oliver, A. M., & Mejía-Teniente, L. (2016). Capsaicin: from plants to a cancer-suppressing agent. *Molecules, 21*(8), 931.

Chen, F., Zhong, Z., Tan, H. Y., Wang, N., & Feng, Y. (2020). The underlying mechanisms of Chinese herbal medicine-induced apoptotic cell death in human cancer. *Programmed Cell Death,* 3.

Cruz–Correa, M., Shoskes, D. A., Sanchez, P., Zhao, R., Hylind, L. M., Wexner, S. D., & Giardiello, F. M. (2006). Combination treatment with curcumin and quercetin of adenomas in familial adenomatous polyposis. *Clinical Gastroenterology and Hepatology, 4*(8), 1035–1038.

Degenhardt, K., Mathew, R., Beaudoin, B., Bray, K., Anderson, D., Chen, G., Mukherjee, C., Shi, Y., Gélinas, C., & Fan, Y. (2006). Autophagy promotes tumor cell survival and restricts necrosis, inflammation, and tumorigenesis. *Cancer Cell, 10*(1), 51–64.

Di Meo, F., Margarucci, S., Galderisi, U., Crispi, S., & Peluso, G. (2019). Curcumin, gut microbiota, and neuroprotection. *Nutrients, 11*(10), 2426.

Dikic, I., & Elazar, Z. (2018). Mechanism and medical implications of mammalian autophagy. *Nature Reviews Molecular Cell Biology, 19*(6), 349–364.

Dorai, T., Cao, Y., Dorai, B., Buttyan, R., & Katz, A. E. (2001). Therapeutic potential of curcumin in human prostate cancer. III. Curcumin inhibits proliferation, induces apoptosis, and inhibits angiogenesis LNCaP prostate cancer cells *in vivo. The Prostate, 47*(4), 293–303.

Elmore, S. (2007). Apoptosis: a review of programmed cell death. *Toxicologic Pathology, 35*(4), 495–516. https://doi.org/10.1080/01926230701320337.

Galluzzi, L., Baehrecke, E. H., Ballabio, A., Boya, P., Bravo-San Pedro, J. M., Cecconi, F., Choi, A. M., Chu, C. T., Codogno, P., & Colombo, M. I. (2017). Molecular definitions of autophagy and related processes. *The EMBO Journal, 36*(13), 1811–1836.

Galluzzi, L., Pietrocola, F., Bravo-San Pedro, J. M., Amaravadi, R. K., Baehrecke, E. H., Cecconi, F., Codogno, P., Debnath, J., Gewirtz, D.

A., & Karantza, V. (2015). Autophagy in malignant transformation and cancer progression. *The EMBO Journal*, *34*(7), 856–880.

Galluzzi, L., Pietrocola, F., Levine, B., & Kroemer, G. (2014). Metabolic control of autophagy. *Cell*, *159*(6), 1263–1276.

Garufi, A., Pistritto, G., Cirone, M., & D'Orazi, G. (2016). Reactivation of mutant p53 by capsaicin, the major constituent of peppers. *Journal of Experimental and Clinical Cancer Research*, *35*(1). https://doi.org/10.1186/s13046-016-0417-9.

Gong, C., Bauvy, C., Tonelli, G., Yue, W., Delomenie, C., Nicolas, V., Zhu, Y., Domergue, V., Marin-Esteban, V., & Tharinger, H. (2013). Beclin 1 and autophagy are required for the tumorigenicity of breast cancer stem-like/progenitor cells. *Oncogene*, *32*(18), 2261–2272.

Greenshields, A. L., Doucette, C. D., Sutton, K. M., Madera, L., Annan, H., Yaffe, P. B., Knickle, A. F., Dong, Z., & Hoskin, D. W. (2015a). Piperine inhibits the growth and motility of triple-negative breast cancer cells. *Cancer Letters*, *357*(1), 129–140.

Greenshields, A. L., Doucette, C. D., Sutton, K. M., Madera, L., Annan, H., Yaffe, P. B., Knickle, A. F., Dong, Z., & Hoskin, D. W. (2015b). Piperine inhibits the growth and motility of triple-negative breast cancer cells. *Cancer Letters*, *357*(1), 129–140.

Greenshields, A. L., Doucette, C. D., Sutton, K. M., Madera, L., Annan, H., Yaffe, P. B., Knickle, A. F., Dong, Z., & Hoskin, D. W. (2015c). Piperine inhibits the growth and motility of triple-negative breast cancer cells. *Cancer Letters*, *357*(1), 129–140.

Gupta, S. C., Patchva, S., & Aggarwal, B. B. (2013). Therapeutic roles of curcumin: lessons learned from clinical trials. *The AAPS Journal*, *15*(1), 195. https://doi.org/10.1208/S12248-012-9432-8

Gupta, S. C., Sung, B., Kim, J. H., Prasad, S., Li, S., & Aggarwal, B. B. (2013). Multitargeting by turmeric, the golden spice: from kitchen to clinic. *Molecular Nutrition & Food Research*, *57*(9), 1510–1528.

H Sarkar, F., Li, Y., Wang, Z., & Padhye, S. (2010). Lesson learned from nature for the development of novel anti-cancer agents: implication of isoflavone, curcumin, and their synthetic analogs. *Current Pharmaceutical Design*, *16*(16), 1801–1812.

Hanahan, D., & Weinberg, R. A. (2011). Hallmarks of cancer: the next generation. *Cell*, *144*(5), 646–674.

Hejazi, J., Rastmanesh, R., Taleban, F.-A., Molana, S.-H., Hejazi, E., Ehtejab, G., & Hara, N. (2016). Effect of curcumin supplementation during radiotherapy on oxidative status of patients with prostate cancer:

a double blinded, randomized, placebo-controlled study. *Nutrition and Cancer, 68*(1), 77–85.

Hengartner, M. O. (2000). The biochemistry of apoptosis. *Nature 2000 407:6805, 407*(6805), 770–776. https://doi.org/10.1038/35037710.

Hermann, R., & von Richter, O. (2012). Clinical evidence of herbal drugs as perpetrators of pharmacokinetic drug interactions. *Planta Medica, 78*(13), 1458–1477.

Huang, W., Chen, Z., Wang, Q., Lin, M., Wu, S., Yan, Q., Wu, F., Yu, X., Xie, X., & Li, G. (2013). Piperine potentiates the antidepressant-like effect of trans-resveratrol: involvement of monoaminergic system. *Metabolic Brain Disease, 28*, 585–595.

Jeong, C.-H., Bode, A. M., Pugliese, A., Cho, Y.-Y., Kim, H.-G., Shim, J.-H., Jeon, Y.-J., Li, H., Jiang, H., & Dong, Z. (2009). [6]-Gingerol suppresses colon cancer growth by targeting leukotriene A4 hydrolase. *Cancer Research, 69*(13), 5584–5591.

Johnson, J. J. (2011). Carnosol: a promising anti-cancer and anti-inflammatory agent. *Cancer Letters, 305*(1), 1–7.

Johnson, J. J., Nihal, M., Siddiqui, I. A., Scarlett, C. O., Bailey, H. H., Mukhtar, H., & Ahmad, N. (2011). Enhancing the bioavailability of resveratrol by combining it with piperine. *Molecular Nutrition & Food Research, 55*(8), 1169–1176.

Jones, E., Michael, S., & Sittampalam, G. S. (2016). Basics of assay equipment and instrumentation for high throughput screening. *Assay Guidance Manual [Internet]*.

Jurenka, J. S. (2009). Anti-inflammatory properties of curcumin, a major constituent of Curcuma longa: a review of preclinical and clinical research. *Alternative Medicine Review, 14*(2).

Kaefer, C. M., & Milner, J. A. (2008). The role of herbs and spices in cancer prevention. *The Journal of Nutritional Biochemistry, 19*(6), 347–361.

Kakarala, M., Brenner, D. E., Korkaya, H., Cheng, C., Tazi, K., Ginestier, C., Liu, S., Dontu, G., & Wicha, M. S. (2010). Targeting breast stem cells with the cancer preventive compounds curcumin and piperine. *Breast Cancer Research and Treatment, 122*, 777–785.

Khor, T. O., Keum, Y.-S., Lin, W., Kim, J.-H., Hu, R., Shen, G., Xu, C., Gopalakrishnan, A., Reddy, B., & Zheng, X. (2006). Combined inhibitory effects of curcumin and phenethyl isothiocyanate on the growth of human PC-3 prostate xenografts in immunodeficient mice. *Cancer Research, 66*(2), 613–621.

Kimmelman, A. C., & White, E. (2017). Autophagy and Tumor Metabolism. *Cell Metabolism*, *25*(5), 1037–1043. https://doi.org/10.1016/J. CMET.2017.04.004.

Knight, A. (2008). Systematic reviews of animal experiments demonstrate poor contributions toward human healthcare. *Reviews on Recent Clinical Trials*, *3*(2), 89–96.

Koppikar, S. J., Choudhari, A. S., Suryavanshi, S. A., Kumari, S., Chattopadhyay, S., & Kaul-Ghanekar, R. (2010). Aqueous cinnamon extract (ACE-c) from the bark of Cinnamomum cassia causes apoptosis in human cervical cancer cell line (SiHa) through loss of mitochondrial membrane potential. *BMC Cancer*, *10*, 1–12.

Kotecha, R., Takami, A., & Espinoza, J. L. (2016). Dietary phytochemicals and cancer chemoprevention: a review of the clinical evidence. *Oncotarget*, *7*(32), 52517.

Kotecha, R., Takami, A., & Espinoza, J. L. (2021). Oncotarget 2016, 7, 52517. *Google Scholar (b) BP George, R. Chandran, H. Abrahamse Antioxidants*, *10*, 1455.

Kroemer, G., Mariño, G., & Levine, B. (2010). Autophagy and the integrated stress response. *Molecular Cell*, *40*(2), 280–293.

Kundu, J. K., & Surh, Y.-J. (2012). Emerging avenues linking inflammation and cancer. *Free Radical Biology and Medicine*, *52*(9), 2013–2037.

Kunnumakkara, A. B., Bordoloi, D., Harsha, C., Banik, K., Gupta, S. C., & Aggarwal, B. B. (2017). Curcumin mediates anticancer effects by modulating multiple cell signaling pathways. *Clinical Science*, *131*(15), 1781–1799.

Kwon, H.-K., Hwang, J.-S., So, J.-S., Lee, C.-G., Sahoo, A., Ryu, J.-H., Jeon, W. K., Ko, B. S., Im, C.-R., & Lee, S. H. (2010). Cinnamon extract induces tumor cell death through inhibition of NFκB and AP1. *BMC Cancer*, *10*, 1–10.

Lai, L., Fu, Q., Liu, Y., Jiang, K., Guo, Q., Chen, Q., Yan, B., Wang, Q., & Shen, J. (2012). Piperine suppresses tumor growth and metastasis *in vitro* and *in vivo* in a 4T1 murine breast cancer model. *Acta Pharmacologica Sinica*, *33*(4), 523–530.

Lee, E., & Surh, Y.-J. (1998). Induction of apoptosis in HL-60 cells by pungent vanilloids,[6]-gingerol and [6]-paradol. *Cancer Letters*, *134*(2), 163–168.

Levine, B., & Klionsky, D. J. (2017). Autophagy wins the 2016 Nobel Prize in Physiology or Medicine: Breakthroughs in baker's yeast fuel advances in biomedical research. *Proceedings of the National Academy of Sciences*, *114*(2), 201–205.

Levine, B., & Kroemer, G. (2008). Autophagy in the pathogenesis of disease. *Cell, 132*(1), 27–42. https://doi.org/10.1016/J.CELL.2007.12.018.

Levy, J. M. M., Towers, C. G., & Thorburn, A. (2017). Targeting autophagy in cancer. *Nature Reviews Cancer, 17*(9), 528–542.

Li, B., Takeda, T., Tsuiji, K., Wong, T. F., Tadakawa, M., Kondo, A., Nagase, S., & Yaegashi, N. (2013). Curcumin induces cross-regulation between autophagy and apoptosis in uterine leiomyosarcoma cells. *International Journal of Gynecologic Cancer, 23*(5).

Liu, C., Cao, F., Tang, Q.-Z., Yan, L., Dong, Y.-G., Zhu, L.-H., Wang, L., Bian, Z.-Y., & Li, H. (2010). Allicin protects against cardiac hypertrophy and fibrosis via attenuating reactive oxygen species-dependent signaling pathways. *The Journal of Nutritional Biochemistry, 21*(12), 1238–1250.

Liu, F., Liu, W., & Tian, S. (2014). Artificial neural network optimization of Althaea rosea seeds polysaccharides and its antioxidant activity. *International Journal of Biological Macromolecules, 70*, 100–107.

Liu, R. H. (2003). Health benefits of fruit and vegetables are from additive and synergistic combinations of phytochemicals. *The American Journal of Clinical Nutrition, 78*(3), 517S–520S.

Maiuri, M. C. (2007). Zalckvar E, Kimchi A, Kroemer G. Self-eating and self-killing: crosstalk between autophagy and apoptosis. *Nat Rev Mol Cell Biol, 8*, 741–752.

Maiuri, M. C., Tasdemir, E., Criollo, A., Morselli, E., Vicencio, J. M., Carnuccio, R., & Kroemer, G. (2009). Control of autophagy by oncogenes and tumor suppressor genes. *Cell Death & Differentiation, 16*(1), 87–93.

Miller, K. D., Nogueira, L., Mariotto, A. B., Rowland, J. H., Yabroff, K. R., Alfano, C. M., Jemal, A., Kramer, J. L., & Siegel, R. L. (2019). Cancer treatment and survivorship statistics, 2019. *CA: A Cancer Journal for Clinicians, 69*(5), 363–385. https://doi.org/10.3322/CAAC.21565

Mizushima, N., & Komatsu, M. (2011). Autophagy: renovation of cells and tissues. *Cell, 147*(4), 728–741. https://doi.org/10.1016/J.CELL.2011.10.026

Mizushima, N., Levine, B., Cuervo, A. M., & Klionsky, D. J. (2008). Autophagy fights disease through cellular self-digestion. *Nature, 451*(7182), 1069–1075.

Mo, J., Jung, J., Yoon, J., Hong, J., Kim, M., Ann, E., Seo, M., Choi, Y., & Park, H. (2010). DJ-1 modulates the p38 mitogen-activated protein kinase pathway through physical interaction with apoptosis signal-regulating kinase 1. *Journal of Cellular Biochemistry*, *110*(1), 229–237.

Mori, A., Lehmann, S., O'Kelly, J., Kumagai, T., Desmond, J. C., Pervan, M., McBride, W. H., Kizaki, M., & Koeffler, H. P. (2006). Capsaicin, a component of red peppers, inhibits the growth of androgen-independent, p53 mutant prostate cancer cells. *Cancer Research*, *66*(6), 3222–3229.

Mould-Quevedo, J. F., García-Peña, C., Contreras-Hernández, I., Juárez-Cedillo, T., Espinel-Bermúdez, C., Morales-Cisneros, G., & Sánchez-García, S. (2009). Direct costs associated with the appropriateness of hospital stay in elderly population. *BMC Health Services Research*, *9*(1), 1–8.

Mulcahy Levy, J. M., & Thorburn, A. (2020). Autophagy in cancer: moving from understanding mechanism to improving therapy responses in patients. *Cell Death & Differentiation*, *27*(3), 843–857.

Pammolli, F., Magazzini, L., & Riccaboni, M. (2011). The productivity crisis in pharmaceutical R&D. *Nature Reviews Drug Discovery*, *10*(6), 428–438.

Park, S.-Y., Kim, J.-Y., Lee, S.-M., Jun, C.-H., Cho, S.-B., Park, C.-H., Joo, Y., Kim, H.-S., Choi, S.-K., & Rew, J.-S. (2014). Capsaicin induces apoptosis and modulates MAPK signaling in human gastric cancer cells. *Molecular Medicine Reports*, *9*(2), 499–502.

Pattingre, S., Tassa, A., Qu, X., Garuti, R., Liang, X. H., Mizushima, N., Packer, M., Schneider, M. D., & Levine, B. (2005). Bcl-2 antiapoptotic proteins inhibit Beclin 1-dependent autophagy. *Cell*, *122*(6), 927–939.

Pommier, P., Hu, Y., Baron, M.-H., Chapet, O., & Balosso, J. (2010). L'hadronthérapie: les ions carbone. *Bulletin Du Cancer*, *97*(7), 819–829.

Prakobwong, S., Gupta, S. C., Kim, J. H., Sung, B., Pinlaor, P., Hiraku, Y., Wongkham, S., Sripa, B., Pinlaor, S., & Aggarwal, B. B. (2011). Curcumin suppresses proliferation and induces apoptosis in human biliary cancer cells through modulation of multiple cell signaling pathways. *Carcinogenesis*, *32*(9), 1372–1380.

Prasad, S., & Aggarwal, B. B. (2011). Turmeric, the golden spice. *Herbal Medicine: Biomolecular and Clinical Aspects,* 2nd Edition.

Prasad, S., & Tyagi, A. K. (2015). Ginger and its constituents: role in prevention and treatment of gastrointestinal cancer. *Gastroenterology Research and Practice*, *2015*.

Prasad, S., Tyagi, A. K., & Aggarwal, B. B. (2014). Recent developments in delivery, bioavailability, absorption and metabolism of curcumin: the golden pigment from golden spice. *Cancer Research and Treatment: Official Journal of Korean Cancer Association, 46*(1), 2–18.

Ravindran, J., Prasad, S., & Aggarwal, B. B. (2009). Curcumin and cancer cells: how many ways can curry kill tumor cells selectively? *The AAPS Journal, 11*, 495–510.

Reeta, V., & Kalia, S. (2022). Turmeric: a review of its' effects on human health. *J Med Plants Stud, 10*(4), 61–63.

Rhode, J., Fogoros, S., Zick, S., Wahl, H., Griffith, K. A., Huang, J., & Liu, J. R. (2007). Ginger inhibits cell growth and modulates angiogenic factors in ovarian cancer cells. *BMC Complementary and Alternative Medicine, 7*, 1–9.

Ronaldson-Bouchard, K., & Vunjak-Novakovic, G. (2018). Organs-on-a-chip: a fast track for engineered human tissues in drug development. *Cell Stem Cell, 22*(3), 310–324.

Ryan, J. L., Heckler, C. E., Ling, M., Katz, A., Williams, J. P., Pentland, A. P., & Morrow, G. R. (2013). Curcumin for radiation dermatitis: a randomized, double-blind, placebo-controlled clinical trial of thirty breast cancer patients. *Radiation Research, 180*(1), 34–43.

Ryan, J. L., Heckler, C. E., Roscoe, J. A., Dakhil, S. R., Kirshner, J., Flynn, P. J., Hickok, J. T., & Morrow, G. R. (2012). Ginger (Zingiber officinale) reduces acute chemotherapy-induced nausea: a URCC CCOP study of 576 patients. *Supportive Care in Cancer, 20*(7), 1479–1489.

Scott, A. M., Wolchok, J. D., & Old, L. J. (2012). Antibody therapy of cancer. *Nature Reviews. Cancer, 12*(4), 278–287. https://doi.org/10.1038/NRC3236

Shanmugam, M. K., Lee, J. H., Chai, E. Z. P., Kanchi, M. M., Kar, S., Arfuso, F., Dharmarajan, A., Kumar, A. P., Ramar, P. S., & Looi, C. Y. (2016). Cancer prevention and therapy through the modulation of transcription factors by bioactive natural compounds. *Seminars in Cancer Biology, 40*, 35–47.

Shanmugam, M. K., Rane, G., Kanchi, M. M., Arfuso, F., Chinnathambi, A., Zayed, M. E., Alharbi, S. A., Tan, B. K. H., Kumar, A. P., & Sethi, G. (2015). The multifaceted role of curcumin in cancer prevention and treatment. *Molecules, 20*(2), 2728–2769.

Sharma, N., Jain, A., Bahudar, S., & Oberoi, S. S. (2021). Efficacy of curcumin and piperine as antioxidant adjuvant to intralesional dexamethasone injection for management of oral submucous fibrosis: a clinical trial. *Journal of Orofacial Sciences, 13*(2), 129–135.

Shobha, G., Joseph, T., Majeed, M., Rajendran, R., & Srinivas, P. (1998). Influence of piperine on the pharmacokinetics of curcumin in animals and human volunteers. *Plant Med*, *64*, 353.

Singh, R., & Lillard Jr, J. W. (2009). Nanoparticle-based targeted drug delivery. *Experimental and Molecular Pathology*, *86*(3), 215–223.

Sironi, D., Christensen, M., Rosenberg, J., Bauer-Brandl, A., & Brandl, M. (2017). Evaluation of a dynamic dissolution/permeation model: mutual influence of dissolution and barrier-flux under non-steady state conditions. *International Journal of Pharmaceutics*, *522*(1–2), 50–57.

Srinivasan, K. (2014). Antioxidant potential of spices and their active constituents. *Critical Reviews in Food Science and Nutrition*, *54*(3), 352–372.

Stratton, M. R., Campbell, P. J., & Futreal, P. A. (2009). The cancer genome. *Nature*, *458*(7239), 719–724. https://doi.org/10.1038/NATURE07943.

Sung, H., Ferlay, J., Siegel, R. L., Laversanne, M., Soerjomataram, I., Jemal, A., & Bray, F. (2021). Global Cancer Statistics 2020: GLOBOCAN Estimates of Incidence and Mortality Worldwide for 36 Cancers in 185 Countries. *CA: A Cancer Journal for Clinicians*, *71*(3), 209–249. https://doi.org/10.3322/CAAC.21660.

Tapsell, L. C., Hemphill, I., Cobiac, L., Patch, C. S., Sullivan, D. R., Fenech, M., Roodenrys, S., Keogh, J. B., Clifton, P. M., Williams, P. G., Fazio, V. A., & Inge, K. E. (2006). Health benefits of herbs and spices: the past, the present, the future. *The Medical Journal of Australia*, *185*(S4). https://doi.org/10.5694/J.1326-5377.2006.TB00548.X.

Tasdemir, E., Maiuri, M. C., Galluzzi, L., Vitale, I., Djavaheri-Mergny, M., D'amelio, M., Criollo, A., Morselli, E., Zhu, C., & Harper, F. (2008). Regulation of autophagy by cytoplasmic p53. *Nature Cell Biology*, *10*(6), 676–687.

Toden, S., Okugawa, Y., Buhrmann, C., Nattamai, D., Anguiano, E., Baldwin, N., Shakibaei, M., Boland, C. R., & Goel, A. (2015). Novel evidence for curcumin and boswellic acid–induced chemoprevention through regulation of miR-34a and miR-27a in colorectal cancer. *Cancer Prevention Research*, *8*(5), 431–443.

Wang, B., Avorn, J., & Kesselheim, A. S. (2013). Clinical and regulatory features of drugs not initially approved by the FDA. *Clinical Pharmacology & Therapeutics*, *94*(6), 670–677.

Wang, N., Wang, Z.-Y., Mo, S.-L., Loo, T. Y., Wang, D.-M., Luo, H.-B., Yang, D.-P., Chen, Y.-L., Shen, J.-G., & Chen, J.-P. (2012). Ellagic acid, a phenolic compound, exerts anti-angiogenesis effects via VEGFR-2 signaling pathway in breast cancer. *Breast Cancer Research and Treatment, 134*, 943–955.

White, E. (2012). Deconvoluting the context-dependent role for autophagy in cancer. *Nature Reviews Cancer, 12*(6), 401–410.

Wirawan, E., Vande Walle, L., Kersse, K., Cornelis, S., Claerhout, S., Vanoverberghe, I., Roelandt, R., De Rycke, R., Verspurten, J., & Declercq, W. (2010). Caspase-mediated cleavage of Beclin-1 inactivates Beclin-1-induced autophagy and enhances apoptosis by promoting the release of proapoptotic factors from mitochondria. *Cell Death & Disease, 1*(1), e18–e18.

Xiao, X., Chen, B., Liu, X., Liu, P., Zheng, G., Ye, F., Tang, H., & Xie, X. (2014). Diallyl disulfide suppresses SRC/Ras/ERK signaling-mediated proliferation and metastasis in human breast cancer by up-regulating miR-34a. *PLoS One, 9*(11), e112720.

Yaffe, P. B., Power Coombs, M. R., Doucette, C. D., Walsh, M., & Hoskin, D. W. (2015). Piperine, an alkaloid from black pepper, inhibits growth of human colon cancer cells via G1 arrest and apoptosis triggered by endoplasmic reticulum stress. *Molecular Carcinogenesis, 54*(10), 1070–1085.

Yamagata, K. (2019). Metabolic syndrome: preventive effects of dietary flavonoids. *Studies in Natural Products Chemistry, 60*, 1–28.

Zhang, Q., Liu, J., Zhang, M., Wei, S., Li, R., Gao, Y., Peng, W., & Wu, C. (2019). Apoptosis induction of fibroblast-like synoviocytes is an important molecular-mechanism for herbal medicine along with its active components in treating rheumatoid arthritis. *Biomolecules, 9*(12), 795.

Zhang, W., Ha, M., Gong, Y., Xu, Y., Dong, N., & Yuan, Y. (2010). Allicin induces apoptosis in gastric cancer cells through activation of both extrinsic and intrinsic pathways. *Oncology Reports, 24*(6), 1585–1592.

Chapter 5

Role of Spices in Cancer Cell Cycle Arrest

Shallu Saini,[a] **Kanupriya Vashishth,**[b]
Nidarshana Chaturvedi Parashar,[a] **Gaurav Parashar,**[c]
Seema Ramniwas,[d] **Gurpreet Kaur Bhatia,**[e] **Moyad Shahwan,**[f,g]
and Hardeep Singh Tuli[a]

[a]*Department of Biosciences and Technology,*
Maharishi Markandeshwar (Deemed to be University), Mullana, Ambala, India
[b]*Advance Cardiac Centre Department of Cardiology, PGIMER Chandigarh, India*
[c]*Division of Biomedical and Life Sciences, School of Science,*
Navrachana University, Vadodara, India
[d]*University Centre for Research and Development,*
University Institute of Pharmaceutical Sciences,
Chandigarh University, Mohali India
[e]*Department of Physics, Maharishi Markandeshwar (Deemed to be University),*
Mullana, Ambala, India
[f]*Department of Clinical Sciences, College of Pharmacy and Health Sciences,*
Ajman University, Ajman, United Arab Emirates
[g]*Centre of Medical and Bio-Allied Health Sciences Research,*
Ajman University, Ajman, United Arab Emirates

hardeep.biotech@gmail.com

5.1   Introduction

Since ancient times, there has been a long tradition of using herbs and spices as a key component in culinary preparation. Although they play a significant part in flavor improvement, herbs, and

Anticancer Spices: Dietary Input to Health
Edited by Hardeep Singh Tuli
Copyright © 2025 Jenny Stanford Publishing Pte. Ltd.
ISBN 978-981-5129-28-1 (Hardcover), 978-1-003-53466-2 (eBook)
www.jennystanford.com

spices are also valued for their therapeutic and medical properties, which have long been recognized (Kaefer et al., 2008; Kunnumakkara et al., 2018). According to numerous studies (Kammath et al., 2021; Aggarwal et al., 2009; Singh Tuli et al., 2022), common spices like curcumin, garlic, ginger, pepper, saffron, cinnamon, and star anise play a significant part in preventing and treating many chronic diseases like diabetes, heart disease, inflammatory diseases, and acting as antioxidants. Over the past 20 years, research has also focused on their involvement in the prevention and treatment of cancer. The economic cost of cancer, one of the major causes of death in the globe, has affected both developed and developing nations (Zheng et al., 2016; Tuli et al., 2023; Chhikara et al., 2023). The search for efficient and less harmful treatment choices is still ongoing due to the limited success with the already existing therapeutic options and the short life expectancy of cancer patients as a result of the multifarious character of cancer (Vashishth et al., 2023; Srinivasan, 2017). In recent years, the rising incidence and frequency of malignancies have been linked to lifestyle and food choices. Focus has been placed on dietary modifications and the use of herbal ingredients to prevent and treat cancer (Singh et al., 2022; Nicastro et al., 2015). In various *in vivo* and *in vitro* studies conducted on various types of cancers, culinary spices have demonstrated promising results with respect to various anticancer properties, such as anti-angiogenic, pro-apoptotic, anti-inflammatory, and cell cycle arrest (de Lima et al., 2018; Bhandari et al., 2015; Zhang et al., 2013). The importance of frequently used spices as cutting-edge therapeutic possibilities for the prevention and treatment of cancer is highlighted in the current chapter.

5.2   Progression and Mechanism of Cancer

According to WHO projections, cancer was the first or second leading cause of death in 112 out of 183 countries in 2019 (Chhikara et al., 2023), making it a significant worldwide health concern. The primary cause of death from cancer is lung cancer, which accounts for 18% of all cancer-related deaths, followed by colorectal, liver, and stomach cancers, which account for 9.4%, 8.3%, and 7.7%, respectively. 6.9% of all fatalities globally are caused by female breast cancer (Tran et al., 2022; Deo et al., 2022). Hereditary, internal stress and environmental effects are significant risk factors for cancer development; nevertheless, the development of cancer varies from patient to patient, depending on the kind of cancer and is influenced by the environment (Hanahan et al., 2011). Loss of growth regulation is one of the eight traits that distinguish cancer. The functioning of anti-apoptotic proteins, transcription factors, cell cycle proteins, protein kinases, growth signaling pathways, etc., can be modulated by inflammatory agents, tumor promoters, environmental carcinogens, and other factors, according to studies (Krakhmal et al., 2015; Greten et al., 2019). Once cancer has taken hold, it possesses eight biological traits that are frequently referred to as its hallmarks, including ongoing proliferative signaling, resistance to growth inhibitors, escape from them, resistance to cell death, adoption of replicative immortality, reprogramming of energy metabolism, induction of angiogenesis, invasion, and metastasis, as well as evading immune defense mechanisms (He et al., 2007). The development of new anticancer agents, targets, and strategies can benefit from the discovery of strategies to suppress the altered cells and phenotypes. The lack of cell cycle control has been linked in studies to unchecked cancer cell proliferation (Vashishth et al., 2023). It has been shown that cancer cells express cyclins and CDKs abnormally, and cell death can be caused if this abnormal phenomenon is prevented and their transcriptions can be halted. With this in mind, it is possible to position cell cycle inhibitors and inhibitors of cell signaling as reasonable targets for cancer therapy together with the identification of suitable treatments for various cancer types (Williams et al., 2012; Sherr et al., 2017; Icard et al., 2019).

5.3 Chemo Protective Properties of Spices in Cell Cycle Arrest

5.3.1 Turmeric/Curcumin

Turmeric, a popular yellow spice used in cuisine all over the world, is primarily composed of curcumin. Despite being a significant spice in the bulk of Asian foods. Additionally, turmeric preparations are recognized to provide therapeutic benefits (Bengmark et al., 2009). The anti-inflammatory, cardioprotective, antioxidant, anticancer, and preventative characteristics of curcumin are among its therapeutic and medical benefits (Jurenka et al., 2009). Studies on several malignancies, including those of the mouth, lung, skin, intestine, and breast, have demonstrated the therapeutic potential of curcumin by producing cell cycle arrest, decreasing angiogenesis, and inhibiting tumor spread (Devassy et al., 2015). Curcumin can cause cell cycle arrest in the GS/S and G2/M phases as well as arrest the downstream signaling cascades, according to studies done on various breast cancer cell lines. Additionally, studies have shown that curcumin has antiproliferative properties by inhibiting cyclin D1 and other Wnt/-catenin pathway elements in cancer cell lines (Choudhuri et al., 2005; Aggarwal et al., 2003). It has been demonstrated that curcumin prevents the growth of cancer by activating the intrinsic and extrinsic apoptotic pathways. For instance, in some breast cancer studies, apoptosis mediated by curcumin can be mediated through both p53-dependent and independent pathways (Panda et al., 2017; Mbese et al., 2019). Different studies on cancer cells have shed light on the antiapoptotic effect of curcumin. Curcumin's synergistic effects in combination therapy have also been proven by researchers (Keyvani–Ghamsari et al., 2020; Abadi et al., 2022). Studies on pancreatic cancer cells have demonstrated the cell cycle arrest and apoptotic potential of curcumin when combined with a small test compound tolfenamic acid (TA) combination therapy is advantageous because it targets various phases of the cell cycle and downstream effector molecules in pancreatic cancer cells. It was shown that the combination produced cell cycle arrest G0/G1, as well as impacting the S-phase of the cell cycle (Basha et al., 2013). Studies on non-small lung cancer (NSLCL) cell lines revealed that treatment with curcumin made the cell population more susceptible to cisplatin therapy by downregulating cyclin D1 and activating caspase-9. The consideration of curcumin as an adjuvant in chemotherapy treatment approaches via the p21/APaf pathways (Jin et al., 2015; Panda et al., 2017). Although curcumin has a low bioavailability and is a potential therapeutic option for cancer treatment, it is urgent to find viable solutions to the bioavailability problems and investigate ways to expand the use of curcumin as an anticancer agent (Panda et al., 2017).

5.3.2 Pepper

Studies on various cancers have examined the therapeutic and cancer-protective benefits of pepper and its derivatives. It is known that pepper-derived alkaloids, including piperlongumine (PL), piperine, and others, have the ability to suppress the expression of cyclin A, B, and D, which stops cancer cells from going through the G1/S and G2/M transition and causes apoptosis. Various relevant studies showed that (Aumeeruddy et al., 2019; Yaffe et al., 2015; Zhang et al., 2015; Jeong et al., 2019) pepper and its extracts cause cell cycle arrest mediated by p53. Grinevicius et al.'s research showed that subjecting MCF-7 cells to ethanolic extracts of *Piper nigrum* triggered the p53-mediated G1/S checkpoint regulation, which delayed and slowed down the cell cycle's advancement and induced apoptosis (Grinevicius et al., 2016). Another study on gastric cancer by Duan C. et al. showed that treatment with PL increased GADD45, an important molecule involved in cell cycle regulation and proliferation in gastric cancer. Through the modification of and interactions with partner proteins, the study showed that PL-mediated overexpression of GADD45 resulted in the downregulation of cyclin B1 and G2 arrest (Duan et al., 2016). In their study, Fofaria et al. showed that treatment with piperine caused ROS-induced G1 cell cycle arrest in human melanoma cells by activating Chk1 and inducing apoptosis (Fofaria et al., 2104). Piperine also possesses anticancer qualities, according to studies on hormone-dependent breast cancer cells and triple-negative breast cancer cells (TNBC). Piperine produced caspase-dependent apoptosis and markedly decreased the expression of proteins associated with the G1 and G2 phases of the cell cycle as well as the proportion of cells in the G2 phase (Greenshields et al., 2015). Studies showing combined docetaxel and piperine administration have shown improved docetaxel anti-tumor activity (Ding et al., 2020). One effective strategy for treating many cancers is to employ spices like pepper and its extract as an auxiliary and additional therapy (Turrini et al., 2020). However, further clinical investigations are required to support the *in vitro* findings and non-clinical findings in order to produce reliable data.

5.3.3 Cinnamon

Cinnamon has been a popular spice since antiquity. The benefits of the spice and its extracts in enhancing human health have been the subject of much research. Additionally, cinnamon and its derivatives have been shown in studies to have anti-proliferative cancer-preventing and cancer-protective qualities. Numerous studies have demonstrated the dose-dependent reduction of cancer cell viability by cinnamon (Sadeghi et al., 2019; Hossain et al., 2022; Kwon et al., 2010). Few non-clinical studies have shown that oral or intra-tumor administration of cinnamon extracts (CE) accelerated CD8+ T cell cytolytic activities and cytolytic mediators like TNF-a, IFN-, up-regulated perforin and granzymes B and C levels, inducing apoptosis and thereby significantly reducing tumor cell proliferation (Dutta et al., 2018). In a study by Cabello et al. on melanoma cell lines, it was shown that CE dramatically suppressed the overexpression of several growth factors, such as TGF-a, VEGF-a, FGF, and EFG, in a dose-dependent manner, consequently reducing cell proliferation (Cabello et al., 2009). Additionally, the essential oil of cinnamon suppressed the activities of epidermal growth factor receptor tyrosine kinase (EGFR-TK) and its downstream signaling in an in-vitro study on laryngeal squamous cell carcinoma cell line conducted by Yang et al., leading to a significant decrease in tumor burden (Yang et al., 2015). Numerous research has shed insight into how cinnamon and its extracts can change the cell cycle phase in various tumor cell lines. For instance, a study on Jurkat, Wurzburg, and U937 cells revealed that CE operated in a conciliatory manner, depending on which cell cycle phase is being arrested. It was shown that CE considerably reduced the population in all three cell lines at the G0/G1 phase, while Wurzburg cells showed the greatest inhibition during this phase. The study also showed that Wurzburg cells had the highest rate of cell cycle arrest at G2/M when compared to other cells. Eugenol, one of cinnamon's active ingredients, has been shown in studies to significantly alter the cell cycle of cancer cells at various stages (Sadeghi et al. 2019; Schoene et al., 2005). In a study by Nile et al., colon cancer cell lines treated with different doses of eugenol showed a significant improvement in cell cycle arrest in a time-dependent manner (Nile et al., 2023). In another work by Ghosh et al., the co-treatment of eugenol with 2-methoxyestradiol markedly boosted the rate of cell cycle arrest at the G2/M phase in prostate cancer cells, indicating the enhanced synergistic effect of the combination therapy (Ghosh et al., 2009). According to research by Kwon et al. (2010), cinnamon and its extracts have also been demonstrated to cause apoptosis in various cancer cell lines by activating caspase-3, speeding up DNA breakage and the production of ROS, and lowering levels of Bcl-2, BcL-xL, and survivin. Additionally, CE has been found to increase the levels of proapoptotic proteins like Bax and aid in DNA fragmentation, proteolytic cleavage of caspase-3 and caspase-9 from their respective proformas, increasing the apoptotic rate in various cancer cell lines when used alone or in combination therapy with known anticancer compounds (Larasati et al., 2014). To go from the bench to the bedside, the encouraging *in vitro* findings on the use of cinnamon and its extract in cancer prevention and treatment demand a translational strategy.

5.3.4 Garlic

The Liliaceae family plant *Allium sativum*, also known as garlic, includes a variety of compounds that have been reported to harbor anticancer potential (Pandey et al., 2023). One of the lipid-soluble molecules is diallyl disulfide (DADS), which is largely present in garlic, and has shown anticancer properties mediated through its ability to inhibit cell proliferation as reported *in vitro* in prostate cancer cells. In PC-3 cells, a dose-dependent cell cycle arrest may have been the action mechanism (Arunkumar et al., 2006). Additionally, diallyl trisulfide (DATS), one of the bioactive components of garlic, can stop the growth of SGC-7901 gastric cancer cells and the G2/M phase of the cell cycle. Additionally, S-allyl-cysteine (SAC) can stop the cell cycle at the G1/S phase in the human ovarian cancer cell line A2780.

Furthermore, it has been observed that SAC and DATS can cause cell cycle arrest in A2780 ovarian cancer cells and SGC-7901 gastric cancer cells in the G2/M and G1/S phases, respectively (Jiang et al., 2017)]. The explanation for the identification of possible mechanisms has been explored using the treatment of garlic extract in EJ bladder cancer cells. It was reported that garlic extract treatment inhibited Cdc25C and Cdc2 phosphorylation and cyclinB1 mediated through induction of p21WAF1, ataxia-telangiectasia mutation, and checkpoint kinase 2 (Shin et al., 2017).

5.3.5 Onion

Through a variety of mechanisms of action, the flavonoid compound quercetin found in onions (*Allium cepa*) has been shown to exhibit anticancer efficacy as reported across different cancer types such as colorectal, ovarian, breast, stomach, lung, leukemia, and melanoma (Harris et al., 2015; Pang et al., 2019). Onion extracts modulate or target multiple pathways to exert their anticancer effect including but not limited to the membrane potential of mitochondria, activation of p53, and arresting cell cycle, preferably in the S-phase (Paesa et al., 2022). However, the extract has been reported to initiate apoptosis in the A549 cell line possibly mediated through cell cycle arrest in the G2/M phase (Wu et al., 2006). One interesting finding is that onion extracts have been shown to respond more favorably and effectively in resistant triple-negative breast cancer cells (MDA-MB-231) when compared to sensitive ER+ (MCF-7) cell lines. These results suggest that onion extracts are a good source of flavonoids with potential anticancer properties (Fragis et al., 2018).

5.3.6 Ginger

According to research by Xu et al. (2020), 6-gingerol, the primary biochemical and pharmacological constituent of ginger, exhibits anticancer effects against a number of cancers. 6-gingerol action has been reported to be linked with the expression of wild-type p53 as shown in BxPC-3 pancreatic cells. According to Park et al.

(2006), 6-gingerol possesses the ability to induce cell cycle arrest at phase G1, and it has also been found to have anticancer properties against gastrointestinal cancer. Furthermore, studies using mice have shown that the anti-tumor effects of ginger and its active components, namely, 6-gingerol and 6-shogaol, also work against cancers of the gastrointestinal tract. In renal cell carcinoma, it has been reported that 6-gingerol, a bioactive substance, can stop the cell cycle and inhibit cell development possibly by activating the AKT-GSK 3/-cyclin D1 axis (Xu et al., 2020). Another study examined how 6-gingerol affected cervical cancer (HeLa) cell lines and human oral cancer (SCC4, KB) in the presence or absence of cisplatin, wortmannin, and rapamycin. Their research suggests that 6-gingerol may have greater ameliorative effects in the treatment of cervical and oral cancer when used alone or in conjunction with cisplatin and PI-3 K inhibitor. Thus, by interrupting the cell cycle and causing apoptosis, 6-gingerol emerges to be a safe and efficient chemotherapeutic/chemo-protective drug that impacts cervical cancer and human oral cells (Kapoor et al., 2016).

5.3.7   Cardamon

Takahashi et al. (2011) and Qin et al. (2012) suggest cardamonin, a chalcone derived from the spice cardamom, exhibits anticancer and anti-inflammatory properties. Cardamonin is effective against nasopharyngeal cancer (NPC) due to its ability to induce mechanisms of controlled cell death and cell cycle arrest at the G2/M phase, as reported in one of the investigations. Similar findings were also documented in triple-negative breast cancer (TNBC) cells, which were caused by changes in cleaved caspase-3, cyt-C, Bcl-2, Bax, and PARP (Shrivastava et al., 2017). Apart from the abovementioned targets, the bioactive substance also leads to the nuclear translocation of the genes p21, p27, and bim, which are targets of Forkhead box O3 (FOXO3a), which subsequently induces apoptosis (Niu et al., 2020). In oral cell carcinoma, it has been shown that cardamom extract can induce DNA damage, which is beyond repair, which subsequently leads to cell cycle arrest and apoptosis [Zaki et al., 2022]. Moreover, studies have demonstrated that cardamom extract damaged DNA irreparably, causing cell cycle arrest and a buildup of cells in this stage of the cell cycle before apoptosis in oral squamous cell carcinoma also [Zaki et al., 2022].

5.3.8 Saffron

The dried flower styles (stigmata) of *Crocus sativus L.*, saffron, are frequently used as spices and have been used since long as conventional medicine across many continents, civilizations, and cultures (Chryssanthi et al., 2011). Studies in pancreatic cancer cells have also been done to determine how crocin, another essential component of the saffron plant, caused the BxPC-3 cells to undergo apoptosis. It was demonstrated that BxPC-3 cells gradually lost viability following dose-dependent therapy, most likely as a result of cell cycle arrest in the G1 phase (Bakshi et al., 2010). In a rat model with liver cancer, saffron also encouraged cell growth inhibition via cell cycle arrest. Also, saffron has been reported to show an anticancer mechanism that involves causing cell cycle arrest, according to a number of earlier research. In an *in vivo* investigation, saffron promoted cell cycle arrest in a liver cancer-bearing rat model. Additionally, research has shown that the natural substance saffron may cause cell death in HepG2 and HeLa cells, where programmed cell death, or apoptosis, plays a significant role (Tavakkol-Afshari et al., 2008). As a result, saffron is a promising chemotherapeutic medicine for cancer treatment in the future.

5.4 Current Obstacles and Upcoming Plans

There have been studies done on the broad therapeutic potential of spices in cancer. However, there are still a lot of issues with developing the clinical use of herbs and spices. It has been noted that there is a lack of established language, a lack of uniformity in the concentrations of goods made from herbs and spices, and variation in the descriptions of these items. A key challenge in developing an efficient clinical application of widely accessible herbs and spices is the lack of consistent and reliable information on the chemical profiles or active components. Additionally, it has been noticed that there are not many clinical studies to back up the clinical and therapeutic effects of spices and their extracts on cancer, which tends to create questions about what is known and is not known about them. However, the evidence and results on the use of frequently used spices as anti-tumor agents are intriguing and deserve more focus. However, greater focus and thorough research are required to uncover the biological impact and influence of risk factors such as genetic makeup and nutrient-nutrient interactions of the regularly utilized species to treat cancer. To maximize their therapeutic potential and create a standardized treatment option, it is urgent to identify biomarkers, their impact, and their susceptibility to commonly used culinary spices. It has also been argued and emphasized that future research should be focused on identifying key signaling molecules that could be potential targets of spices in cancer treatment. To further understand how certain malignancies react to various spices, more extensive research is required. Future cancer treatments will have additional avenues to explore thanks to the urgently required translational strategy to identify suitable species as prospective cancer targets.

References

Abadi AJ, Mirzaei S, Mahabady MK, Hashemi F, Zabolian A, Hashemi F, Raee P, Aghamiri S, Ashrafizadeh M, Aref AR, Hamblin MR. Curcumin and its derivatives in cancer therapy: potentiating antitumor activity of cisplatin and reducing side effects. *Phytotherapy Research*. 2022 Jan; 36(1):189–213.

Aggarwal BB, Kumar A, Bharti AC. Anticancer potential of curcumin: preclinical and clinical studies. *Anticancer Research*. 2003 Jan 1; 23(1/A):363–98.

Aggarwal BB, Van Kuiken ME, Iyer LH, Harikumar KB, Sung B. Molecular targets of nutraceuticals derived from dietary spices: potential role in suppression of inflammation and tumorigenesis. *Experimental Biology and Medicine*. 2009 Aug; 234(8):825–49.

Arunkumar A, Vijayababu MR, Srinivasan N, Aruldhas MM, Arunakaran J. Garlic compound, diallyl disulfide induces cell cycle arrest in prostate cancer cell line PC-3. *Molecular and Cellular Biochemistry.* 2006 Aug; 288:107–13.

Aumeeruddy MZ, Mahomoodally MF. Combating breast cancer using combination therapy with 3 phytochemicals: piperine, sulforaphane, and thymoquinone. *Cancer.* 2019 May 15; 125(10):1600–11.

Bakshi H, Sam S, Rozati R, Sultan P, Islam T, Rathore B, Lone Z, Sharma M, Triphati J, Saxena RC. DNA fragmentation and cell cycle arrest: a hallmark of apoptosis induced by crocin from Kashmiri saffron in a human pancreatic cancer cell line. *Asian Pac J Cancer Prev.* 2010 Jan 1; 11(3):675–9.

Basha R, Connelly SF, Sankpal UT, Nagaraju GP, Patel H, Vishwanatha JK, Shelake S, Tabor-Simecka L, Shoji M, Simecka JW, El-Rayes B. Small molecule tolfenamic acid and dietary spice curcumin treatment enhances antiproliferative effect in pancreatic cancer cells via suppressing Sp1, disrupting NF-kB translocation to nucleus and cell cycle phase distribution. *The Journal of Nutritional Biochemistry.* 2016 May 1; 31:77–87.

Bengmark S, Mesa MD, Gil A. Plant-derived health-the effects of turmeric and curcuminoids. *Nutricion Hospitalaria.* 2009; 24(3):273–81.

Bhandari PR. Crocus sativus L.(saffron) for cancer chemoprevention: a mini review. *Journal of Traditional and Complementary Medicine.* 2015 Apr 1; 5(2):81–7.

Cabello CM, Bair III WB, Lamore SD, Ley S, Bause AS, Azimian S, Wondrak GT. The cinnamon-derived Michael acceptor cinnamic aldehyde impairs melanoma cell proliferation, invasiveness, and tumor growth. *Free Radical Biology and Medicine.* 2009 Jan 15; 46(2):220–31.

Chhikara BS, Parang K. Global Cancer Statistics 2022: the trends projection analysis. *Chemical Biology Letters.* 2023; 10(1):451.

Choudhuri T, Pal S, Das T, Sa G. Curcumin selectively induces apoptosis in deregulated cyclin D1-expressed cells at G2 phase of cell cycle in a p53-dependent manner. *Journal of Biological Chemistry.* 2005 May 20; 280(20):20059–68.

Chryssanthi DG, Dedes PG, Karamanos NK, Cordopatis P, Lamari FN. Crocetin inhibits invasiveness of MDA-MB-231 breast cancer cells via downregulation of matrix metalloproteinases. *Planta Medica.* 2011 Jan; 77(02):146–51.

de Lima RM, Dos Reis AC, de Menezes AA, Santos JV, Filho JW, Ferreira JR, de Alencar MV, da Mata AM, Khan IN, Islam A, Uddin SJ. Protective and therapeutic potential of ginger (Zingiber officinale) extract and [6]-gingerol in cancer: a comprehensive review. *Phytotherapy Research*. 2018 Oct; 32(10):1885–907.

de Souza Grinevicius VM, Kviecinski MR, Mota NS, Ourique F, Castro LS, Andreguetti RR, Correia JF, Wilhem Filho D, Pich CT, Pedrosa RC. Piper nigrum ethanolic extract rich in piperamides causes ROS overproduction, oxidative damage in DNA leading to cell cycle arrest and apoptosis in cancer cells. *Journal of Ethnopharmacology*. 2016 Aug 2; 189:139–47.

Deo SV, Sharma J, Kumar S. GLOBOCAN 2020 report on global cancer burden: challenges and opportunities for surgical oncologists. *Annals of Surgical Oncology*. 2022 Oct; 29(11):6497–500.

Devassy JG, Nwachukwu ID, Jones PJ. Curcumin and cancer: barriers to obtaining a health claim. *Nutrition Reviews*. 2015 Mar 1; 73(3): 155–65.

Ding Y, Ding Y, Wang Y, Wang C, Gao M, Xu Y, Ma X, Wu J, Li L. Soluplus®/ TPGS mixed micelles for co-delivery of docetaxel and piperine for combination cancer therapy. *Pharmaceutical Development and Technology*. 2020 Jan 2; 25(1):107–15.

Duan C, Zhang B, Deng C, Cao Y, Zhou F, Wu L, Chen M, Shen S, Xu G, Zhang S, Duan G. Piperlongumine induces gastric cancer cell apoptosis and G2/M cell cycle arrest both *in vitro* and *in vivo*. *Tumor Biology*. 2016 Aug; 37(8):10793–804.

Dutta A, Chakraborty A. Cinnamon in anticancer armamentarium: a molecular approach. *Journal of Toxicology*. 2018 Mar 29; 2018.

Fofaria NM, Kim SH, Srivastava SK. Piperine causes G1 phase cell cycle arrest and apoptosis in melanoma cells through checkpoint kinase-1 activation. *PloS One*. 2014 May 7; 9(5):e94298.

Fragis M, Murayyan AI, Neethirajan S. Cytotoxic activity and anti-cancer potential of Ontario grown onion extracts against breast cancer cell lines. *Functional Foods in Health and Disease*. 2018 Mar 31; 8(3):159–74.

Ghosh R, Ganapathy M, Alworth WL, Chan DC, Kumar AP. Combination of 2-methoxyestradiol (2-ME2) and eugenol for apoptosis induction synergistically in androgen independent prostate cancer cells. *The Journal of Steroid Biochemistry and Molecular Biology*. 2009 Jan 1; 113(1–2):25–35.

Greenshields AL, Doucette CD, Sutton KM, Madera L, Annan H, Yaffe PB, Knickle AF, Dong Z, Hoskin DW. Piperine inhibits the growth and motility of triple-negative breast cancer cells. *Cancer Letters*. 2015 Feb 1; 357(1):129–40.

Greten FR, Grivennikov SI. Inflammation and cancer: triggers, mechanisms, and consequences. *Immunity*. 2019 Jul 16; 51(1):27–41.

Hanahan D, Weinberg RA. Hallmarks of cancer: the next generation. *Cell*. 2011 Mar 4; 144(5):646–74.

Harris S, Brunton N, Tiwari U, Cummins E. Human exposure modelling of quercetin in onions (Allium cepa L.) following thermal processing. *Food Chemistry*. 2015 Nov 15; 187:135–9.

He M, Rosen J, Mangiameli D, Libutti SK. Cancer development and progression. *Microarray Technology and Cancer Gene Profiling*. 2007 Jan; 1:117–33.

Hossain MS, Kader MA, Goh KW, Islam M, Khan MS, Harun-Ar Rashid M, Ooi DJ, Melo Coutinho HD, Al-Worafi YM, Moshawih S, Lim YC. Herb and spices in colorectal cancer prevention and treatment: a narrative review. *Frontiers in Pharmacology*. 2022 Jun 30; 13:865801.

Hurtado M, Sankpal UT, Ranjan A, Maram R, Vishwanatha JK, Nagaraju GP, El-Rayes BF, Basha R. Investigational agents to enhance the efficacy of chemotherapy or radiation in pancreatic cancer. *Critical Reviews in Oncology/Hematology*. 2018 Jun 1; 126:201–7.

Icard P, Fournel L, Wu Z, Alifano M, Lincet H. Interconnection between metabolism and cell cycle in cancer. *Trends in Biochemical Sciences*. 2019 Jun 1; 44(6):490–501.

Jeong CH, Ryu H, Kim DH, Cheng WN, Yoon JE, Kang S, Han SG. Piperlongumine induces cell cycle arrest via reactive oxygen species accumulation and IKKβ suppression in human breast cancer cells. *Antioxidants*. 2019 Nov 14; 8(11):553.

Jiang X, Zhu X, Huang W, Xu H, Zhao Z, Li S, Li S, Cai J, Cao J. Garlic-derived organosulfur compound exerts antitumor efficacy via activation of MAPK pathway and modulation of cytokines in SGC-7901 tumor-bearing mice. *International Immunopharmacology*. 2017 Jul 1; 48:135–45.

Jin H, Qiao F, Wang Y, Xu Y, Shang Y. Curcumin inhibits cell proliferation and induces apoptosis of human non-small cell lung cancer cells through the upregulation of miR-192-5p and suppression of PI3K/Akt signaling pathway. *Oncology Reports*. 2015 Nov 1; 34(5):2782–9.

Jurenka JS. Anti-inflammatory properties of curcumin, a major constituent of Curcuma longa: a review of preclinical and clinical research. *Alternative Medicine Review*. 2009 Jun 1; 14(2).

Kaefer CM, Milner JA. The role of herbs and spices in cancer prevention. *The Journal of Nutritional Biochemistry*. 2008 Jun 1; 19(6):347–61.

Kammath AJ, Nair BPS, Nath LR. Curry versus cancer: potential of some selected culinary spices against cancer with *in vitro*, *in vivo*, and human trials evidences. *Journal of Food Biochemistry*. 2021 Mar; 45(3):e13285.

Kapoor V, Aggarwal S, Das SN. 6-Gingerol mediates its anti-tumor activities in human oral and cervical cancer cell lines through apoptosis and cell cycle arrest. *Phytotherapy Research*. 2016 Apr; 30(4):588–95.

Keyvani-Ghamsari S, Khorsandi K, Gul A. Curcumin effect on cancer cells' multidrug resistance: an update. *Phytotherapy Research*. 2020 Oct; 34(10):2534–56.

Krakhmal NV, Zavyalova MV, Denisov EV, Vtorushin SV, Perelmuter VM. Cancer invasion: patterns and mechanisms. *Acta Naturae (англоязычная версия)*. 2015; 7(2 (25)):17–28.

Kunnumakkara AB, Sailo BL, Banik K, Harsha C, Prasad S, Gupta SC, Bharti AC, Aggarwal BB. Chronic diseases, inflammation, and spices: how are they linked? *Journal of Translational Medicine*. 2018 Dec; 16(1) 1–25.

Kwon HK, Hwang JS, So JS, Lee CG, Sahoo A, Ryu JH, Jeon WK, Ko BS, Im CR, Lee SH, Park ZY. Cinnamon extract induces tumor cell death through inhibition of NFκB and AP1. *BMC Cancer*. 2010 Dec; 10:1–0.

Kwon HK, Hwang JS, So JS, Lee CG, Sahoo A, Ryu JH, Jeon WK, Ko BS, Im CR, Lee SH, Park ZY. Cinnamon extract induces tumor cell death through inhibition of NFκB and AP1. *BMC Cancer*. 2010 Dec; 10:1–0.

Larasati YA, Putri DD, Utomo RY, Hermawan A, Meiyanto E. Combination of cisplatin and cinnamon essential oil inhibits HeLa cells proliferation through cell cycle arrest. *Journal of Applied Pharmaceutical Science*. 2014 Dec 29; 4(12):014–9.

Mbese Z, Khwaza V, Aderibigbe BA. Curcumin and its derivatives as potential therapeutic agents in prostate, colon and breast cancers. *Molecules*. 2019 Nov 30; 24(23):4386.

Nicastro HL, Ross SA, Milner JA. Garlic and onions: their cancer prevention properties. *Cancer Prevention Research*. 2015 Mar 1; 8(3):181–9.

Nile A, Shin J, Park GS, Lee S, Lee JH, Lee KW, Kim BG, Han SG, Saini RK, Oh JW. Cinnamaldehyde-rich cinnamon extract induces cell death in colon cancer cell lines HCT 116 and HT-29. *International Journal of Molecular Sciences*. 2023 May 3; 24(9):8191.

Niu P, Li J, Chen H, Zhu Y, Zhou J, Shi D. Anti-proliferative effect of cardamonin on mTOR inhibitor-resistant cancer cells. *Molecular Medicine Reports.* 2020 Mar 1; 21(3):1399–407.

Paesa M, Nogueira DP, Velderrain-Rodríguez G, Esparza I, Jiménez-Moreno N, Mendoza G, Osada J, Martin-Belloso O, Rodríguez-Yoldi MJ, Ancín-Azpilicueta C. Valorization of onion waste by obtaining extracts rich in phenolic compounds and feasibility of its therapeutic use on colon cancer. *Antioxidants.* 2022 Apr 7; 11(4):733.

Panda AK, Chakraborty D, Sarkar I, Khan T, Sa G. New insights into therapeutic activity and anticancer properties of curcumin. *Journal of Experimental Pharmacology.* 2017 Mar; 31:31–45.

Panda AK, Chakraborty D, Sarkar I, Khan T, Sa G. New insights into therapeutic activity and anticancer properties of curcumin. *Journal of Experimental Pharmacology.* 2017 Mar; 31:31–45.

Pandey P, Khan F, Alshammari N, Saeed A, Aqil F, Saeed M. Updates on the anticancer potential of garlic organosulfur compounds and their nanoformulations: plant therapeutics in cancer management. *Frontiers in Pharmacology.* 2023 Mar 20; 14:1154034.

Pang B, Xu X, Lu Y, Jin H, Yang R, Jiang C, Shao D, Liu Y, Shi J. Prediction of new targets and mechanisms for quercetin in the treatment of pancreatic cancer, colon cancer, and rectal cancer. *Food & Function.* 2019; 10(9):5339–49.

Park YJ, Wen J, Bang S, Park SW, Song SY. 6-Gingerol induces cell cycle arrest and cell death of mutant p53-expressing pancreatic cancer cells. *Yonsei Medical Journal.* 2006 Oct 31; 47(5):688–97.

Qin Y, Sun CY, Lu FR, Shu XR, Yang D, Chen L, She XM, Gregg NM, Guo T, Hu Y. Cardamonin exerts potent activity against multiple myeloma through blockade of NF-κB pathway *in vitro. Leukemia Research.* 2012 Apr 1; 36(4):514–20.

Sadeghi S, Davoodvandi A, Pourhanifeh MH, Sharifi N, ArefNezhad R, Sahebnasagh R, Moghadam SA, Sahebkar A, Mirzaei H. Anti-cancer effects of cinnamon: insights into its apoptosis effects. *European Journal of Medicinal Chemistry.* 2019 Sep 15; 178:131–40.

Schoene NW, Kelly MA, Polansky MM, Anderson RA. Water-soluble polymeric polyphenols from cinnamon inhibit proliferation and alter cell cycle distribution patterns of hematologic tumor cell lines. *Cancer Letters.* 2005 Dec 8; 230(1):134–40.

Sherr CJ, Bartek J. Cell cycle–targeted cancer therapies. *Annual Review of Cancer Biology.* 2017 Mar 6; 1:41–57.

Shin SS, Song JH, Hwang B, Noh DH, Park SL, Kim WT, Park SS, Kim WJ, Moon SK. HSPA6 augments garlic extract-induced inhibition of proliferation, migration, and invasion of bladder cancer EJ cells: implication for cell cycle dysregulation, signaling pathway alteration, and transcription factor-associated MMP-9 regulation. *PLoS One.* 2017 Feb 10; 12(2): e0171860.

Shrivastava S, Jeengar MK, Thummuri D, Koval A, Katanaev VL, Marepally S, Naidu VG. Cardamonin, a chalcone, inhibits human triple negative breast cancer cell invasiveness by downregulation of Wnt/β-catenin signaling cascades and reversal of epithelial–mesenchymal transition. *Biofactors.* 2017 Mar; 43(2):152–69.

Singh N, Yadav SS. Ethnomedicinal uses of Indian spices used for cancer treatment: a treatise on structure-activity relationship and signaling pathways. *Current Research in Food Science.* 2022 Oct 11.

Singh Tuli H, Rath P, Chauhan A, Sak K, Aggarwal D, Choudhary R, Sharma U, Vashishth K, Sharma S, Kumar M, Yadav V. Luteolin, a potent anticancer compound: from chemistry to cellular interactions and synergetic perspectives. *Cancers.* 2022 Oct 31; 14(21):5373.

Srinivasan K. Antimutagenic and cancer preventive potential of culinary spices and their bioactive compounds. *PharmaNutrition.* 2017 Sep 1; 5(3):89–102.

Takahashi A, Yamamoto N, Murakami A. Cardamonin suppresses nitric oxide production via blocking the IFN-γ/STAT pathway in endotoxin-challenged peritoneal macrophages of ICR mice. *Life Sciences.* 2011 Aug 29; 89(9–10):337–42.

Tavakkol-Afshari J, Brook A, Mousavi SH. Study of cytotoxic and apoptogenic properties of saffron extract in human cancer cell lines. *Food and Chemical Toxicology.* 2008 Nov 1; 46(11):3443–7.

Tran KB, Lang JJ, Compton K, Xu R, Acheson AR, Henrikson HJ, Kocarnik JM, Penberthy L, Aali A, Abbas Q, Abbasi B. The global burden of cancer attributable to risk factors, 2010–19: a systematic analysis for the Global Burden of Disease Study 2019. *The Lancet.* 2022 Aug 20; 400(10352):563–91.

Tuli HS, Kaur J, Vashishth K, Sak K, Sharma U, Choudhary R, Behl T, Singh T, Sharma S, Saini AK, Dhama K. Molecular mechanisms behind ROS regulation in cancer: a balancing act between augmented tumorigenesis and cell apoptosis. *Archives of Toxicology.* 2023 Jan; 97(1):103–20.

Turrini E, Sestili P, Fimognari C. Overview of the anticancer potential of the "king of spices" piper nigrum and its main constituent piperine. *Toxins*. 2020 Nov 26; 12(12):747.

Vashishth K, Ranjan S, Joshi H, Singh T, Yerer Aycan MB, Tuli HS. Translational therapeutic targets: from bench to clinical trials. *InOncology: Genomics, Precision Medicine and Therapeutic Targets*. 2023 Jul 1 (pp. 265–274); Singapore: Springer Nature Singapore.

Williams GH, Stoeber K. The cell cycle and cancer. *The Journal of Pathology*. 2012 Jan; 226(2):352–64.

Wu XJ, Stahl T, Hu Y, Kassie F, Mersch-Sundermann V. The production of reactive oxygen species and the mitochondrial membrane potential are modulated during onion oil–induced cell cycle arrest and apoptosis in A549 cells. *The Journal of Nutrition*. 2006 Mar 1; 136(3):608–13.

Xu S, Zhang H, Liu T, Yang W, Lv W, He D, Guo P, Li L. 6-Gingerol induces cell-cycle G1-phase arrest through AKT–GSK 3β–cyclin D1 pathway in renal-cell carcinoma. *Cancer Chemotherapy and Pharmacology*. 2020 Feb; 85:379–90.

Yaffe PB, Power Coombs MR, Doucette CD, Walsh M, Hoskin DW. Piperine, an alkaloid from black pepper, inhibits growth of human colon cancer cells via G1 arrest and apoptosis triggered by endoplasmic reticulum stress. *Molecular Carcinogenesis*. 2015 Oct; 54(10): 1070–85.

Yang XQ, Zheng H, Ye Q, Li RY, Chen Y. Essential oil of Cinnamon exerts anti-cancer activity against head and neck squamous cell carcinoma via attenuating epidermal growth factor receptor-tyrosine kinase. *J BUON*. 2015 Nov 1; 20(6):1518–25.

Zhang J, Zhu X, Li H, Li B, Sun L, Xie T, Zhu T, Zhou H, Ye Z. Piperine inhibits proliferation of human osteosarcoma cells via G2/M phase arrest and metastasis by suppressing MMP-2/-9 expression. *International Immunopharmacology*. 2015 Jan 1; 24(1):50–8.

Zhang Z, Wang CZ, Wen XD, Shoyama Y, Yuan CS. Role of saffron and its constituents on cancer chemoprevention. *Pharmaceutical Biology*. 2013 Jul 1; 51(7):920–4.

Zheng J, Zhou Y, Li Y, Xu DP, Li S, Li HB. Spices for prevention and treatment of cancers. *Nutrients*. 2016 Aug 12; 8(8):495.

Zheng J, Zhou Y, Li Y, Xu DP, Li S, Li HB. Spices for prevention and treatment of cancers. *Nutrients*. 2016 Aug 12; 8(8):495.

Chapter 6

Anti-Angiogenic Effects of Spices on Cancer

Neha Atale[a] and Vibha Rani[b]

[a]*Department of Cardiothoracic Surgery,*
Division of Lung Transplant & Lung Failure,
Thomas E. Starzl Transplantation Institute,
University of Pittsburgh, Pennsylvania, USA
[b]*Department of Biotechnology,*
Jaypee Institute of Information Technology,
Noida, Uttar Pradesh, India

vibha.rani@jiit.ac.in

6.1 Introduction

Spices are known for their culinary qualities and food flavoring, additionally, they have the ability to prevent cancer. The health benefits of spices are due to the presence of active components, responsible for anti-angiogenesis, proliferation, and apoptosis [1, 2]. Along with these, they have various properties such as antioxidant, antibacterial, and immune modulatory. Since oxidative stress, inflammatory stress, and immunological response have been linked to the origin, development, and spread of malignancies, spices may thus be utilized to prevent or cure cancer [3–5].

Anticancer Spices: Dietary Input to Health
Edited by Hardeep Singh Tuli
Copyright © 2025 Jenny Stanford Publishing Pte. Ltd.
ISBN 978-981-5129-28-1 (Hardcover), 978-1-003-53466-2 (eBook)
www.jennystanford.com

Currently, cancer leads to 8.2 million fatalities and 14 million new cases, and it is predicted that the number of novel cases will rise by over 70% during the following two decades. Chemotherapy, radiation, and surgery are the main forms of treatment. [6]. Chemotherapy alone could be useful for a tiny tumor; however, surgery and radiation alone are only effective when the tumor is circumscribed and small in size. Additionally, they may cause certain negative effects. Since spices are a potential source of active components, there is a significant need for novel anticancer medications with fewer adverse effects. They may prevent cancer by interfering with the process of angiogenesis and inhibiting their growth factors.

Angiogenesis is the process of the growth of fresh blood vessels from the vasculature that already exists. Endothelial cell invasion, proliferation, migration, and differentiation into naive arteries are different steps of its development [7]. A critical stage in the development of a tumor is thought to be the acquisition of an angiogenic phenotype [8, 9]. Blood vessels contribute to tumors in order to supply them with the oxygen and nutrients they require as well as to remove metabolic waste. Additionally, growth factors secreted by endothelial cells promote the formation of tumors in an autocrine and paracrine way [10]. Neoplastic cells enter the bloodstream at a higher rate when angiogenesis begins, which makes metastasis easier [11]. Some investigations suggested that neovascularization is required for solid tumors to go from an in situ carcinoma to an invasive malignancy. As a result, the prevention of angiogenesis is a very efficient method for the cure of many malignancies [12].

As per the mechanism, angiogenesis is interfered with by targeting various markers and growth factors such as NO, VEGF, and MMPs, which take part in endothelial cell maintenance. Cancer cells, fibroblasts, and macrophages that infiltrate the tumor microenvironment produce specific cytokines and enzymes [13, 14]. Spices with therapeutic purposes precisely inhibit the growth of new blood vessels in tumors without significantly harming healthy tissues or causing severe side effects. Presently, the use of spices as VEGF pathway inhibitors in angiogenesis is recognized as a clinically effective anticancer therapeutic method.

Other angiogenic inhibitors have some toxicity issues such as bevacizumab [15]. Therefore, we focus on natural sources as angiogenic inhibitors and discuss the role of spices in the prevention of angiogenesis in this chapter. Table 6.1 indicates the target of spices and their active components for inhibition of angiogenesis.

6.2 Spices: Natural Sources Against Cancer

6.2.1 Black Cumin

Black cumin *Nigella sativa* is widely used in Indian and Eastern cuisines because of its aroma and taste. The seeds comprise different phytocomponents such as thymoquinone and dithymoquinone thymohydroquinone (nigellone) etc. [16]. Thymoquinone had a significant role in the prevention of tumor progression and angiogenesis in various models [17]. It is a healthy spice regularly used in rice and other foods and also its oil and aqueous extracts contain anti-inflammatory, antimicrobial, hypoglycemic, immune booster, and anticancer properties [18, 19]. The study on HepG2 and MOLT4 cancer cell line experiments showed its cytotoxic and anticancer effects. Aqueous and ethanol extracts of cumin seeds showed cytotoxic antiproliferative effects on cancer cells [20].

In human glioblastoma cells U-87, thymoquinone administration led to lowering FAK levels, ERK phosphorylation, and matrix metalloproteinases (MMP-2 and 9) secretion, which results in inhibition of migration. Other reports also confirmed its antimetastatic role in reducing cancer cell proliferation and migration through decreasing ERK1/2 phosphorylation [21]. Thymoquinone therapy suppresses TWIST1 promoter expression and lowers its expression in breast cancer cell lines, which prevents cells from migrating, invading, and metastasizing through the epithelial-mesenchymal transition (EMT). Thymoquinone reduced PI3K/AKT signaling and decreased mTOR activity in bladder cancer in addition to interfering with EMT [22]. Numerous research investigated the role of cumin seed oil in the inhibition of human fibrosarcoma cell line HT1080 development [23].

In a breast cancer study, the methanolic extract of cumin showed enhancement in the expression of apoptotic caspases, showing its anticancer activity [24]. It also diminished the JAK2 and STAT3 expression and increased the ROS level, further promoting apoptosis. It inhibited the activity of NF-kB, IL-8, PI3K/AKT, and MAPK [25, 26]. Thymoquinone suppressed the development of human prostate tumors at low doses with essentially no chemotoxic side effects. In a mouse model of xenografted human prostate cancer (PC3), it inhibited tumor angiogenesis. In addition, researchers found that endothelial cells were more vulnerable to the effects of thymoquinone on cancer cell function compared to PC3 cancer cells [17]. Thymoquinone had an inhibitory effect on VEGF-induced ERK activation but not on VEGF receptor 2 activation. Therefore, it can be stated that black cumin is a promising anticancer spice, however, further studies should be conducted.

6.2.2 Black Pepper

Black pepper (*Piper nigrum*) is a widely used seed in various recipes. Piperine, a key component of black pepper, has shown anticancer and anti-angiogenic activities. The administration of piperine inhibits *in vitro* proliferation, migration, and tube synthesis by HUVECs, the suppression of breast cancer cell-induced angiogenesis, and collagen-induced angiogenic activity by rat aorta explants in chick embryos. Piperine hindered the PI3K/Akt signaling cascade that potentiates angiogenesis [27]. The TRPV1 cation channel was inactivated by piperine to reduce angiogenesis [28].

The coarse extract of piperine-free *P. nigrum* (PFPE) was also found to inhibit breast cancer. In breast cancer-prone rats, PFPE was observed to increase p53 and decrease the levels of the estrogen receptor, E-cad, MMP-9, MMP-2, c-Myc, and VEGF. Methanol and dichloromethane extracts of the plant's fruits were analyzed for inhibition of breast cancer cell lines like MCF-7 [29]. Furthermore, the extract suppresses angiogenesis by downregulating VEGF and reducing migration/invasion by lowering matrix metalloproteinase (MMP)-2 and -9 in cancer [30].

Table 6.1 Target of spices and their active components for inhibition of angiogenesis

Spices	Active component	Target	Cancer cells
Black cumin (*N. sativa*)	Thymoquinone	VEGF↓, NF-kB↓, IL-8↓, PI3K/AKT↓, and MAPK↓	Hep G2, MOLT 4, HT-1080,
Black pepper (*P. nigrum*)	Piperine	E-cad↓, MMP-9↓, MMP-2↓, c-Myc↓, and VEGF↓	HUVEC, MCF-7
Cinnamon (*C. zeylanicum*)	Procyanidin	VEGFR-2↓, AKT↓, MAPK↓, VEGFR1/Flt1↓	HUVEC
Clove (*S. aromaticum*)	Eugenol, Sesquiterpene	VEGF↓, VEGFR1↓, TIMP-2↓, and RECK ↓	HT-29, Hep G2, 3LL
Galangal (*A. officinarum*)	Galangin	Akt↓, p70S6K↓, HIF-1α↓, VEGF↓	HT-1080
Garlic (*A. sativum*)	Allicin, alliin	GSH↓, VEGF↓	MCF-7, HCC-70, CAM model
Ginger (*Z. officinale*)	Gingerol, shogaol, paradols	MAPK↓, AP-1↓, p-VEGFR2↓, VE-cadherin↓	MCF-7
Oregano (*O. vulgare*)	Caryophyllene oxide	MMP-1, Collagen I, PAI-1, TIMP 1 and 2	Cancer cells, Chick chorioallantoic membrane
Red pepper (*C. annum*)	Capsaicin	p38↓, MAPK↓, and PKB ↓, MMP9 ↓	HUVEC, EC
Turmeric (*C. longa*)	Curcumin	MMP9↓, MMP2↓, VEGF↓, CXCL-1, CXCL-2, IL-6	MCF-7

6.2.3 Cinnamon

Cinnamon, *Cinnamomum zeylanicum* is enriched with procyanidins and has beneficial effects on cancer management [31]. Procyanidins were found to inhibit EGFR2 kinase activity, while a few reports showed its inhibition in a chick chorioallantoic membrane as well [32]. Various components of cinnamon extract such as type A procyanidin trimer and tetramers, potentially diminished VEGFR-2 kinase activity in endothelial cells, which results in the prevention of endothelial cell angiogenesis *in vitro*, as well as blood vessel formation *in vivo* [33].

AKT and MAPK phosphorylation caused by TPA was reduced by cinnamon extract. Gene expression studies in HUVEC demonstrated that treatment with cinnamon extract inhibited TPA-induced protein kinase C, PKC, as well as suppression of VEGFR1/Flt1 and VEGFR2/KDR/Flk1 mRNA expression [34]. The findings imply that PKC-dependent activation of MAPK mediates the action of cinnamon extract against angiogenesis. Further research will be needed to determine to confirm the role of cinnamon extract in anti-angiogenic activity.

6.2.4 Clove

Clove (*Syzygium aromaticum*) is a well-known spice in traditional Asian and Indian medicine. It has plenty of bioactive components, namely, desquiterpenes, caryophyllene, tannins, and eugenol [35]. Clove oil has effective antibacterial and analgesic properties. Eugenol, a clove component, has a distinctive odor and has been found in some anticancer formulations [36]. Oxidative stress markers such as inducible iNOS and COX-2 were found to be reduced in dimethylbenz[a]anthracen (DMBA) and eugenol-treated mice, showing its anticarcinogenic effect [37]. Using a tumor xenograft model called HT-29, the effects of ethyl acetate extract of clove (EAEC) and its bioactive component were studied *in vivo*. The element of EAEC that is responsible for its anticancer action has been identified as oleanolic acid (OA). Both EAEC and OA exhibit cytotoxicity against various human cancer cell lines [38].

Eugenol treatment inhibited cell proliferation and angiogenesis in gastric cancer as demonstrated by changes in MMPs actions, VEGF, VEGFR1, TIMP-2, and RECK expression. Eugenol treatment caused apoptosis to be triggered by the mitochondrial membrane potential loss by changing Apaf-1 and caspases [39]. Eugenol is a great contender for halting the spread of cancer since it has the potential to maintain the ratio of pro- and antiapoptotic proteins and the balance of angiogenesis-promoting proteins. Eugenol doses showed inhibition in various cancer cell lines such as HL-60, HepG2, and 3LL, and increased the expression of caspase 9 and caspase 3 [40].

6.2.5 Galangal

Galangal (*Alpinia officinarum*) is also an Asian spice and used for medicinal purposes. Galangin, a biocomponent from galangal, shows anticancer effects. Galangin was found to promote autophagy in cancer cells, by regulating TGF-β receptor pathway [41]. Additionally, MMP-9 breaks down type IV collagen in the basement membrane and is a key player in the development of tumors and inflammation. PMA-induced MMP-9 expression, which was inhibited by galangin through downregulating NF-κB, and AP-1-stimulated MMP-9 expression was silenced by galangin in HT-1080 cells [42]. Reports showed that galangin inhibited Akt/p70S6K/HIF-1α pathway and further downregulated the VEGF expression, however, more studies are needed [43].

6.2.6 Garlic

Garlic (*Allium sativum*) has organo-sulfur compounds, which have anticancer activity. The sulfur compounds in garlic have beneficial effects by lowering reactive species stress, neutralizing carcinogens, and enhancing immunological response. Allicin along with garlic powder prohibited the growth of breast cancer cells and growth arrest [44]. In both MCF-7 and HCC-70 (triple-negative) breast cancer cells, the growth-inhibitory effect of allicin was strongly correlated with decreasing glutathione levels [45]. Both of the cancer cells showed more severe cytotoxicity and antiproliferative activity in response to allicin, which decreased mitochondrial membrane potential, induced apoptosis, and increased the expression of caspases [46].

In the CAM model, alliin showed effective suppression of VEGF-induced angiogenesis. The anti-inflammatory effects of alliin on FGF2-induced EC tube formation and angiogenesis were greatly improved by the antioxidant vitamins C and E. The effects of alliin on preventing angiogenesis are influenced by cellular NO and p53 [47].

6.2.7 Ginger

Ginger (*Zingiber officinale*) rhizome is a well-known spice of Southern Asia [42, 43]. The volatile oil, which contains several monoterpenoids and sesquiterpenoids, gives the substance a distinctive smell [48]. The gingerols in fresh rhizomes are what give them their pungent flavor like 6-gingerol (1-[40-hydroxy30-methoxyphenyl]-5-hydroxy-3-decanoate). Dried rhizomes have a pungent flavor because they contain shogaols, including 6-shogaol, which are synthesized after the degradation of gingerols. Terpenoids, alkanes, paradols, and diarylheptanoids are the other compounds found in ginger [49]. According to studies, ginger's phenolic constituents, such as gingerols, shogaols, and paradols, have anti-inflammatory, antioxidant, and antitumor activities [50].

According to studies, 6-gingerol has a lethal impact on human colon cancer cells by activating MAP Kinase. The antiproliferation effect of 6-gingerol on human skin cell lines was observed in interfering MAPK and AP-1 signaling pathways [51]. By altering the PI3K/AKT signaling pathway, 6-gingerol works in conjunction with chemotherapy, notably cisplatin, to attack gastric cancer cells. As a result, cell cycle arrest occurs at the G1 phase. 6-gingerol has an anti-angiogenesis impact by hindering the micro-vessel development and stabilizing the p-VEGFR2/VE-cadherin complex [52]. Additionally, some other investigations have shown that 6-gingerol has an inhibitory impact on the inhibition of endothelial cell tube development, preventing the tumor's blood supply.

6.2.8   Oregano

The plant oregano (*Origanum vulgare*), which contains carvacrol, thymol, and several other anticancer chemicals, is widely included in the Mediterranean Diet [53]. Caryophyllene oxide, a sesquiterpene derived from the essential oils of medicinal herbs like oregano, had an anticancer impact by inhibiting the STAT3 activation pathway [54]. Oregano aqueous leaf extract showed inhibition of angiogenesis by lowering blood vessel formation in the chick chorioallantoic membrane. A number of tissue-remodeling indicators, including collagen I, collagen III, the EGFR, MMP-1, PAI-1, and TIMP 1 and 2 were also strongly reduced by OEO [55].

6.2.9   Red Chili Pepper

Red chili pepper (*Capsicum annuum*) contains capsaicin, which has anti-angiogenic properties [56]. Endothelial cells, when treated with capsaicin showed a reduction in proliferation, migration, and tube formation *in vivo*. It also prevented vessel sprouting in a Matrigel assay in mice and downregulating p38 MAPK, and PKB activation [57]. Further, capsaicin enhanced the breaking down of HIF 1α a critical marker of hypoxia, which increases VEGF production [58]. Capsaicin enhanced breast cancer cell death by hindering the NOTCH pathway [59].

Other bioactive components such as capsinoids and dihydrocapsiate also helped in increasing anti-angiogenic activities in various studies [60]. Capsiate and dihydrocapsiate suppressed VEGF-associated endothelial permeability and cell-to-cell junction synthesis [61]. The anticancer activity of capsaicin is associated with the decreased expression of cyclin D1, which diminished the Rb activation, further promoting the G1 check of HUVEC. Molecular docking studies revealed the binding of capsaicin and capsiate to Src kinase in a hydrophobic cleft; however, wet lab studies should be performed to further reveal the distinct mechanism [62].

6.2.10 Turmeric

Turmeric (*Curcuma longa*) is a well-known compound for its antioxidant and anti-inflammatory properties [63]. This spice is mild-flavored and typically found in Indian curry blends. It contains yellow colored compound curcumin, which contributes to its chemo-preventative and immunological activities. *In vitro* studies showed that curcumin may have several beneficial effects and have some clinical utility in patients with prostate cancer, gastrointestinal, and other cancers.

Curcumin intervenes with several signaling pathways, including NF-κB, MAPK, and EGFR pathways [63]. Dysfunctional NF-κB activity has been observed in cancer cells as well as in xenografts, and the NF-κB pathway induces angiogenesis and metastasis. Curcumin stops NF-κB activation and thus downregulates cancer-related genes, such as Bcl-2 and IL-6 [64], and also chemokine markers like CXCL-1 and CXCL-2 [65]. Treatment with curcumin reduced tumor volume and cell growth in breast cancer xenografts while also inhibiting angiogenesis.

Further studies revealed that it also inhibited the process of angiogenesis by reducing VEGF expression and regulated by the PI3k/AKT pathway [66]. In order to prevent cancer, chemicals having antioxidant qualities and curcumin may snare free radicals. Several cellular and preclinical studies have shown that curcumin reduces free radicals and active oxygen species, by preventing DNA damage brought on by oxidative factors like ionizing radiation [67]. Curcumin is also provided with chemotherapy drugs like 5-fluorouracil, doxorubicin, and cisplatin as combination therapy and boosts the synergistic impact, suppressing cancer malignancies [68]. Curcumin was also found to decrease VEGF-A expression in *in vitro* investigations. In a mouse model of human breast cancer, curcumin has been demonstrated to drastically reduce the expression of VEGFR2/3 and prevent angiogenesis [69]. According to Carroll et al., co-administration of curcumin with medroxyprogesterone acetate (MPA) can lower VEGF levels in the mammary glands of treated mice by 34% [70].

Curcumin also negatively regulates the expression of the VEGF and MMP9 expression, which is closely associated with angiogenesis. Demethoxycurcumin, a structural analog of curcumin, has shown inhibition against MMP-9 activity [71]. It interferes with the function of both MMP2 and MMP9, responsible for angiogenic switch, and repair ECM function.

6.3 Role of Spices as Nanomedicine for Health Benefits

Nanotechnology and herbal medicine are used to overcome the toxicity and bioavailability of active compounds. The functional characteristics of nanoparticles are improved by their tiny size and high surface-to-volume ratio. Anticancer activities of MCF-7, cumin seed extract, chemically produced silver nanoparticles (AgNPs), and biosynthesized (Bio-AgNPs) nanoparticles were examined [72]. To extend the effects of these medications for treating health issues and to get beyond the constraints of oral bioavailability, cinnamon and cumin (Ci-Cu) dual drug-loaded poly(D,L-lactide-co-glycolide) nanoparticles were developed [73]. Piperine was coupled with monoclonal antibodies against CD133 (mAbCD133) and nanoliposomes to improve its bioavailability [74]. The bioavailability of piperine was dramatically enhanced by cancer stem cell targeting manufactured nano liposomal technique.

The anticancer potential of curcumin has been constrained by its poor bioavailability. Thus, curcumin was nano-formulated to improve its therapeutic effectiveness in ovarian cancer. Dimethylbenz(a)anthracene (DMBA)-induced ovarian cancer in rats was treated with curcumin nanoparticles and cisplatin. Ovarian tumor volume and weight were significantly reduced after the treatment of cisplatin and nanocurcumin. Cisplatin and nanocurcumin were used to lower IL-6 levels, JAK expression, and STAT3 phosphorylation. Inhibiting proliferation via downregulating the PI3K/Akt and JAK/STAT3 signaling pathways, nanocurcumin combined with cisplatin offers therapeutic promise in ovarian cancer models [75]. *In vitro* testing on garlic nanoparticles (G-AgNPs) was done against the breast cancer cell lines MCF-7 and G-AgNPs showed anticancer efficacy [76]. Figure 6.1 shows the anti-angiogenic properties of spices.

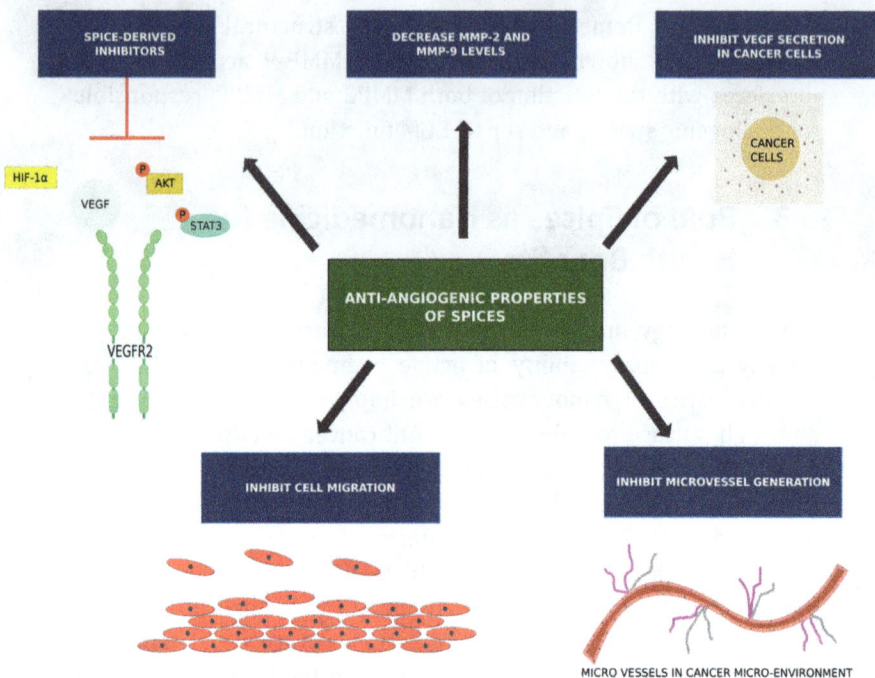

Figure 6.1 Angiogenic properties of spices.

6.4 Conclusion

Spices, as a part of our regular diet, may decrease the cancer risk. This chapter reveals the effect of spices on various cancer cells and shows an anti-angiogenesis effect. Various mechanisms of cancer cell proliferation, apoptosis, angiogenesis, and immunocompetence could be affected by mentioned spices, which ultimately hinder the tumor activity. The possibility of a synergistic impact that might improve the anticancer effect of conventional therapy increases when a variety of spices are present in a single meal. The crucial function of bio-nanoparticles in the treatment of many forms of cancer is produced by extracts from culinary spices and found to be useful against cancer. Further research is required to design anticancer diets with the ideal spice to enhance the anti-angiogenesis mechanism.

Acknowledgment

We acknowledge the University of Pittsburgh and Jaypee Institute of Information Technology for their infrastructural support.

Conflict of Interest

Authors declare no conflict of interest.

List of Abbreviations

APAF-1:	Apoptotic peptidase activating factor 1
CAM:	Chick chorioallantoic membrane
COX-2:	Cyclooxygenase-2
CXCL-1:	C-X-C motif chemokine ligand 1
CXCL-2:	C-X-C motif chemokine ligand 2
DMBA:	Dimethylbenz[a]anthracen
EAEC:	Ethyl acetate extract of clove
EC:	Endothelial cells
EMT:	Epithelial-mesenchymal transition
ERK:	Extracellular signal-regulated kinase 1
FAK:	Focal adhesion kinase
FGF:	Fibroblast growth factors
6-gingerol:	(1-[40-hydroxy30-methoxyphenyl]-5-hydroxy-3-decanoate)
HIF 1α:	Hypoxia inducible factor 1 α
HUVEC:	Human umbilical vein endothelial cells
3-LL:	Lewis lung carcinoma
MAPK:	Mitogen-activated protein kinases
MMPs:	Matrix metalloproteinases
mAbCD133:	Monoclonal antibodies against CD133
mTOR:	Mammalian target of rapamycin
NP:	Nanoparticle
NF-κB:	Nuclear factor-kappaB
NO:	Nitric oxide
OA:	Oleanolic acid
OEO:	Oregano essential oil

PFPE:	Piperine free *P. nigrum*
PKB:	Protein kinase B
PMA:	Phorbol 12-myristate 13-acetate
RECK:	Reversion-inducing cysteine-rich protein with Kazal motifs
STAT3:	Signal transducer and activator of transcription 3
TIMP-2:	Tissue inhibitor of metalloproteinases 2
TPA:	Tissue-type plasminogen activator
TRPV-1:	Transient receptor potential vanilloid 1
TWIST-1:	Twist family bHLH transcription factor 1
VEGF:	Vascular endothelial growth factor
VEGFR2/ KDR/Flk-1:	Vascular endothelial growth factor receptor 2
VEGFR-1/Flt-1:	Vascular endothelial growth factor receptor-1

References

1. Zheng, J., Zhou, Y, Li, Y., Xu, D. P., Li, S., and L,i H. B. (2016). Spices for prevention and treatment of cancers. *Nutrients.*, 8, pp. 495–530.

2. Rubio, L., Motilva M. J., and Romero, M. P. (2013). Recent advances in biologically active compounds in herbs and spices: A review of the most effective antioxidant and anti-inflammatory active principles. *Crit Rev Food Sci Nutr,* 53, pp. 943–953.

3. Zhou, Y., Li, Y., Zhou, T., Zheng, J., Li, S., and Li, H. B. (2016). Dietary natural products for prevention and treatment of liver cancer. *Nutrients.*, 8, pp. 156–179.

4. Deng, G. F., Xu, X. R., Guo, Y. J., Xia, E. Q., Li, S., Wu, S., Chen, F., Ling, W. H., and Li, H.B. (2012). Determination of antioxidant property and their lipophilic and hydrophilic phenolic contents in cereal grains. *J Funct Foods.*, 4, pp. 906–914.

5. Butt, M. S., Naz, A., Sultan, M. T., Qayyum, M. M. Anti-oncogenic perspectives of spices/herbs: A comprehensive review. (2013). *Excli J.*, 12, pp. 1043–1065.

6. Schirrmacher, V. (2019). From chemotherapy to biological therapy: A review of novel concepts to reduce the side effects of systemic cancer treatment. *Int J Oncol.*, 54, pp. 407–419.

7. Lamalice, L, Boeuf, F. L., and Huot, J. (2007). Endothelial cell migration during angiogenesis. *Circ Res.*, 100, pp. 782–794.

8. Lugano, R., Ramachandran, M., and Dimberg, A. (2020). Tumor angiogenesis: Causes, consequences, challenges, and opportunities. *Cell Mol Life Sci.*, 77, pp. 1745–1770.

9. Atale, N. and Rani V. (2020). "Angiogenesis: A therapeutic target for cancer" in *Drug targets in cellular processes of cancer: From nonclinical to preclinical models*, 1st Ed., Springer, pp. 165–183.

10. Atale, N. and Rani V. (2022). "Role of nanotherapeutics in inhibiting cancer angiogenesis: A novel perspective" in *Nanotherapeutics in cancer,* 1st Ed., Taylor & Francis, pp. 1–23.

11. Bielenberg, D. R. and Zetter, B. R. (2015). The contribution of angiogenesis to the process of metastasis. *Cancer J.*, 21, pp. 67–73.

12. Katayama, Y., Uchino, J., Chihara, Y., Tamiya, N., Kaneko, Y., Yamada, T., and Takayama, K. (2019). Tumor neovascularization and developments in therapeutics. *Cancers.*, 11, pp. 316–332.

13. Jiang, B. H. and Liu, L. Z. (2009). PI3K/pTEN signaling in angiogenesis and tumorigenesis. *Adv Cancer Res.,* 102, pp. 19–65.

14. Raskov, H., Orhan, A., Gaggar, S., and Gögenur, I. (2021). Cancer-associated fibroblasts and tumor-associated macrophages in cancer and cancer immunotherapy. *Front Oncol.*, 11, pp. 668731.

15. El-Kenawi, A. E. and El-Remessy, A. B. (2013). Angiogenesis inhibitors in cancer therapy: Mechanistic perspective on classification and treatment rationales. *Br J Pharmacol.*, 170, pp. 712–729.

16. Ahmad, A., Husain, A., Mujeeb, M., Khan, S. A., Najmi, A. K., Siddique, N. A., Damanhouri, Z. A., and Anwar, F. (2013). A review on therapeutic potential of *Nigella sativa*: A miracle herb. *Asian Pac J Trop Biomed.*, 3, pp. 337–352.

17. Yi, T., Cho, S. G, Yi, Z., Pang, X., Rodriguez, M., Wang, Y., Sethi, G., Aggarwal, B. B., and Liu, M. (2008). Thymoquinone inhibits tumor angiogenesis and tumor growth through suppressing AKT and extracellular signal-regulated kinase signaling pathways. *Mol Cancer Ther.*, 7, pp.1789–1796.

18. Almatroodi, S. A., Almatroudi, A., Alsahli, M. A., Khan, A. A., and Rahmani, A. H. (2020). Thymoquinone, an active compound of *Nigella sativa*: Role in prevention and treatment of cancer. *Curr Pharm Biotechnol.,* 21, pp. 1028–1041.

19. Hossain, M. S., Sharfaraz, A., Dutta, A., Ahsan, A., Masud, M. A., Ahmed, I. A., et al. (2021). A review of ethnobotany, phytochemistry, antimicrobial pharmacology and toxicology of *Nigella sativa* L. *Biomed Pharmacother.,* 143, pp. 112182–1121207.

20. Swamy, S. M. K. and Tan, B. K. H. (2000). Cytotoxic and immunopotentiating effects of ethanolic extract of *Nigella sativa* L. seeds. *J Ethanopharmacol*, 70, pp. 1–7.

21. Kolli-Bouhafs, K., Boukhari, A., Abusnina, A., Velot, E., Gies, J. P., Lugnier, C., and Rondé, P. (2012). Thymoquinone reduces migration and invasion of human glioblastoma cells associated with FAK, MMP-2 and MMP-9 down-regulation. *Invest New Drugs.*, 30, pp. 2121–2131.

22. Khan, M. A., Tania, M., Wei, C., Mei, Z., Fu, S., Cheng, J., Xu, J., and Fu, J. (2015). Thymoquinone inhibits cancer metastasis by downregulating TWIST1 expression to reduce epithelial to mesenchymal transition. *Oncotarget.*, 6, pp. 19580–19591.

23. Khan, M. A., Chen, H. C., Tania, M., and Zhang, D. Z. (2011). Anticancer activities of *Nigella sativa* (black cumin). *Afr J Trad Complement Altern Med.*, 8, pp. 226–232.

24. Majdalawieh, A. F. and Fayyad, M. W. (2016). Recent advances on the anti-cancer properties of *Nigella sativa*, a widely used food additive. *J Ayurveda Integr Med.*, 7, pp. 173–180.

25. Lu, B., Shinohara, E. T., Edwards, E., Geng, L., Tan, J., and Hallahan, D. E. (2005). The use of tyrosine kinase inhibitors in modifying the response of tumor microvasculature to radiotherapy. *Technol Cancer Res Treat.*, 4, pp. 691–698.

26. Perona, R. (2006). Cell signalling: Growth factors and tyrosine kinase receptors. *Clin Transl Oncol.*, 8, pp. 77–82.

27. Doucette, C. D., Hilchie, A. L., Liwski, R., and Hoskin, D. W. (2013). Piperine, a dietary phytochemical, inhibits angiogenesis. *J Nutr Biochem.*, 24, pp. 231–239.

28. Negri, S., Faris, P., Rosti V., Antognazza, M. R, Lodola, F., and Moccia, F. (2020). Endothelial TRPV1 as an emerging molecular target to promote therapeutic angiogenesis. *Cell.*, 9, pp. 134–163.

29. Sriwiriyajan, S., Tedasen, A., Lailerd, N., Boonyaphiphat, P., Nitiruangjarat, A., Deng, Y., and Graidist, P. (2016). Anticancer and cancer prevention effects of piperine-free *Piper nigrum* extract on N-nitrosomethylurea-induced mammary tumorigenesis in rats. *Cancer Prev Res.*, 9, pp. 74–82.

30. Den, Y., Sriwiriyajan, S., Tedasen, A., Hiransai, P., and Graidist, P. (2016). Anti-cancer effects of *Piper nigrum* via inducing multiple molecular signaling *in vivo* and *in vitro*. *J Ethnopharmacol.*, 188, pp. 87–95.

31. Rao, P. V. and Gan, S. H. (2014). Cinnamon: A multifaceted medicinal plant. *Evid Based Complement Alternat Med.*, 2014, pp. 642942–642954.

32. Daveri, E., Adamo, A. M., Alfine, E., Zhu, W., and Oteiza, P.I. (2021). Hexameric procyanidins inhibit colorectal cancer cell growth through both redox and non-redox regulation of the epidermal growth factor signaling pathway. *Redox Biol.*, 38, pp. 101830–101841.

33. Lu, J., Zhang, K., Nam, S., Anderson, R. A., Jove, R., and Wen, W. (2010). Novel angiogenesis inhibitory activity in Cinnamon extract blocks VEGFR2 kinase and downstream signaling. *Carcinogenesis*, 31, pp. 481–488.

34. Bansode, R. R., Leung, T., Randolph, P., Williams, L. L., Ahmedna, M. (2013). Cinnamon extract inhibits angiogenesis in zebrafish and human endothelial cells by suppressing VEGFR1, VEGFR2, and PKC-mediated MAP kinase. *Food Sci Nutr.*, 1, pp. 74–82.

35. Batiha, G. E., Alkazmi, L. M., Wasef, L. G., Beshbishy, A. M., Nadwa, E. H., and Rashwan, E. K. (2020). *Syzygium aromaticum L.* (Myrtaceae): Traditional uses, bioactive chemical constituents, pharmacological and toxicological activities. *Biomolecules.*, 10, pp. 202–218.

36. Zari, A. T., Zari, T. A., and Hakeem, K. R. (2021). Anticancer properties of eugenol: A review. *Molecules.*, 26, pp. 7407–7424.

37. Kaur, G., Athar, M., and Alam, M. S. (2010). Eugenol precludes cutaneous chemical carcinogenesis in mouse by preventing oxidative stress and inflammation and by inducing apoptosis. *Mol Carcinog.*, 49, pp. 290–301.

38. Liu, H., Schmitz, J. C., Wei, J., Cao, S., Beumer, J. H., Strychor, S., Cheng, L., Liu, M., Wang, C., Wu, N., Zhao, X., Zhang, Y., Liao, J., Chu, E., and Lin, X. (2014). Clove extract inhibits tumor growth and promotes cell cycle arrest and apoptosis. *Oncol Res.*, 21(5), pp. 247–59.

39. Manikandan, P., Murugan, R. S., Priyadarsini, R. V., Vinothini, G., and Nagini, S. (2010). Eugenol induces apoptosis and inhibits invasion and angiogenesis in a rat model of gastric carcinogenesis induced by MNNG. *Life Sci.,* 86, pp. 936–941.

40. Jaganathan, S. K. and Supriyanto, E. (2010). Antiproliferative and molecular mechanism of eugenol-induced apoptosis in cancer cells. *Molecules.*, 17(6), pp. 6290–304.

41. Tuli, H. S., Sak, K., Adhikary, S., Kaur, G., Aggarwal, D., Kaur, J., Kumar, M., Parashar, N. C., Parashar, G., Sharma, U., and Jain, A. (2022). Galangin: A metabolite that suppresses anti-neoplastic activities

through modulation of oncogenic targets. *Exp Biol Med (Maywood).,* 247(4), pp. 345–359.

42. Choi, Y. J., Lee, Y. H., and Lee, S.T. (2015). Galangin and kaempferol suppress phorbol-12-myristate-13-acetate-induced matrix metalloproteinase-9 expression in human fibrosarcoma HT-1080 cells. *Mol. Cells.,* 38, pp. 151–155.

43. Huang, H., Chen, A. Y., Rojanasakul, Y., Ye, X., Rankin, G. O., and Chen, Y.C. (2015). Dietary compounds galangin and myricetin suppress ovarian cancer cell angiogenesis. *J Funct Foods.,* 15, pp. 464–475.

44. Omar, S. H. and Al-Wabel, N. A. (2010). Organosulfur compounds and possible mechanism of garlic in cancer. *Saudi Pharm J.,* 18(1), pp. 51–58.

45. Pandey, P., Khan, F., Alshammari, N., Saeed, A., Aqil, F., and Saeed, M. (2023). Updates on the anticancer potential of garlic organosulfur compounds and their nanoformulations: Plant therapeutics in cancer management. *Front Pharmacol.,* 14, 1154034, pp. 1–11.

46. Jun, Z., Suzuki, M., Xiao, J., Wen, J., Talbot, S. G., and Li, G. C., et al. (2009). Comparative effects of natural and synthetic diallyl disulfide on apoptosis of human breast-cancer MCF-7 cells. *Biotechnol. Appl. Biochem.,* 52, pp. 113–119.

47. Mousa, A. S. and Mousa, S. A. (2005). Anti-angiogenesis efficacy of the garlic ingredient alliin and antioxidants: Role of nitric oxide and p53. *Nutr Cancer.,* 53, pp. 104–10.

48. Mao, Q. Q., Xu, X. Y., Cao, S. Y., Gan, R. Y., Corke, H., Beta, T., and Li, H. B. (2019). Bioactive compounds and bioactivities of ginger (*Zingiber officinale* Roscoe). *Foods.,* 8, pp. 185.

49. Bischoff-Kont, I. and Fürst, R. (2021). Benefits of ginger and its constituent 6-shogaol in inhibiting inflammatory processes. *Pharmaceuticals (Basel).,* 14, pp. 571.

50. Rahmani, A. H., Shabrmi, F. M., and Aly, S. M. (2014). Active ingredients of ginger as potential candidates in the prevention and treatment of diseases via modulation of biological activities. *Int J Physiol Pathophysiol Pharmacol.,* 6, pp. 125–36.

51. Radhakrishnan, E. K., Bava, S. V., Narayanan, S. S., Nath, L. R., Thulasidasan, A. K., Soniya, E. V., and Anto, R. J. (2014). [6]-gingerol induces caspase-dependent apoptosis and prevents PMA-induced proliferation in colon cancer cells by inhibiting MAPK/AP-1 signaling. *PLoS One.,* 9(8), pp. e104401.

52. Zhong, W., Yang, W., and Qin, Y. et al. (2019). 6-Gingerol stabilized the p-VEGFR2/VE-cadherin/β-catenin/actin complex promotes microvessel normalization and suppresses tumor progression. *J Exp Clin Cancer Res.*, 38, 285, pp. 1–24.

53. Zinno, P., Guantario, B., Lombardi, G., Ranaldi, G., Finamore, A., Allegra, S., Mammano, M.M., Fascella, G., Raffo, A., and Roselli, M. (2023). Chemical composition and biological activities of essential oils from origanum vulgare genotypes belonging to the carvacrol and thymol chemotypes. *Plants.*, 12, 1344, pp. 1–24.

54. Fidyt, K., Fiedorowicz, A., Strządała, L., and Szumny, A. (2016). β-caryophyllene and β-caryophyllene oxide-natural compounds of anticancer and analgesic properties. *Cancer Med.*, 5, pp. 3007–3017.

55. Paderes, N. M. (2020). Antiangiogenic activity of oregano (*Origanum vulgare*) aqueous extract in-vivo through chick chorioallantoic membrane (CAM) assay. *Sys Rev Pharm.*, 11(6), pp. 1222–1227.

56. Friedman, J. R., Richbart, S. D., Merritt, J. C., Brown, K. C., Denning, K. L., Tirona, M. T., Valentovic, M. A., Miles, S. L., and Dasgupta, P. (2019). Capsaicinoids: Multiple effects on angiogenesis, invasion and metastasis in human cancers. *Biomed Pharmacother.*, 118, 109317, pp. 1–17.

57. Min, J. K., Han, K. Y., Kim, E. C., Kim, Y. M., Lee, S. W., Kim, O. H., Kim, K. W., Gho, Y. S., and Kwon, Y. G. (2004). Capsaicin inhibits *in vitro* and *in vivo* angiogenesis. *Cancer Res.*, 64, pp. 644–651.

58. Patel, P. S., Yang, S., Li, A., Varney, M. L., and Singh, R. K. (2002). Capsaicin regulates vascular endothelial cell growth factor expression by modulation of hypoxia inducing factor-1alpha in human malignant melanoma cells. *J Cancer Res Clin Oncol.*, 128, pp. 461–468.

59. Shim, Y. and Song, J. M. (2015). Quantum dot nanoprobe-based high-content monitoring of notch pathway inhibition of breast cancer stem cell by capsaicin. *Mol Cell Probes.*, 29, pp. 376–381.

60. Chilczuk, B., Marciniak, B., Stochmal, A., Pecio, Ł., Kontek, R., Jackowska, I., and Materska, M. (2020). Anticancer potential and capsianosides identification in lipophilic fraction of sweet pepper (*Capsicum annuum* L.). *Molecules.*, 25(13), pp. 3097.

61. Pyun, B. J., Choi, S., Lee, Y., Kim, T. W., Min, J. K., Kim, Y., Kim, B. D., Kim, J. H., Kim, T. Y., Kim, Y. M., and Kwon, Y. G. (2008). Capsiate, a nonpungent capsaicin-like compound, inhibits angiogenesis and vascular permeability via a direct inhibition of Src kinase activity. *Cancer Res.*, 68, pp. 227–235.

62. Min, J. K., Han, K. Y., Kim, E. C., Kim, Y. M., Lee, S. W., Kim, O. H., Kim, K. W., Gho, Y. S., and Kwon, Y. G. (2004). Capsaicin inhibits *in vitro* and *in vivo* Angiogenesis, *Cancer Res.,* 64, pp. 644–651.

63. Sharifi-Rad, J., Rayess, Y. E., Rizk, A. A., Sadaka, C., Zgheib, R., Zam, W., Sestito, S., Rapposelli, S., Neffe-Skocińska, K., Zielińska, D., Salehi, B., Setzer, W. N., Dosoky, N. S., Taheri, Y., El Beyrouthy, M., Martorell, M., Ostrander, E. A., Suleria, H. A. R., Cho, W. C., Maroyi, A., and Martins, N. (2020). Turmeric and its major compound curcumin on health: bioactive effects and safety profiles for food, pharmaceutical, biotechnological and medicinal applications. *Front Pharmacol.,* 11, pp. 1–23.

64. Farghadani, R. and Naidu, R. (2021). Curcumin: Modulator of key molecular signaling pathways in hormone-independent breast cancer. *Cancers (Basel).,* 13 (14), 3427, pp. 1–29.

65. Wang, W., Nag, S. A., and Zhang, R. (2015). Targeting the NFκB signaling pathways for breast cancer prevention and therapy. *Curr Med Chem.,* 22(2), pp. 264–289.

66. Fu, Z., Chen, X., Guan, S., Yan, Y., Lin, H., and Hua, Z. C. (2015). Curcumin inhibits angiogenesis and improves defective hematopoiesis induced by tumor-derived VEGF in tumor model through modulating VEGF-VEGFR2 signaling pathway. *Oncotarget.,* 6(23), pp. 19469–19482.

67. Mansouri, K., Rasoulpoor, S., and Daneshkhah, A. et al. (2020). Clinical effects of curcumin in enhancing cancer therapy: A systematic review. *BMC Cancer.,* 20, 791, pp. 1–11.

68. Tan, B. L. and Norhaizan, M. E. (2019). Curcumin combination chemotherapy: The implication and efficacy in cancer. *Molecules.,* 24(14), 2527, pp. 1–21.

69. Bimonte, S., Barbieri, A., Palma, G., Rea, D., Luciano, A., D'Aiuto, M., Arra, C., and Izzo, F. (2015). Dissecting the role of curcumin in tumour growth and angiogenesis in mouse model of human breast cancer. *Biomed Res Int.,* 878134, pp. 1–7.

70. Carroll, C. E., Benakanakere, I., Besch-Williford, C., Ellersieck, M. R., and Hyder, S. M. (2010). Curcumin delays development of medroxyprogesterone acetate-accelerated 7,12-dimethylbenz[a] anthracene-induced mammary tumors. *Menopause.,* 17, pp. 178–84.

71. Wilken, R., Veena, M. S., Wang, M. B., and Srivatsan, E. S. (2011). Curcumin: A review of anti-cancer properties and therapeutic activity in head and neck squamous cell carcinoma. *Mol Cancer.,* 10, 12, pp. 1–19.

72. Dinparvar, S., Bagirova, M., Allahverdiyev, A. M., Abamor, E. S., Safarov, T., Aydogdu, M., and Aktas, D. (2020). A nanotechnology-based new approach in the treatment of breast cancer: Biosynthesized silver nanoparticles using Cuminum cyminum L. seed extract. *J Photochem Photobio.*, 208, pp. 111902: 1–8.

73. Sangal, A., Rattan, S., and Maurya, M.R. et al. (2023). Novel formulation for co-delivery of cinnamon- and cumin-loaded polymeric nanoparticles to enhance their oral bioavailability. *Biotech.*, 13, 63, pp. 1–8.

74. Thao, D. T., Minh, L. N., Anh, T. T. M., Thi Nga, N., Hue, P. T. K., and Van Kiem, P. (2021). The improved anticancer activities of piperine nanoliposome conjugated cd133 monoclonal antibody against NTERA-2 cancer stem cells. *Natural Product Communications.*, 16(2), pp. 1–7.

75. Sandhiutami, N. M. D., Arozal, W., Louisa, M., Rahmat, D., and Wuyung, P. E. (2021). Curcumin nanoparticle enhances the anticancer effect of cisplatin by inhibiting PI3K/AKT and JAK/STAT3 pathway in rat ovarian carcinoma induced by DMBA. *Front Pharmacol.*, 11, pp. 603235–603245.

76. Vijayakumar, S., Malaikozhundan, B., Saravanakumar, K., Durán-Lara, E. F., Wang, M. H., and Vaseeharan, B. (2019). Garlic clove extract assisted silver nanoparticle – Antibacterial, antibiofilm, antihelminthic, anti-inflammatory, anticancer and ecotoxicity assessment. *J Photochem Photobiol B: Biol.*, 198, pp. 12–19.

Chapter 7

Antimetastatic Action of Spices

Shallu Saini,[a] Hemant Joshi,[b] Seema Ramniwas,[c] Moyad Shahwan,[d,e] Gurpreet Kaur Bhatia,[f] and Hardeep Singh Tuli[a]

[a]*Department of Biosciences and Technology,*
Maharishi Markandeshwar (Deemed to be University), Mullana, Ambala, India
[b]*School of Biotechnology, Jawaharlal Nehru University, New Delhi, India*
[c]*University Centre for Research and Development,*
University Institute of Pharmaceutical Sciences, Chandigarh University,
Mohali, India
[d]*Department of Clinical Sciences, College of Pharmacy and Health Sciences,*
Ajman University, Ajman, United Arab Emirates
[e]*Centre of Medical and Bio-Allied Health Sciences Research,*
Ajman University, Ajman, United Arab Emirates
[f]*Department of Physics, Maharishi Markandeshwar (Deemed to be University),*
Mullana, Ambala, India

shalucool37@gmail.com

7.1 Introduction

Metastasis is a multiscale, multi-component process that incorporates several concurrent, partially overlapping subprocesses. The main factor in cancer lethality is metastasis, which is the process by which cancer cells spread from a primary lesion to distal organs. Numerous biological pathways are involved in the dissemination of cells from a primary tumor (Suhail et al.,

Anticancer Spices: Dietary Input to Health
Edited by Hardeep Singh Tuli
Copyright © 2025 Jenny Stanford Publishing Pte. Ltd.
ISBN 978-981-5129-28-1 (Hardcover), 978-1-003-53466-2 (eBook)
www.jennystanford.com

2019). These include penetrating the stroma or cooperating with it, evading immune monitoring by thwarting, or utilizing their anti-tumorigenic mechanisms, manipulating the tissue microenvironment, and developing resistance to therapeutic intervention (Deng et al., 2016). Spices have been used as flavoring agents in food and as conventional medicine for centuries. The bioactive component of spices is mainly responsible for exerting some specific pharmacological actions. Numerous studies have reported the antioxidant, anti-inflammatory, and immune system modulation activities of spices might be responsible for exerting anti-proliferative, anti-angiogenic, anti-metastatic, apoptosis-promoting functions, and potentiating the efficacy of conventional cancer treatments to cure various types of cancers, such as breast, colon, prostate, stomach, lung, and liver cancers (Vasanthi et al., 2010). Indian spices have been used for thousands of years and are well-known for adding flavor, color, and aroma to food, but their medicinal benefits are less frequently acknowledged. Thousands of studies conducted over the past 20 years have shown that spices include phytochemicals that may protect against a number of chronic diseases, including cancer, diabetes, cardiovascular, pulmonary, neurological, and autoimmune diseases (Aggarwal et al., 2008).

Phytochemicals from different spices, such as turmeric (curcumin), red pepper (capsaicin), cloves (eugenol), ginger (zerumbone), fennel (anethole), kokum (gambogic acid), fenugreek (diosgenin), and black cumin (thymoquinone), have been related to the ability to prevent cancer. We should concentrate on health measures including prevention, early detection, and efficient therapies in order to reduce cancer mortality (Bandyopadhyay 2014). Spices have a big impact on human health thanks to their bioactives. In addition to other health benefits, they have the potential to fight cancer. Among the natural chemopreventive bioactives that can slow, delay, or reverse multi-stage carcinogenesis, spice-derived phytochemicals have received a lot of attention recently (Srinivasan 2017). Turmeric, garlic, ginger, and black cumin are among the spices with documented anticarcinogenic properties in cancer animal models. Many prescription medications used in the clinical treatment of cancer patients come from real plant species. Additionally, it is becoming clearer how these spices exert their anticancer benefits (Saraswathi et al., 2020).

7.2   Mechanism of Cancer Metastasis

Metastasis is the process by which cancer cells spread from their originating location to an additional organ. In fact, cancer metastasis is to blame for the most therapeutic failures, as patients pass away from the many tumor growths, making it one of the most intriguing stages in the pathophysiology of the disease (Fidler 1975).

There are five key stages in the growth of tumor metastasis: 1. invasion of primary tumor cells into surrounding tissue and blood and/or lymphatic vessels; 2. release of tumor cell emboli into circulation; 3. arrest of the emboli in small vascular channels of different organs; 4. invasion of primary tumor cells into the wall of the arresting vessel and multiplication; and 5. growth of vascularized stroma into the new tumor as proliferating tumor cells invade the distant organ (Fig. 7.1) (Joshi et al., 2023; San Juan et al., 2019; Zeidman, 1957). Metastases, or secondary tumor growths, are the result of the halted tumor emboli's final development. The invasion, embolization, arrest, and emboli formation processes can then start up again.

Proteolytic disruption of the basement membrane by tumor cells can lead to spread and overt malignancy. Extracellular matrix protease activity is often tightly regulated by specific localization, autoinhibition, and tissue-secreted inhibitors. To overcome this strict control and unleash proteolytic activity on the basement membrane and interstitial extracellular matrix, cancerous cells employ a variety of strategies. Extracellular proteases can produce a wide variety of bioactive cleaved peptides in addition to promoting tumor invasion. These goods have the ability to control tumor angiogenesis, cancer cell survival and proliferation, and migration. Complicating matters, some matrix metalloproteinases' (MMPs) pleiotropic activities may actually inhibit tumor growth. The significant joint abnormalities that MMP inhibitors generated in clinical trials, which have thus far prevented the effective use of these drugs in anticancer therapy, are evidence of the physiological importance of MMPs (Gupta et al., 2006).

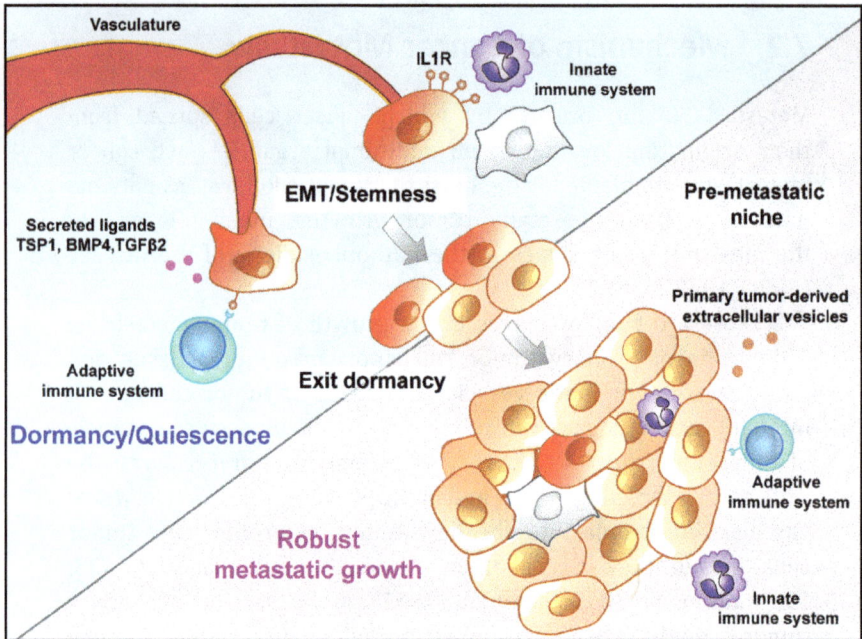

Figure 7.1 Mechanism of initiation and progression of events that promote tumor metastasis (San Juan et al., 2019).

7.3 Preclinical Studies of Spices for Cancer Metastasis

It investigated the phytochemical analysis of 31 spices and the traditional usage of 46 spices. According to the study's findings, curcumin is one of the bioactive that has been studied the most in terms of *in vitro*, *in vivo*, clinical, and SAR anticancer studies, while other bioactives like 1,8-cineole, trans-anethole, diosgenin, and trigonelline have been studied the least or not at all for these purposes (Singh et al., 2022). It was reported that the dietary chemopreventive agent thymoquinone (TQ), found in black seed, is promising (Fig. 7.2). The study considered the effects of thymoquinone (TQ) on HCT-116 human colon cancer cells and found that TQ slows colon cancer cell growth, which is associated with cell cycle G1 phase arrest (Gali-Muhtasib et al., 2004). The anticancer activity of the various *Cinnamomum tamala* extracts was examined in a mouse tumor model produced by fibrosarcoma. The most effective anticancer agent among the several extracts was found in the petroleum ether fraction of the methanol extract (Fig. 7.2). Despite the inhibition of topoisomerase-I enzyme activity, the fraction has dramatically slowed down tumor development and proliferation (Thanekar et al., 2016).

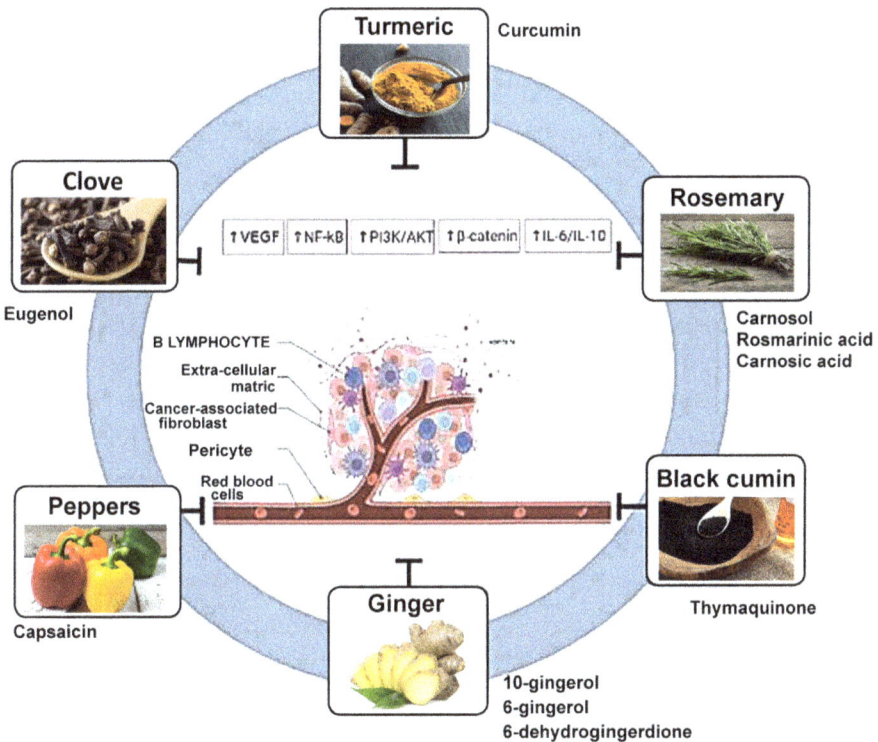

Figure 7.2 Anti-cancerous mechanisms of various spices and their bioactives (Talib et al., 2022).

Capsaicin, one of the main components of red pepper, was tested *in vitro* against three ATL cell lines. Treatment with capsaicin slowed the proliferation of ATL cells in a way that depended on the dose and the passage of time. Apoptosis and cell cycle arrest were principally responsible for the inhibitory effect (Fig. 7.2) (Zhang et al., 2003).

Ginger's aqueous extract was tested on albino Wistar rats that had gastric cancer brought on by N-nitroso N-methyl urea (MNU) (Fig. 7.2). By dramatically reducing the pathogenic alterations brought on by inflammation and oxidative stress, extract supplementation has finally stopped the growth of the tumor (Mansingh et al., 2020). It was investigated how triple-negative breast cancer (TNBC) cells invade and spread in the presence of curcumin. By using the transwell assay, colony formation, and wound healing, the effect of curcumin on TNBC cells was discovered. The study's findings demonstrated that curcumin prevented TNBC cells from proliferating, invading, migrating, and forming mammospheres (Li et al., 2022).

7.4 Clinical Trials

In a previous study, it was investigated the viability and acceptability of docetaxel and curcumin together in 14 people who had metastatic breast cancer succumbed to it during the phase 1 trial. Curcumin was ingested starting at 500 mg and increased until a hazardous level was reached (Bayet-Robert et al., 2010). Only 8 patients out of 14 had quantifiable lesions, according to the RECIST (Response Evaluation Criteria in Solid Tumors) data. Most patients showed signs of improvement. On the side effects of platinum-based adjuvant treatment for ovarian cancer, ginger's impact was examined (Bayet-Robert et al., 2010). A total of 49 participants participated in the trial and received 2 gm of ginger pills. Results showed that ginger medication considerably lowered the harmful effects of chemotherapy and significantly reduced the number of illnesses. These actions have been linked to gingerol and shogaol, which can now be further researched for their potential to prevent cancer (Shokri et al., 2017).

7.5   Safety and Bioavailability

The term "bio-safety of spices" describes the defense of living things against the toxins emitted by spices. Since spices and their bioactives are generally regarded as harmless, they are frequently used in the proper quantities to prepare a variety of cuisines. They function in a dose-dependent way (Singh et al., 2022). For instance, the National Cancer Institute has classified curcuminoids as generally recognized as safe (GRAS). Up to 12 g of curcumin per day is often safe with only moderate side effects. The number of micronutrients and phytocompounds that are absorbed, delivered to their target organs/tissues, where they are metabolized, and then eliminated is known as bioavailability. However, because it would require *in vivo* testing, it is not practical to calculate the predicted amount of physiologically accessible phytochemicals in people (Gupta et al., 2017).

7.6   Conclusion

Spices are well known for exerting various pharmacological actions in which anti-cancerous activity is the most studied one. Curcumin and thymoquinone are two good examples of spices for which most of the research about their anti-cancerous activities has already gained fame. Several spices showed anti-tumorigenic activities under *in vitro* and *in vivo* studies by possessing anti-proliferative, anti-invasion, anti-metastatic, anti-angiogenic, cell cycle growth arrest, and apoptosis-promoting functions. Metastasis is the main hallmark of cancer cells and the prevention of this process can be done by using several spices to inhibit the tumor cells' progression and dissemination in distant tissues. In this chapter, we summarized the mechanism of tumor metastasis, pre-clinical and clinical studies of the anti-metastatic action of spices, and later on, the safety and biological availability of spices are discussed in brief. Despite gaining much popularity as an anti-cancer agent, bioactive components of spices are still not commercially available in the market as a potential anti-cancer drug. Therefore, to overcome this issue, numerous studies are needed to explore the protective effects, safety, bioavailability, pharmacodynamics, and pharmacokinetic profiles of these bioactive components by conducting pre-clinical and clinical studies.

References

Aggarwal, B. B., Kunnumakkara, A. B., Harikumar, K. B., Tharakan, S. T., Sung, B., & Anand, P. (2008). Potential of spice-derived phytochemicals for cancer prevention. *Planta medica*, 74(13), 1560–1569.

Bandyopadhyay, D. (2014). Farmer to pharmacist: Curcumin as an anti-invasive and antimetastatic agent for the treatment of cancer. *Frontiers in Chemistry*, 2, 113.

Bayet-Robert, M., Kwiatowski, F., Leheurteur, M., Gachon, F., Planchat, E., Abrial, C., ... & Chollet, P. (2010). Phase I dose escalation trial of docetaxel plus curcumin in patients with advanced and metastatic breast cancer. *Cancer Biology & Therapy*, 9(1), 8–14.

Deng, Y. I., Verron, E., & Rohanizadeh, R. (2016). Molecular mechanisms of anti-metastatic activity of curcumin. *Anticancer Research*, 36(11), 5639–5647.

Fidler, I. J. (1975). Mechanisms of cancer invasion and metastasis. In *Biology of Tumors: Surfaces, Immunology, and Comparative Pathology*, pp. 101–131. Boston, MA: Springer US.

Gali-Muhtasib, H., Diab-Assaf, M., Boltze, C., Al-Hmaira, J., Hartig, R., Roessner, A., & Schneider-Stock, R. (2004). Thymoquinone extracted from black seed triggers apoptotic cell death in human colorectal cancer cells via a p53-dependent mechanism. *International journal of oncology*, 25(4), 857–866.

Gupta, A. P., Khan, S., Manzoor, M. M., Yadav, A. K., Sharma, G., Anand, R., & Gupta, S. (2017). Anticancer curcumin: natural analogues and structure-activity relationship. *Studies in Natural Products Chemistry*, 54, 355–401.

Gupta, G. P., & Massagué, J. (2006). Cancer metastasis: Building a framework. *Cell*, 127(4), 679–695.

Joshi, H., Kumar, G., Tuli, H. S., & Mittal, S. (2022). Inhibition of cancer cell metastasis by nanotherapeutics: Current achievements and future trends. In *Nanotherapeutics in Cancer*, pp. 161–209. Jenny Stanford Publishing.

Li, M., Guo, T., Lin, J., Huang, X., Ke, Q., Wu, Y., & Hu, C. (2022). Curcumin inhibits the invasion and metastasis of triple negative breast cancer via Hedgehog/Gli1 signaling pathway. *Journal of Ethnopharmacology*, 283, 114689.

Mansingh, D. P., Pradhan, S., Biswas, D., Barathidasan, R., & Vasanthi, H. R. (2020). Palliative role of aqueous ginger extract on N-nitroso-N-methylurea-induced gastric cancer. *Nutrition and Cancer*, 72(1), 157–169.

R Vasanthi, H., & P Parameswari, R. (2010). Indian spices for healthy heart-an overview. *Current Cardiology Reviews*, 6(4), 274–279.

San Juan, B. P., Garcia-Leon, M. J., Rangel, L., Goetz, J. G., & Chaffer, C. L. (2019). The complexities of metastasis. *Cancers*, 11(10), 1575.

Saraswathi, K., Arumugam, P., & Sivaraj, C. (2020). Pharmacological activities of differential parts of selected Essential Indian Spices. *Journal of Pharmacognosy and Phytochemistry*, 9(2), 2024–2033.

Shokri, F., Gharebaghi, P. M., Esfahani, A., Sayyah-Melli, M., Shobeiri, M. J., Ouladsahebmadarek, E., & Ghojazadeh, M. (2017). Comparison of the complications of platinum-based adjuvant chemotherapy with and without ginger in a pilot study on ovarian cancer patients. *Int J Womens Health Reprod Sci*, 5(4), 324–31.

Singh, N., & Yadav, S. S. (2022). Ethnomedicinal uses of Indian spices used for cancer treatment: A treatise on structure-activity relationship and signaling pathways. *Current Research in Food Science*.

Srinivasan, K. (2017). Antimutagenic and cancer preventive potential of culinary spices and their bioactive compounds. *Pharma Nutrition*, 5(3), 89–102.

Suhail, Y., Cain, M. P., Vanaja, K., Kurywchak, P. A., Levchenko, A., & Kalluri, R. (2019). Systems biology of cancer metastasis. *Cell Systems*, 9(2), 109–127.

Talib, W. H., AlHur, M. J., Al Naimat, S., Ahmad, R. E., Al-Yasari, A. H., Al-Dalaeen, A., ... & Mahmod, A. I. (2022). Anticancer effect of spices used in Mediterranean diet: Preventive and therapeutic potentials. *Frontiers in Nutrition*, 9, 905658.

Thanekar, D., Dhodi, J., Gawali, N., Raju, A., Deshpande, P., Degani, M., & Juvekar, A. (2016). Evaluation of antitumor and anti-angiogenic activity of bioactive compounds from Cinnamomum tamala: *In vitro*, *in vivo* and in silico approach. *South African Journal of Botany*, 104, 6–14.

Zeidman, I. (1957). Metastasis: A review of recent advances. *Cancer Research*, 17(3), 157–162.

Zhang, J., Nagasaki, M., Tanaka, Y., & Morikawa, S. (2003). Capsaicin inhibits growth of adult T-cell leukemia cells. *Leukemia Research*, 27(3), 275–283.

Chapter 8

Anti-Inflammatory and Antioxidant Potential of Spices, with a Special Focus on Cancer Management – Recent Insights

Dhruv Sanjay Gupta,[a] **Rahul Dinkar Shingte,**[a] **Daksh Sanjay Gupta,**[b] **Meena Chintamaneni,**[a] **Ginpreet Kaur,**[a] and **Hardeep Singh Tuli**[c]

[a]*Department of Pharmacology,*
Shobhaben Pratapbhai Patel School of Pharmacy and Technology Management,
SVKM'S NMIMS, Vile Parle-West, Mumbai, India
[b]*Vivekanand Education Society's College of Pharmacy,*
Chembur, Mumbai, Maharashtra, India
[c]*Department of Biosciences and Technology,*
Maharishi Markandeshwar (Deemed to be University), Mullana, Ambala, India

ginpreet.aneja@gmail.com

8.1 Introduction

Cancer is amongst the known severe progressive metabolic syndromes and is one of the leading causes of mortality and morbidity around the globe. Regardless of advancements in clinical diagnosis and prognosis, treatment, and prevention, due to its heterogeneous and complex nature, the lethality of cancer

Anticancer Spices: Dietary Input to Health
Edited by Hardeep Singh Tuli
Copyright © 2025 Jenny Stanford Publishing Pte. Ltd.
ISBN 978-981-5129-28-1 (Hardcover), 978-1-003-53466-2 (eBook)
www.jennystanford.com

persists. According to the WHO, in 2021, an estimated population of 20 million people were diagnosed with cancer and approximately 10 million cancer-related deaths were recorded (Sung et al., 2021). The complicated interwoven pathogenesis that develops at genetic, phenotypic, and pathological levels causes uncontrolled and sustained proliferation of cells producing genetic alterations and mutations within cells resulting in the normal cell transforming into a malignant cell (Hausman, 2019). Additionally, not only its ability to develop resistance against conventional cancer treatments but also its capability to reoccur once treated has made cancer a major health menace in both developing and developed nations (Cui et al., 2018). Over the years, many efforts have been made to develop strategies for the treatment of tumors that involve surgical removal of the tumor, chemotherapy and its combination with radiation therapy, immunotherapy, phototherapy, stem cell transformation, and so on (Chu et al., 2020). These treatments are usually accompanied by fatal side effects and therapeutic inefficiencies, which include compromised bioavailability, high toxicity due to nonspecific action, rapid metabolism, and limitation of use in metastasis (S. Gupta & Shukla, 2022).

The challenge of diminishing the harmful adverse effects of cancer treatments is approached by using a more drug-targeted method facilitating improved drug efficacy and bioavailability. However, the intrinsic properties of cancer stem cells (CSCs) to auto-renew and self-differentiate leads to multiple drug resistance (MDR), and consequently the failure in therapy causes metastasis and reoccurrence of cancer (Bukowski et al., 2020). Along with CSCs, chemoresistance can also occur due to epithelial-to-mesenchymal transition (EMT), ABC transporter-mediated drug efflux, exocytosis of drug-loaded lysosomes, stimulation of DNA damage response proteins, cell signaling pathway deregulations, and epigenetic alterations (Sun et al., 2023). Therefore, developing a novel therapeutic strategy that is more targeted, controlled, and personalized is crucial. This has led to the exploration of plant-based therapeutic strategies. One such example of synergizing phytochemicals along with targeted and controlled CSC-focused nano-therapy is the combination of anti-CD123-curcumin NPs.

In comparison to curcumin NPs, the conjugated CD123 antibody along with curcumin accelerated cellar uptake and stimulated programmed cell death in the KG-1a cell line isolated from the bone marrow of human acute myelogenous leukemia indicating the prominent cytotoxic effect of anti-CD123-curcumin NPs toward re-sensitizing leukemic-CSCs and inhibiting their self-renewal property (Nirachonkul et al., 2021).

Plant-based foods and constituents are a rich source of phytochemicals that have numerous antitumor properties such as promoting apoptosis, inhibiting angiogenesis and cellular migration, reducing inflammation, and neutralizing oxidative stress (Ranjan et al., 2019). However, the therapeutic efficacy of these agents is compromised due to their high hydrophobicity, limited bioavailability, and requirement of high doses (Choudhari et al., 2020). Therefore, encapsulating these phytochemicals into nanocarriers can improve their bioavailability and be an effective drug delivery strategy in malignancy management. One such plant-based ingredient that has widely been used by mankind since early civilization is spices and herbs (Zheng et al., 2016). These fragrant and flavored condiments form the basis of the most popular culinary cuisines. During ancient times, traders would voyage around the world to find lands that produced these pungent plants. It was believed that the ancient Egyptian, Christian, and Islamic communities grew these herbs and spices for their association with temples and daily rituals (Metwaly et al., 2021). During the late 14th century, a Portuguese sailor, Vasco da Gama traveled across India looking for jewels and returned with ginger, pepper, cinnamon, and jewels. Moreover, cinnamon is reported to be one of the oldest spices of the ancient Roman and Greek eras (Ribeiro-Santos et al., 2017). Today, Asia is the biggest contributor to producing of variety of spices and herbs, and the USA is one of the major buyers of these condiments followed by Germany, Japan, and France (Akaberi et al., 2021). The ease of availability and potency of these natural phytochemicals in spices and herbs have made them a useful resource for investigating treatment strategies for various ailments.

8.2 Pathogenesis of Cancer and Intervention Strategies: Key Molecular Markers and Targets

The lethal cascade of carcinogenesis involves several events that eventually lead to sustained molecular malfunction. These events involve cellular transformation, over-proliferation, invasion, angiogenesis, and metastasis, and eventually leading to multi-organ failure (Sarian et al., 2017). The transcription factor, nuclear factor kappa (NF-κB) is one of the significant genes that mediate these processes along with inflammatory chemokines, tumor-promoting proteins, and carcinogens (Xia et al., 2014). Therefore, agents that can inhibit NF-κB are investigated in suppressing tumorigenesis. One of the contributors to cancer pathogenesis is over production of reactive oxidative species (ROS) in the cells altering the tumor microenvironment and stimulating angiogenesis, metastasis, and survival of cancer cells (Liou & Storz, 2010). Additionally, carcinogens, inflammatory mediators, and tumor-promoting proteins induce activation of NF-κB through phosphorylation and ubiquitination that leads to its translocation to the nucleus, thus binding to the DNA. Further, gene products from certain protein expressions regulated by NF-κB contribute to the progression of cancer (J. Chen & Chen, 2013). Another family of transcription factors, STAT (signal transducer and activator of transcription) is known to regulate genetic expressions producing proteins that are involved in cell proliferation, chemoresistance, angiogenesis, and cell survival (Loh et al., 2019). Amongst all seven members, STAT-3 has proven to play a pivotal role in cancer initiation, progression, and metastasis. Gene diagnostical data reveals that unusual phosphorylation of STAT-3 is seen amongst 70% of cancers, mainly non-small cell lung cancer (NSCLC) and breast cancer (Mohrherr et al., 2020). Several studies comparing neoplastic and healthy tissues revealed higher STAT-3 expression in cancerous cells, and hence STAT-3 is considered one of the oncogenic markers in various cancer models. Another common clinical finding among cancer patients is chronic inflammation. It is also known to be one of the major mediators of tumor pathogenesis, also, interestingly all the prominent mediators involved in chronic inflammation are regulated by transcription factors, NF-κB, signal transducer, and activator of transcription-3 (STAT3). The activity of curcumin in inhibiting IL-6-induced activation of STAT-3 and its nuclear translocation was reported in human multiple myeloma cells (Abadi et al., 2022).

The bioactive constituents and their analogs extracted from the dietary spices and herbs have been studied for their anti-neoplastic properties for decades and are currently being tested for their potential in conjugation with chemotherapy in tumor treatment. These constituents are mainly found in higher concentrations in different parts of the plant, e.g., seeds, roots, bark, rhizomes, leaves, flowers, sprouts, fruits, and stems, and show varied pharmacological activities (Choudhari et al., 2020). Several naturally occurring products from spices such as alkaloids, carotenoids, taxanes, terpenoids, lignans, saponins, gums, oils, flavonoids, and biomolecules and their metabolites have proven to play a significant role in anticancer treatment (Iqbal et al., 2017). Numerous preclinical and clinical studies justify the anti-neoplastic potential of phytochemicals alone or in combination with other treatments in the prevention and therapy of not only cancer but also infectious, metabolic, cardiovascular, inflammatory, autoimmune, and neurodegenerative diseases (Islam et al., 2016). The potential of these phytoconstituents extracted from spices as potent anticancer agents has been revealed through promising results reported from preclinical testing. Overall, these biomolecular agents perform their function by either of these mechanisms as outlined in Fig. 8.1; by inhibiting the proteins and enzymes involved in downstream signaling pathways that upregulate the cancer cell proliferation [Cdc2, CDK2 and CDK4 kinases, topoisomerase enzyme, COX-1 (Cyclooxygenase) and COX-2, Bcl-2, cytokines, PI3K, Akt, MAPK/ERK, MMP, TNK, mechanistic target of rapamycin (mTOR)], or by mutation of DNA repair activation proteins (p21, p27, and p53 genes and Bax, Bid, and Bak proteins), or through accelerating the apoptosis by activation of programmed cell death enzymatic cascade (Caspase-3, 7, 8, 9, 10, 12), or by activating the oxidative stress neutralizing enzymes (GSH, GHT, and GPxn) (Michalkova et al., 2021; Pratheeshkumar et al., 2012).

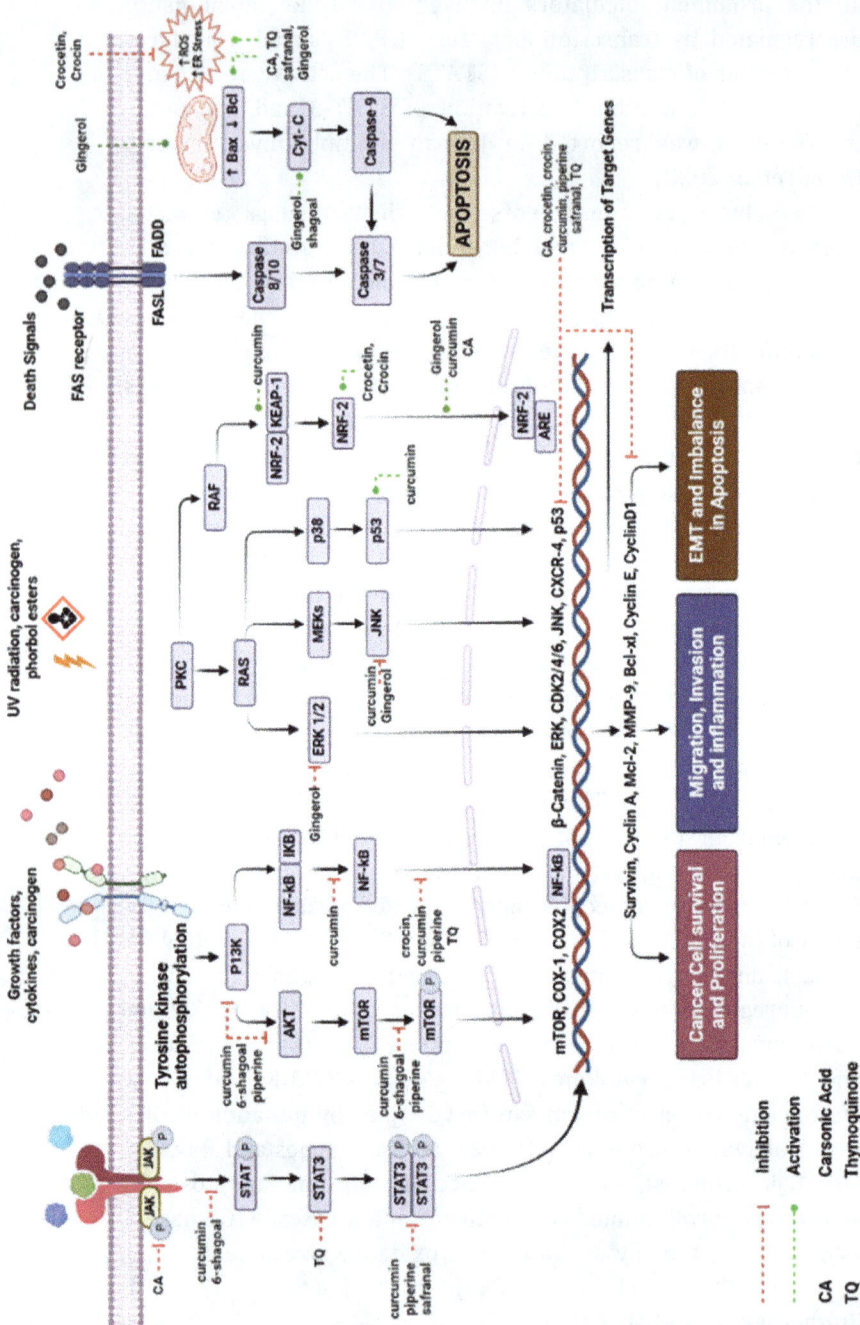

Figure 8.1 General molecular pathogenesis of cancer and molecular targets underlying anticancer potential of spice and herb-derived phytochemicals.

Curcumin, a polyphenolic ingredient obtained from *Curcuma longa L.* is widely known for its antioxidant, anti-inflammatory, and anticancer uses. The anticancer effect of curcumin is studied in preclinical models with breast, lung, colorectal, gastric, lymphoma, multiple myeloma, brain, AML, and bone cancer (Giordano & Tommonaro, 2019). Several clinical studies have demonstrated the impact of curcumin on the treatment of breast cancer. The pathogenesis of breast cancer reveals the role of survival signaling molecules, such as NF-κB, P13K/Akt, and STATs in cancer cell proliferation and curcumin has been reported to inhibit their expression (Wong et al., 2021). This curcumin-mediated inhibition further leads to the silencing of downstream signaling pathways eventually causing downregulation of inflammatory cytokine expression (CXC1 and CXCL2 and controlling the expression of matrix metalloproteinase 9 (MMP-9), urokinase plasminogen activator (uPA), uPA receptor (uPAR), intracellular adhesion molecule 1 (ICAM-1), β-Catenin, and chemokine receptor 4 (CXCR4) (Sakai et al., 2016). The anti-proliferative effect of curcumin studied on breast cancer models reported its anticancer action by inhibiting JAK2/STAT3, NF-κB, PI3K/Akt, mTOR pathway, reducing EMT and further downregulating expression of cyclin D1, and cyclin E, meanwhile inducing tumor-suppressing protein's expressions such as p21, p27, and p53, thereby inhibiting breast cancer stem cells (Hao et al., 2023).

Another phenolic constituent obtained from ginger (*Zingiber officinale* Roscoe), [6]-gingerol is shown to possess tumor-suppressing activity (Prasad & Tyagi, 2015). In human colon cancer cell lines, gingerol inhibited JNK, ERK ½, and p38 downstream signaling pathways, thus blocking the expression of cell survival target genes (Radhakrishnan et al., 2014). The chemopreventive action of gingerol is further enhanced by targeting NRF2 and NF-κB pathways to overcome inflammation and oxidative stress (Schadich et al., 2016). Another phenolic component obtained from ginger, 6-shogoal tested in lung cancer cell line shows its inhibitory effect on mTOR, STAT, and Akt signaling cascade (M. O. Kim et al., 2014). Gingerols and shogoals have also been reported for their pro-apoptotic activity by mediating the outer mitochondrial layer and stimulating the cytochrome-c release resulting in apoptosis induction.

Recent preclinical studies revealed the property of thymoquinone (TQ), a monoterpene obtained from black cumin (*Nigella sativa*) seed oil in reducing tumor weight and size by accelerating apoptotic pathways and inhibiting STAT activation in human gastric cancer cells (Banerjee et al., 2010). Additionally, studies have reported the usefulness of thymoquinone in adjuvant therapy with other cancer-suppressing agents. TQ suppresses cancer cell growth and viability by interfering in MAPK/ERK signaling pathways and neutralizing oxidative stress (Yu & Kim, 2015). The inhibitory action of TQ on various transcription factors like NF-κB and STAT3 further silences the downstream pathways that express several inflammatory mediators, cytokines, pro-angiogenic proteins, and anti-apoptotic agents. The sustained and overactive STAT3 is a prominent finding in various malignancies, TQ exerts a suppressing effect on STAT3 phosphorylation thus downregulating the expression of cancer initiation (Cyclins, CDK4), survival (Survivin, Bcl-2), and migration (MMP-9) target genes (Pal et al., 2021).

Saffron, obtained from stigmas of *Crocus sativus* is an ancient spice and natural food colorant that has been used for centuries. It contains secondary metabolites such as crocins, crocetin, safranal, and picroocrocin. The color of saffron is due to the presence of crocin and crocetin, meanwhile, the odor and aroma are contributed by safranal (Escribano et al., 1996). These carotenoids have revealed various health benefits due to their neuroprotective, anti-inflammatory, antitumor, hepatoprotective, antioxidant, and cardioprotective actions. The chemoprotective action of crocin studied in thioacetamide-induced hepato-carcinogeneic rats primarily reduced the oxidative stress and expression of inflammatory mediators. Crocin enhanced the expression of Nrf2 and its translocation to the nucleus resulting in the generation of phase-2 antioxidant enzymes, thus diminishing oxidative moieties (Elsherbiny et al., 2020). Meanwhile, in the mice colorectal mucosa, crocin administration caused inhibition of NF-κB, thus decreasing the transcription of inflammatory genes, including COX-2, IL-1β, TNF-α, and iNOS (Ashktorab et al., 2019). The Nrf2 enhancing mechanism was consistently seen with both crocin and crocetin when administered in different cancer cell lines, including hepatocellular liver cell line (HepG2), adenocarcinoma ovarian cell epithelial cell line (Sk-ov-3), and adenocarcinoma cervical epithelial cancer cell line (HeLa). However, within HeLa cell lines, crocetin was observed to have higher Nrf2 activation and significantly induced ROS than crocin (Weiskirchen, 2022). Hence, revealing a higher cytotoxic nature of crocetin compared to crocin. Another widely consumed dietary phytochemical constituent that has shown promising anticancer activity in preclinical studies is piperine. Piperine, a nitro-alkaloid is extracted from dried fruit of black pepper (*Piper nigrum L.*) or long pepper (*Piper longum L.*) species (Park et al., 2012). The inhibitory impact of piperine on the growth of prostate cancer cells was seen due to its influence on activated-STAT3 and NF-κB expression (Samykutty et al., 2013).

Additionally, studies revealed that piperine influences cell migration by suppressing the expression of the p13K/Akt/mTOR pathway (Zeng & Yang, 2018). Piperine was found to significantly reduce the PMA-induced MMP-9 expression by blocking PKC-α/ERK ½ activity and subsequently also suppressing the NF-κB activity (Hwang et al., 2011). These clinical studies provide evidence of the potential of piperine as a powerful phytochemical in controlling cancer initiation and migration. Piperine has been investigated with other spice-derived constituents such as a combination of piperine and curcumin was evaluated using an *in vitro* breast cancer stem cell model, and the combination showed inhibitory effects on mammosphere generation, serial passaging, ALDH+, and activates caspase-3 further inducing apoptosis (Kakarala et al., 2010). A study on HER2-overexpressing breast cancer cells revealed that prior administration of piperine improved paclitaxel sensitivity toward the breast cancer cells (Do et al., 2013). Rosemary (*Rosmarinus officinalis L.*) leaves are widely incorporated in cuisines for their prominent flavor and aroma. Over the years, the pharmaceutical and medicinal abilities of rosemary extracts have been investigated. The primary phenolic diterpenes and triterpenes, which include carnosic acid, carnosol, rosmarinic acid, and rosmanol, extracted from this plant are widely studied *in vitro* and *in vivo* for their anticancer activity. Carnosic acid was reported to possess the property to neutralize reactive oxygen radicals (Xiang et al., 2013). Furthermore, *in vitro* studies performed on colon cancer cell lines revealed the anti-proliferative and anti-angiogenic properties of carnosic acid by inhibiting the JAK phosphorylation and induction of apoptotic proteins (Allegra et al., 2020; D.-H. Kim et al., 2016). The antioxidant properties of most of these rosemary extracts are elucidated in several research papers. Additionally, it stimulates antioxidant enzyme expression by stimulating the activation of Nrf-2 (Satoh et al., 2008).

All these findings suggest the chemopreventive and chemoprotective potential of phytochemicals in managing the cascade of cancer. This chapter further summarizes the detailed pieces of evidence on spice and herb-derived phytochemical antitumor activity and their incorporation with nanotechnology to strengthen their pharmacokinetic properties making them a safe, targeted, and controlled system of delivery in cancer management.

8.3   Exploration of Spices with Anticancer Benefits

This section aims to offer a complete overview of various spices of key interest, with significant chemopreventive benefits. For each of the spices discussed, the authors have aimed to provide a brief description of major sources, and actives present along with their benefits, and results from recent pre-clinical studies undertaken.

8.3.1   Turmeric (Curcumin)

Chiefly derived from the rhizome of the plant *Curcuma longa* (a member of the family *Zingiberaceae*), turmeric is an herb, which has several applications in medicine. It finds utility as an anti-inflammatory agent in alleviating colic, chest pains, and arthritis, and is used in the treatment of disorders of the gastrointestinal tract such as inflammation of the stomach lining and hyperacidity, and also acts as a potentially effective therapeutic agent against neurodegenerative diseases, microbial action, and jaundice. The principal curcuminoid of turmeric (curcumin) is chemically a beta-diketone comprising feruloyl groups and also comes under the category of a polyphenol, an aromatic ether, and a diarylheptanoid. Beta-phellandrene, p-cymene, terpinolene, cineole, and myrcene are among the frequently occurring monoterpenes present in turmeric (S. C. Gupta et al., 2013). By means of mechanisms such as DNA methylation, curcumin has shown remarkable epigenetic effects against cancerous cells. In the context of breast cancer cells, curcumin acts as a proapoptotic agent and has demonstrated its effects in preventing malignancy, as represented in *in vitro* and *in vivo* studies, where MCF-7 breast cancer cells showed a markedly increased curcumin uptake as compared to normal cells, accompanied by the inhibition of HDACs such as HDAC1 and HDAC2, in addition to the effects on the expression of miRNAs, both oncogenic and tumor suppressing, resulting in the inhibition of tumor formation and spread, and the prevalence of apoptosis. Clinical trials have shown that curcumin/docetaxel and curcumin/paclitaxel combinations led to a notable tumor reduction percentage as compared to a placebo (Fabianowska-Majewska et al., 2021).

Curcumin has also shown significant usefulness in its targeting of lung cancer cells, such as its ability to diminish the regulation of Bcl-XL, p53, egr-1, and c-myc, the cumulative effect of which is the inhibition of the growth of cells with damaged DNA, apoptosis inducement as well as the upregulation of cyclin-dependent kinase (CDK) inhibitors. The anti-inflammatory and anti-carcinogenic effects of curcumin may be attributed to its role in mitigating COX-2 and 5-LOX, along with the prevention of phosphorylation of cytosolic phospholipase A2. The proliferation of non-small-cell lung cancer cell lines A549 and NCI-H460 has been suppressed by curcumin, by its mediation of cell cycle arrest (Mehta et al., 2014). The condensation polymerization of curcumin yields poly-curcumin, which has shown antitumor effects against the SKOV3 and OVCAR3 ovarian cancer cell lines. Curcumin also enhances the efficacy of cisplatin, a widely used drug in the treatment of ovarian cancer, by bringing about an inhibition of the FA/BRCA pathway, which regulates DNA repair by homologous recombination. Diarylidenyl piperidones (DAPs), structural analogs of curcumin, have exhibited potent anticancer properties, and are notably more cytotoxic to cell lines of ovarian and colon cancer, as compared to other types (Terlikowska et al., 2014). Despite the benefits that it possesses, one of the major drawbacks of curcumin as a therapeutic agent is its low bioavailability, compounded by its chemical instability, high reactivity, and rapid metabolism. Owing to this, derivatives such as curcumin phospholipid complexes, turmeric oils, and curcumin nanoparticles (Lopresti, 2018) must be further investigated in clinical trials. Figure 8.2 showcases the chemical structure of curcumin, the primary active constituent of turmeric.

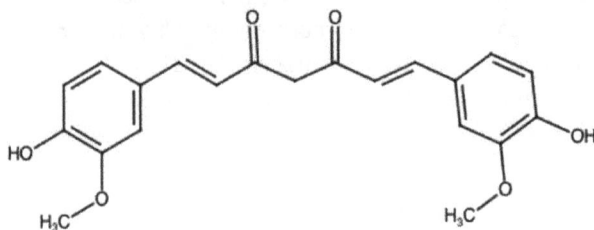

Figure 8.2 Chemical structure of curcumin.

8.3.2 Ginger (Gingerols and Shogaols)

Zingiber officinale Roscoe, commonly referred to as ginger, is a herbaceous perennial plant, the rhizome component of which has been used for its medicinal properties and as a spice for centuries. Ginger's phenolic constituents include gingerols, shogaols, and paradols, of which gingerols and shogaols are found to occur in higher proportions. Its terpene elements are zingiberene, α-curcumene, β-sesquiphellandrene, α-farnesene, and β-bisabolene, which form the primary components of essential oils of ginger (Prasad & Tyagi, 2015). It functions as a potent antioxidant, anti-diabetic, and anti-inflammatory agent. It has shown effects in decreasing serum lipid levels along with blood pressure, in conjunction with its role in suppressing adipogenesis and lipid accumulation. Its cytotoxicity, attributed to its ability to inhibit carcinogenic processes, has been explored in this explored in this section (Mao et al., 2019).

8.3.2.1 Gingerols

A study conducted by Lee et al. showed that the metastasis of MDA-MB-321, an invasive and poorly differentiated epithelial breast cancer cell line, is prevented by [6]-gingerol. This is owing to its role in preventing adhesion to the fibronectin, one of the essential components of the basement membrane. This can be further extrapolated to the role of [6]-gingerol in suppressing the expressions of MMP-2 and MMP-9 proteins, both of which play a role in cancer cell survival and angiogenesis (Lee et al., 2008). In a study by Kim et al., it was found that [6]-gingerol suppresses the expression of H460, A549, and H1299 lung adenocarcinoma cell lines, by bringing about cell membrane disruption along with diminution of cell volume. Furthermore, [6]-gingerol has been found to regulate the HIF-1α/HSP90 pathway, which results in inhibition of cancer cell migration in conditions of normoxia. In *in vivo* studies, [6]-gingerol also showed a reduction in Ki-67 protein levels, which are associated with severe prognosis in lung cancer patients (M. J. Kim et al., 2022). In ovarian cancer cells, [10]-gingerol has demonstrated the ability to arrest the cell cycle at the G2 phase, accompanied by a decrease in the expression of A, B1, and D3 cyclins, which are involved in the G2/M transition and cell cycle progression, as determined in a study by Rasmussen et al. Moreover, [10]-gingerol was found to exert an antitumor effect on 3 different ovarian cancer cell lines, namely, HEY, OVCAR3, and SKOV-3. Future clinical trials may involve the use of [10]-gingerol nanoparticles, in order to amplify its efficacy (Rasmussen et al., 2019). Figure 8.3 details the chemical structure of two widely studied gingerols, 10-gingerol (A) and 6-gingerol (B).

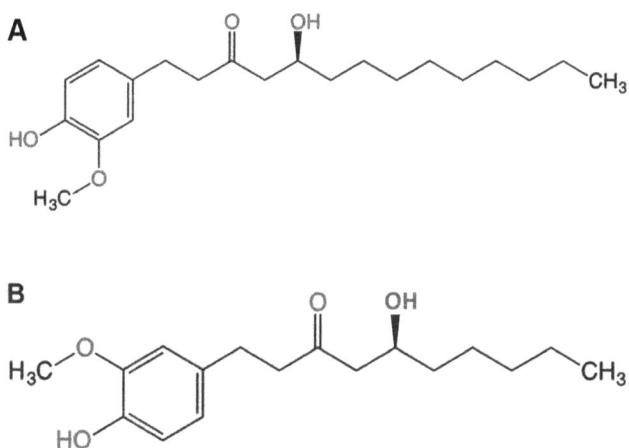

Figure 8.3 Chemical structure of 10-gingerol (A) and 6-gingerol (B).

8.3.2.2 Shogaols

In a study by Ray et al., in the breast cancer cell lines, MCF-7 and MDA-MB-231, [6]-shogaol was found to be effective in monolayer and spheroid culture environments, evident in the decreased levels of cancer stem cell markers-CD44[+]CD24[-]/[low]. It displayed much more efficacy than taxol, along with not exerting any harmful effects on non-cancerous cells (Ray et al., 2015). A study by Bawadood et al. showed that Cyclin D1 and HES1, involved in the notch signaling pathway of cancer cells, were both inhibited by [6]-shogaol (Bawadood et al., 2020). A study by Kim et al. showed that in non-small cell lung cancer, [6]-shogaol, having enhanced activity due to the presence of an α,β-unsaturated carbonyl moiety, was found to inhibit Akt kinase, the abnormal expression of which has been observed in lung cancer and is linked to higher rates of tumorigenesis. This may be attributed to [6]-shogaol's influence on caspase cleavage inducement and reduced STAT3 phosphorylation. [6]-shogaol was also found to reduce the levels of CCL2, a potent adenosine, which plays a role in cancer cell proliferation. Kim et al. conducted a study, wherein in ovarian cancer cell lines, A2780, Caov-3, and SK-OV-3, [6]-shogaol was shown to induce increased levels of lactate dehydrogenase toxicity and caspase-3 activity, both of which are hallmarks of apoptosis. Moreover, [6]-shogaol also regulates apoptosis by its influence on endoplasmic reticulum stress and corresponding Ca^{2+} release (T. W. Kim & Lee, 2023). Thus, [6]-shogaol is a competent candidate for a natural anticancer formulation. Figure 8.4 offers an overview of the chemical structure of 6-shogaol.

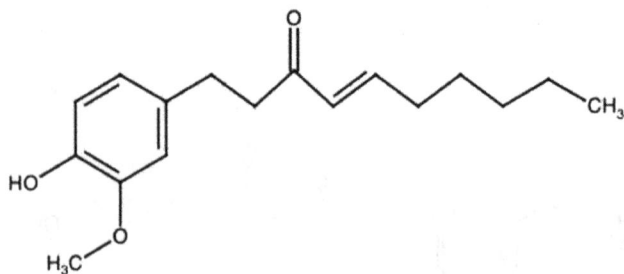

Figure 8.4 Chemical structure of 6-shogaol.

8.3.3   Pepper (Piperine)

Piper Nigrum L., referred to as black pepper in common terminology, is a perennial climbing vine belonging to the family *Piperaceae*, and has been in use as a spice, condiment, and medicinal herb. Rich in vitamins and flavonoids such as quercetin and myricetin, black pepper essential oils comprise β-caryophyllene, sabinene, β-phellandrene, and α-thujene as their major constituents (Ashokkumar et al., 2021).

The primary bioactive component of pepper is piperine, to which many of pepper's therapeutic properties are attributed. Among pepper's pharmacological benefits are its ability to function as an anticonvulsant, antidepressant, anti-allergic, and anti-inflammatory agent, along with its role in promoting CNS development and acting as a cardioprotective compound (Haq et al., 2021). In this section, the anticancer action of piperine has been depicted. In a study by Greenshields et al., it was reported that piperine exerts anticancer effects on HER2-overexpressing SKBR3, BT-474, T-47D, and MDA-MB-468 breast cancer cell lines, as well as MCF-7 cells in mammospheres. Its mechanism is interrelated to the intrinsic pathway of apoptosis, the effects of which are manifested as alteration of the mitochondrial membrane, cytochrome C release into the cytosol, and consequent caspase-9 activation by means of apoptosome formation (Greenshields et al., 2015). In a study by Lai et al., 4T1 mammary carcinoma cells were inhibited by piperine, along with bringing about diminished mRNA expression of MMP-9 and MMP-13, which play a significant role in the invasion and metastasis of breast cancer (Lai et al., 2012). In a study carried out by Lin et al., on the effects of piperine on lung cancer cells, two lung cancer cell lines – A549 and WI38 – were provided a regulated dose of piperine. The outcome of which there was no antitumor activity seen in the WI38 cells, there were significant ramifications seen in the A549 cells, delineated as apoptosis inducement and inhibition of the cell cycle (Lin et al., 2014).

In a murine study carried out on Swiss albino mice by Selvendiran et al., it was revealed that piperine has an antitumor effect on benzo[a]pyrene-induced lung cancer in mice, accompanied by diminished lipid peroxidation and elevated levels of enzymatic and non-enzymatic antioxidants (such as SOD, CAT, and GPx) (Selvendiran et al., 2003). In a study by Wojtowicz et al., involving ovarian cancer cell line W1, piperine was found to increase the sensitivity of drug-resistant cell lines to cytotoxic anticancer drugs such as topotecan and paclitaxel. At a concentration of IC50, piperine was found to suppress cell cycle progression. Furthermore, the normalization of PTPRK levels and decrease in phosphotyrosine levels, both of which reduce drug resistance in cancer cell lines, was attributed to piperine (Wojtowicz et al., 2021). In a study by Si et al., when A2780 ovarian cancer cell lines were exposed to piperine, inhibition of cancer cell proliferation was observed, in addition to bringing about apoptosis, evident via fragmentation of genetic material and condensation of chromatin, brought about via the increase in levels of caspase-3 and caspase-9, indicating the intrinsic apoptotic pathway. Further, piperine also caused apoptosis through the inhibition of the JNK/p38 MAPK signaling pathway, which has pro-tumorigenic functions such as metastasis and angiogenesis (Si et al., 2018). Thus, the alkaloid piperine finds application as a potent anticancer agent. Figure 8.5 depicts the chemical structure of piperine.

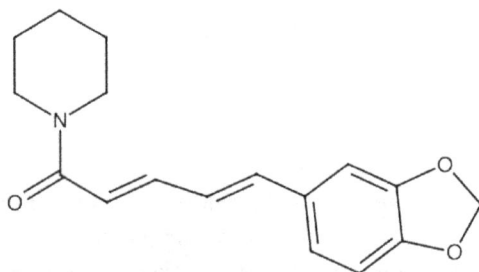

Figure 8.5 Chemical structure of piperine.

8.3.4 Saffron (Crocin, Crocetin and Safranal)

Commonly referred to as "red gold", saffron is derived from the dehydrated stigmas of *Crocus sativus L.*, and finds application as a plant-based medicament, a condiment as well as a coloring agent (Winterhalter & Straubinger, 2000). Composed primarily of flavonoids, monoterpenes, and carotenoids (Caballero-Ortega et al., 2004), the primary bioactive compounds of saffron are cis/trans crocin, crocetin, and safranal. In addition to these, picrocrocin, kaempferol, hydroxy-trimethyl-carboxaldehyde-cyclohexene, β-carotene, γ-carotene, lycopene, and zeaxanthin are also constituents of saffron (Maggi et al., 2020). Saffron's therapeutic action extends to cardiovascular diseases, Parkinson's disease, glaucoma, diabetic retinopathy, Alzheimer's disease, hypertension, and a host of other conditions. In this review, the anticancer effects of saffron's main bioactive constituents have been studied.

8.3.4.1 Crocin

8,8-diapocarotene-8,8-dioic acid, referred to as crocin, is a soluble carotenoid, which has proved to be a potent antitumor agent. In MCF-7 breast cancer cell lines, crocin (at 3.5 mg/ml concentration) was shown to act by stimulating an increased expression of caspase-7 and caspase-9 (involved in apoptotic cell detachment and activation of executioner caspases, respectively), along with tumor suppressors p53 and poly(ADP-ribose) polymerase inhibitors, all of which have a cumulative effect in aiding apoptosis and preventing cancerous cell proliferation (Hoshyar & Mollaei, 2017). In a study by Chen et al., involving A549 and SPC-A1 lung cancer cell lines, crocin was found to have a number of anticarcinogenic effects. Cytomorphological changes such as a change in the cellular refractive index, atrophy, and altered cell shape were observed. A gradual increase in the Bax/Bcl-2 ratio as well as p53 levels was noted, indicative of tumor suppressive characteristics. Furthermore, crocin was found to have synergism with cisplatin and pemetrexed in the treatment of lung cancer (S. Chen et al., 2015). In the case of ovarian cancer, crocin was found to reduce cell cycle progression in the A2780 ovarian cancer cell line, as well as its cisplatin-resistant variant, by means of reduced mRNA expression of MRP1 and MRP2. Moreover, crocin has also depicted inhibitory effects on HO-8910 ovarian cancer cell lines (Veisi et al., 2020).

8.3.4.2 Crocetin

The metabolic product of the carotenoid crocin, crocetin has demonstrated a potent antitumor ability. In a study carried out by Sajjadi et al., the efficacy of crocetin as well as crocin was evaluated in the treatment of N-methyl-N-nitrosourea (NMU)-induced breast cancer in female Wistar albino rats. While both crocin and crocetin were found to reduce tumor volume, latency period, tumor incidence, and mean tumor number at the tumor initiation and tumor promotion stages, crocetin was found to have higher efficacy than crocin due to easier gastrointestinal absorption as well as the lower concentration requirement of crocetin to form complexes with DNA (Bathaie & Sajjadi, 2017).

In lung cancer cell lines such as A549 and VA13, crocetin was found to inhibit the synthesis of nucleic acids as well as colony-forming units, at doses of 100–150 µg/mL (G. Gutheil et al., 2012). In a study carried out by Wang et al., to assess the cytotoxicity of derivatives of crocetin, it was found that in combination with ethylamine/4-Fluorbenzylamine, crocetin inhibited the expression of SKOV-3 ovarian cancer cell lines, with the conjugation enhancing the solubility and anti-inflammatory effects of crocetin (Wang et al., 2020). Thus, crocetin exhibits potential as an effective anticancer treatment option.

8.3.4.3 Safranal

Safranal, a constituent of saffron, is primarily responsible for its aromatic activity and also possesses anticancer benefits. In a study by Zarrineh et al., incorporating sialiomics and proteomics analysis, safranal was found to suppress the growth of MDA-MB-231 breast cancer cell lines (Zarrineh et al., 2022). In a study by Malaekeh-Nikouei et al., safranal was found to inhibit the growth of HeLa (malignant) and L929 (non-malignant) cancer cell lines by preventing an increase in cell size and cell volume. This effect can be further enhanced by the use of nano-liposomal safranal formulations (Malaekeh-Nikouei et al., 2013).

Used in conjunction with topoisomerase inhibitors such as topotecan (TPT), safranal can bring about the apoptosis of NSCLC A549 lung cancer cell lines, and this is advantageous as the administration of safranal before TPT inhibits the increase of TDP1 levels, reducing TPT-induced damage to non-cancerous cells, as determined in a study by Lozon et al. (Lozon et al., 2022). In a study by Ashrafian et al., Safranal was shown to regulate EGFR expression and bring about the expression of pro-apoptotic genes, which makes it an effective candidate as an anticarcinogenic agent (Ashrafian et al., 2022). Figure 8.6 represents the structure of safranal.

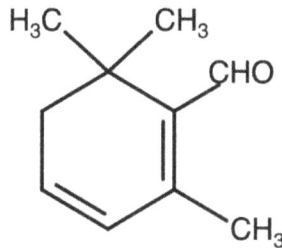

Figure 8.6 Chemical structure of safranal.

8.3.5 Black Cumin (Thymoquinone)

Nigella sativa, an annual flowering plant belonging to the family *Ranunculaceae*, yields seeds known commonly as black cumin, used as a spice and an herbal medicament. The predominant bioactive component of black cumin is thymoquinone (TQ), along with which are present nigellone, thymohydroquinone, carvacrol, and p-cymene. It is also a source of sodium, iron, magnesium, phosphorus, retinol, copper, and zinc (Srinivasan, 2018). Black cumin has numerous functions, manifested in its role as a hepatoprotective compound and an antimicrobial agent, and has established nephroprotective, gastroprotective, and analgesic properties (Khan, 1999).

In a murine study by Shanmugam et al., a mouse model induced with breast cancer was subjected to treatment with TQ, and the rate of osseous metastasis was markedly diminished. The expression of CXCR4, which plays a prominent role in cancer cell survival, was also decreased by the thymoquinone-mediated alteration of the NF-κB pathway, which prevents cancer cell proliferation (Shanmugam et al., 2018).

In another study by Alobaedi et al., TQ was used in conjunction with resveratrol, a polyphenolic stilbene that has demonstrated potent anticancer activity in numerous studies. The combination showed remarkable synergism, owing to an amalgamation of apoptotic effects of TQ and resveratrol, with TQ being involved in increasing the Bax/Bcl2 ratio, whereas the latter was found to alter the ERK1/2 MAP pathway. This was accompanied by a decrease in vascular endothelial growth factor levels and a consequent decrease in angiogenesis, along with increased IFN-γ levels, an important tumor suppressant. Additionally, low toxicity and economic feasibility make the TQ-RES combination an effective anticancer treatment option (Alobaedi et al., 2017).

In a separate study by Alhakamy et al., TQ-loaded soy-phospholipid-based phytosomes were formulated by means of a Box-Behnken design tool, and it was discovered that TQ-phytosomes have greatly improved efficiency as compared to TQ alone, against A549 lung cancer cell lines. This was supported by an increased rate of arrest of cancerous cells at the G0–G1 phase, a higher percentage of apoptotic inducement, nine times higher activation of caspase-3, and a greater rate of generation of reactive oxygen species, thus making phytosomal drug delivery an effective strategy to combat low bioavailability (Alhakamy et al., 2020). Alam et al. conducted a study wherein a synergism of thymoquinone and quercetin (a flavonol), significantly improved early apoptosis rates in NSCLS cells (Alam et al., 2022).

Ha et al., conducted a s study wherein the effects of TQ were determined in ovarian cancer cell lines, in a lysophosphatidic acid (LPA) rich tumor microenvironment. While TQ did not have any significant effects on cancer cell proliferation, it was found that it exhibited remarkable effects in inhibiting the basal as well as the LPA-induced metastasis of OVCAR8, SKOV3, and HeyA8 cell lines (Ha et al., 2020).

Folic acid-thymoquinone-chitosan nanoparticles, formulated in a study by İnce et al., showed significant cell membrane disruption in SKOV3 ovarian cancer cell lines. Moreover, selective targeting of cancer cells was undertaken, which is of great significance in cancer treatment approaches (Ýnce et al., 2020).

Future perspectives show nanobiotechnology as a competent tool to design anticancer agents, in conjunction with phytochemicals like thymoquinone.

8.4 Evidence from Pre-Clinical Studies

The preclinical data obtained from in silico and *in vitro* studies, as well as animal models, necessitates a detailed investigation of the beneficial role of spices as therapeutic agents in the prevention and management of cancer. According to the preclinical studies outlined below, spices were seen to attenuate the risks associated with cancer through multiple mechanisms against oxidative stress and inflammation, and regulating the levels of key biomarkers. Table 8.1 offers an overview of data from the latest pre-clinical studies conducted to study the benefits of spices in the management of cancer.

8.5 Clinical Picture

Table 8.2 offers an encapsulation of recent clinical trials undertaken, to establish the efficacy and safety of the active constituents of the spices discussed in the preceding sections. The applications of these compounds range from antioxidant and anti-inflammatory benefits to the management of challenges and adverse effects associated with chemotherapy, such as nausea and depression. There have been surprisingly few studies that have sought to monitor the effects of dietary consumption of herbs and spices, despite the fact that interest in herbs and spices as therapeutic agents continues to grow exponentially. Although the consumption of spices varies largely across different geographies, this significant group of foodstuffs should not be overlooked, especially given the potential advantages they may have for human health (Haq et al., 2021). These studies warrant the need for a greater number of clinical trials in diverse populations, to obtain a better understanding of the pharmacological benefits of these agents.

Table 8.1 Key insights from recent pre-clinical studies

Compound	Molecular mechanism	Model used	Dose and duration	Outcome	Conclusion	Reference
Actives in ginger ($n = 6$)	Modulation of phosphatidylinositol 3-kinase (PI3K) signaling pathway, protection of healthy cells from free radical damage	In silico study using drug databases and docking software	—	Identification of key targets for cancer management, including proteins involved in apoptosis, such as TP53 and PI3Ks	Actives screened were seen to interact with a variety of biological targets, prompting the need for a greater number of in silico studies to evaluate various bioactives and uncover potential targets for cancer management	[Zhang et al., 2021]
6-gingerol	Cell cycle blockade, mitochondrial membrane damage, triggering of apoptosis, reduction of angiogenesis	Human gastric cancer cell line (AGS)	10–300 µM	Activation of caspase cascade, increased oxidative stress, leading to apoptosis	The metabolic processes brought about in the mitochondria may be explored as a potential target for compounds such as gingerol, chiefly due to the disruption of energy metabolism	[Mansingh et al., 2018]
Curcumin (sourced from turmeric root)	Suppression of cellular proliferation and migration, cytoprotective effects on healthy cells owing to the prevention of cellular invasion	Human colorectal cell lines	2.5–75 µM	Low IC50 values, potent action eliciting desired pharmacological effects at low doses	The potency of curcumin serves as a promising indicator of potential applications in the clinical management of aggressive cancers, including colorectal cancer	[Calibasi-Kocal et al., 2019]

Compound	Molecular mechanism	Model used	Dose and duration	Outcome	Conclusion	Reference
Curcumin	Modulation of mitochondrial membrane activity, decreased levels of proteins involved in autophagy (such as P62)	Female C57BL/6 mice	100 mg/kg/day, i.e., for 15 days	Inhibition of tumor growth and proliferation, induction of ferroptosis	Curcumin was observed to trigger ferroptosis by facilitating the onset of autophagy, indicating enhanced potential for its usage in lung cancer management	[Tang et al., 2021]
Piperine	Activation of apoptotic proteins, triggering of apoptosis, protection of healthy cells from toxicity of synthetic moieties	MCF-7 breast cancer cell line	20, 30 µM of piperine, in combination with cisplatin, over 24 hours	Exertion of a synergistic effect, activation of caspases (chiefly caspase-3 and 9), reduction of blockers of apoptosis such as Bcl-2	Administration of natural agents such as piperine, in combination with chemotherapeutic agents, may enhance their anticancer properties. In addition to this, there is a marked reduction in the toxic effects exerted by these agents, which, in turn, enhances the benefits of co-administration	[Fattah et al., 2021]

Table 8.2 Overview of recently undertaken clinical trials

Dose and duration	Volunteers	Design	Outcome	Conclusion	Reference
Capsules comprising turmeric, red clover, flax seed, and resveratrol (296.4 mg of phenolic/capsule, 3 capsules/day), over a week	26 patients with breast cancer	Randomized, controlled, clinical trial	Exertion of anti-proliferative effects, triggering of cell cycle arrest and apoptosis	Curcuminoids may have benefits as an adjunct therapy, in breast cancer management	(Ávila-Gálvez et al., 2021)
Curcumin (4 g/day), for a week leading up to radiotherapy	40 patients with stage IIB/IIIB cervical carcinoma	Randomized, placebo-controlled controlled, clinical trial	Marked reduction in the levels of survivin, thereby facilitating apoptosis	With a special focus on cervical cancer, curcumin may be harnessed to improve sensitization to radiotherapy, resulting in improved clinical outcomes	[Panahi et al., 2021)
Dietary consumption of spices, including cinnamon, turmeric, garlic, ginger, black pepper, and rosemary	125 patients with early-stage breast cancer	Randomized, controlled trial	Improved dietary adherence, consumption of anti-inflammatory foodstuffs, reduction in consumption of foods promoting inflammation	A combination of patient education and dietary interventions may be useful in the management of breast cancer. The consumption of spices widely used in Mediterranean diets may be a beneficial intervention	[Zuniga et al., 2019)
Ginger (1650 mg/day), for a period of 14 days	15 cancer patients (with varying diagnoses) with anorexia-cachexia syndrome (ACS)	Clinical trial	ACS may be responsible for limiting a variety of treatment options, and ginger supplementation was observed to be	Ginger may be employed in the modulation of gastric motility and may be used to manage adverse	[Bhargava et al., 2020)

Dose and duration	Volunteers	Design	Outcome	Conclusion	Reference
			linked with positive outcomes. Undertaking an electrogastrography in patients revealed improved myoelectric activity, along with reduced nausea	effects associated with chemotherapy, such as nausea	
Jollab (A saffron-based beverage), 60 mL/day for 28 days	75 patients with breast cancer	Randomized, controlled clinical trial	Marked reduction in fatigue over a four-week period	Saffron supplementation may result in improved health outcomes in cancer patients, chiefly due to a reduction in fatigue. This, in turn, results in an improved quality of life	[Mirzaei et al., 2022]
Crocin (active in Saffron), 30 mg/day, over 4 months	72 patients with breast cancer	Randomized, controlled clinical trial	Reduction in stress and anxiety, protection from the onset of depressive episodes, accompanied by a reduction in hypersensitivity and neurological disorders	Saffron may be explored as a promising alternative to synthetic molecules, for the management of anxiety and stress resulting from chemotherapy, and may be explored as an adjunct to conventional therapy	[Salek et al., 2021]
Curcumin (2 g/day) alongside a combination of folinic acid, 5-fluorouracil, and oxaliplatin (FOLFOX)	28 patients with metastatic colorectal cancer (CRC)	Open-labeled, randomized controlled clinical trial	Satisfactory safety and tolerability profile	Curcumin may be employed as an adjunct to synthetic molecules in the management of CRC, in order to improve the overall survival of patients	[Howells et al., 2019]

8.6 Marketed Formulations Comprising Spices as Principal Actives

As the concern with respect to the side effects of chemotherapy and long-term health outcomes continues to grow, there have been new possibilities emerging in the domain of therapeutic alternatives. The dietary supplement market is growing at an unprecedented rate, as it offers an attractive alternative to chemoprevention. Most of the formulations are available as tablets and capsules, comprising phytoconstituent extracts. Table 8.3 offers an overview of the composition of these products, the dose offered, as well as key indications and benefits. It is also interesting to note that several formulations offer a combination of two or more phytoconstituents, to bring about a synergistic action. This, in combination with interventions such as nanoencapsulation and controlled release, offers opportunities for targeted, site-specific delivery, and improved therapeutic outcomes. The authors have offered a perspective on these formulations as they are a cost-effective and accessible line of treatment.

8.7 Conclusion and Future Perspectives

The growing incidence of cancer in developed as well as developing nations is a cause for concern and has prompted the exploration of alternative therapeutic strategies. Spices, with established uses in traditional medicine and practices, have recently come to the forefront, owing to a wide variety of health benefits offered by their actives. Over the course of the chapter, the authors have aimed to highlight the pressing need for exploring adjunct therapeutic strategies, to combat challenges such as drug resistance, toxicity, and adverse effects. In addition to this, the pathogenesis of cancer was discussed, with a special focus on key molecular markers and potential targets for phytochemicals. Various spices such as curcumin, pepper, cumin, ginger, and saffron have been discussed in detail, to give readers an understanding of their key roles in the management of inflammation and oxidative stress. Any discussion with respect

Table 8.3 Composition of products, dose offered, as well as key indications and benefits

Composition	Product	Dose	Indication and key benefits
Turmeric (curcumin) + black pepper	Sandhu herbals	1500 mg (curcumin) + 10 mg (*Piper nigrum*)	Immune support, overall improvement in health, lowered inflammation
Ginger root extract	Nature's Truth ginger root supplement (quick-release capsules)	550 mg	Dietary support, lowered inflammation, improved gut health
Turmeric (curcumin) + black pepper	Innate vitality	1800 mg	Antioxidant and anti-inflammatory benefits
Ginger + curcumin	Gaia zingiber with curcumin liquid-filled capsules	Ginger root extract (60 mg) + turmeric root extract (25 mg)	Lowered inflammation and oxidative stress, overall health improvement, immunomodulation
Turmeric (curcumin)	Solgar turmeric root extract capsules	300 mg	Lowering of oxidative stress, improved health outcomes
Black ginger (*Kaempferia parviflora*) extract	Swanson black ginger extract capsules	100 mg	Improved circulation, enhanced bioavailability due to encapsulation, reduction in inflammation, and damaging effects of free radicals
Ginger + rosemary	New chapter Ginger Force capsules	Ginger (96 mg) + rosemary (5 mg)	Improved digestive health, reduction in inflammation, immune benefits
Saffron extract	Life extension-optimized saffron capsules	88.25 mg	Dietary supplements, lowered oxidative stress, immune support
Black cumin seed oil	Amazing herbs cumin seed oil soft-gel capsules	500 mg	Rich source of essential fatty acid, improved redox balance, reduction in inflammatory markers
Black cumin seed	Swanson black cumin seed capsules	400 mg	Immune health supports microbial balance

to novel therapeutic interventions would remain incomplete without evidence from pre-clinical and clinical studies, and an attempt has been made to offer recent updates from such studies. However, the widespread usage and clinical translation of these actives from a clinical perspective remains limited, owing to a number of drawbacks. Some of these include poor stability and aqueous solubility, limiting systemic bioavailability. Various research efforts have attempted to address this gap by employing novel drug delivery systems, including but not limited to nanoparticles, microspheres, and micellar delivery. There exists a need for standardization of these platforms, in order to minimize the possibility of variability and ensure largely uniform therapeutic benefits with a satisfactory safety profile. Moving forward, the authors believe that a greater number of clinical trials would aid the assessment of newer actives, and strengthen our understanding of compounds with established pharmacological benefits. The domain of spices in disease management continues to offer exciting opportunities for research, and tapping into it would entail economic benefits, improved quality of life of patients, and a significant reduction in disease burden, all of which are pressing needs that must be met.

References

Abadi, A. J., Mirzaei, S., Mahabady, M. K., Hashemi, F., Zabolian, A., Hashemi, F., Raee, P., Aghamiri, S., Ashrafizadeh, M., Aref, A. R., Hamblin, M. R., Hushmandi, K., Zarrabi, A., & Sethi, G. (2022). Curcumin and its derivatives in cancer therapy: Potentiating antitumor activity of cisplatin and reducing side effects. *Phytotherapy Research: PTR*, *36*(1), 189–213. https://doi.org/10.1002/ptr.7305.

Akaberi, M., Sahebkar, A., & Emami, S. A. (2021). Turmeric and Curcumin: From Traditional to Modern Medicine. In P. C. Guest (Ed.), *Studies on Biomarkers and New Targets in Aging Research in Iran* (Vol. 1291, pp. 15–39). Springer International Publishing. https://doi.org/10.1007/978-3-030-56153-6_2.

Alam, S., Mohammad, T., Padder, R. A., Hassan, Md. I., & Husain, M. (2022). Thymoquinone and quercetin induce enhanced apoptosis in non-small cell lung cancer in combination through the Bax/Bcl2 cascade.

Journal of Cellular Biochemistry, 123(2), 259–274. https://doi. org/10.1002/jcb.30162.

Alhakamy, N. A., Badr-Eldin, S. M., A. Fahmy, U., Alruwaili, N. K., Awan, Z. A., Caruso, G., Alfaleh, M. A., Alaofi, A. L., Arif, F. O., Ahmed, O. A. A., & Alghaith, A. F. (2020). Thymoquinone-loaded soy-phospholipid-based phytosomes exhibit anticancer potential against human lung cancer cells. *Pharmaceutics, 12*(8), 761. https://doi.org/10.3390/ pharmaceutics12080761.

Allegra, A., Tonacci, A., Pioggia, G., Musolino, C., & Gangemi, S. (2020). Anticancer activity of *Rosmarinus officinalis L.*: Mechanisms of action and therapeutic potentials. *Nutrients, 12*(6), 1739. https://doi. org/10.3390/nu12061739.

Alobaedi, O. H., Talib, W. H., & Basheti, I. A. (2017). Antitumor effect of thymoquinone combined with resveratrol on mice transplanted with breast cancer. *Asian Pacific Journal of Tropical Medicine, 10*(4), 400–408. https://doi.org/10.1016/j.apjtm.2017.03.026.

Ashktorab, H., Soleimani, A., Singh, G., Amr, A., Tabtabaei, S., Latella, G., Stein, U., Akhondzadeh, S., Solanki, N., Gondré-Lewis, M. C., Habtezion, A., & Brim, H. (2019). Saffron: The golden spice with therapeutic properties on digestive diseases. *Nutrients, 11*(5), 943. https://doi. org/10.3390/nu11050943.

Ashokkumar, K., Murugan, M., Dhanya, M. K., Pandian, A., & Warkentin, T. D. (2021). Phytochemistry and therapeutic potential of black pepper [*Piper nigrum (L.)*] essential oil and piperine: A review. *Clinical Phytoscience, 7*(1), 52. https://doi.org/10.1186/s40816-021-00292-2.

Ashrafian, S., Zarrineh, M., Jensen, P., Nawrocki, A., Rezadoost, H., Ansari, A. M., Farahmand, L., Ghassempour, A., & Larsen, M. R. (2022). Quantitative phosphoproteomics and acetylomics of safranal anticancer effects in triple-negative breast cancer cells. *Journal of Proteome Research, 21*(11), 2566–2585. https://doi.org/10.1021/acs. jproteome.2c00168.

Ávila-Gálvez, M. Á., González-Sarrías, A., Martínez-Díaz, F., Abellán, B., Martínez-Torrano, A. J., Fernández-López, A. J., Giménez-Bastida, J. A., & Espín, J. C. (2021). Disposition of dietary polyphenols in breast cancer patients' tumors, and their associated anticancer activity: The particular case of curcumin. *Molecular Nutrition & Food Research, 65*(12), 2100163. https://doi.org/10.1002/mnfr.202100163.

Banerjee, S., Padhye, S., Azmi, A., Wang, Z., Philip, P. A., Kucuk, O., Sarkar, F. H., & Mohammad, R. M. (2010). Review on molecular and therapeutic potential of thymoquinone in cancer. *Nutrition and Cancer, 62*(7), 938–946. https://doi.org/10.1080/01635581.2010.5 09832.

Bathaie, S. Z., & Sajjadi, M. (2017). Comparative study on preventive effect of saffron carotenoids, crocin and crocetin, in NMU-induced breast cancer in rat. *Cell J (Yakhteh), 19*(1). https://doi.org/10.22074/cellj.2016.3901.

Bawadood, A. S., Al-Abbasi, F. A., Anwar, F., El-Halawany, A. M., & Al-Abd, A. M. (2020). 6-Shogaol suppresses the growth of breast cancer cells by inducing apoptosis and suppressing autophagy via targeting notch signaling pathway. *Biomedicine & Pharmacotherapy, 128*, 110302. https://doi.org/10.1016/j.biopha.2020.110302.

Bhargava, R., Chasen, M., Elten, M., & MacDonald, N. (2020). The effect of ginger (*Zingiber officinale* Roscoe) in patients with advanced cancer. *Supportive Care in Cancer, 28*(7), 3279–3286. https://doi.org/10.1007/s00520-019-05129-w.

Bukowski, K., Kciuk, M., & Kontek, R. (2020). Mechanisms of multidrug resistance in cancer chemotherapy. *International Journal of Molecular Sciences, 21*(9), 3233. https://doi.org/10.3390/ijms21093233.

Caballero-Ortega, H., Pereda-Miranda, R., Riverón-Negrete, L., Hernández, J. M., Medécigo-Ríos, M., Castillo-Villanueva, A., & Abdullaev, F. I. (2004). Chemical composition of saffron (Crocus sativus l.) from four countries. *Acta Horticulturae, 650*, 321–326. https://doi.org/10.17660/ActaHortic.2004.650.39.

Calibasi-Kocal, G., Pakdemirli, A., Bayrak, S., Ozupek, N. M., Sever, T., Basbinar, Y., Ellidokuz, H., & Yigitbasi, T. (2019). Curcumin effects on cell proliferation, angiogenesis and metastasis in colorectal cancer. *Journal of B.U.ON.: Official Journal of the Balkan Union of Oncology, 24*(4), 1482–1487.

Chen, J., & Chen, Z. J. (2013). Regulation of NF-κB by ubiquitination. *Current Opinion in Immunology, 25*(1), 4–12. https://doi.org/10.1016/j.coi.2012.12.005.

Chen, S., Zhao, S., Wang, X., Zhang, L., Jiang, E., Gu, Y., Shangguan, A. J., Zhao, H., Lv, T., & Yu, Z. (2015). Crocin inhibits cell proliferation and enhances cisplatin and pemetrexed chemosensitivity in lung cancer cells. *Translational Lung Cancer Research, 4*(6), 775–783. https://doi.org/10.3978/j.issn.2218-6751.2015.11.03.

Choudhari, A. S., Mandave, P. C., Deshpande, M., Ranjekar, P., & Prakash, O. (2020). Phytochemicals in cancer treatment: From preclinical studies to clinical practice. *Frontiers in Pharmacology*, *10*, 1614. https://doi.org/10.3389/fphar.2019.01614.

Chu, D.-T., Nguyen, T. T., Tien, N. L. B., Tran, D.-K., Jeong, J.-H., Anh, P. G., Thanh, V. V., Truong, D. T., & Dinh, T. C. (2020). Recent progress of stem cell therapy in cancer treatment: Molecular mechanisms and potential applications. *Cells*, *9*(3), 563. https://doi.org/10.3390/cells9030563.

Cui, Q., Wang, J.-Q., Assaraf, Y. G., Ren, L., Gupta, P., Wei, L., Ashby, C. R., Yang, D.-H., & Chen, Z.-S. (2018). Modulating ROS to overcome multidrug resistance in cancer. *Drug Resistance Updates*, *41*, 1–25. https://doi.org/10.1016/j.drup.2018.11.001.

Do, M. T., Kim, H. G., Choi, J. H., Khanal, T., Park, B. H., Tran, T. P., Jeong, T. C., & Jeong, H. G. (2013). Antitumor efficacy of piperine in the treatment of human HER2-overexpressing breast cancer cells. *Food Chemistry*, *141*(3), 2591–2599. https://doi.org/10.1016/j.foodchem.2013.04.125.

Elsherbiny, N. M., Eisa, N. H., El-Sherbiny, M., & Said, E. (2020). Chemo-preventive effect of crocin against experimentally-induced hepatocarcinogenesis via regulation of apoptotic and Nrf2 signaling pathways. *Environmental Toxicology and Pharmacology*, *80*, 103494. https://doi.org/10.1016/j.etap.2020.103494.

Escribano, J., Alonso, G.-L., Coca-Prados, M., & Fernández, J.-A. (1996). Crocin, safranal and picrocrocin from saffron (Crocus sativus L.) inhibit the growth of human cancer cells *in vitro*. *Cancer Letters*, *100*(1–2), 23–30. https://doi.org/10.1016/0304-3835(95)04067-6.

Fabianowska-Majewska, K., Kaufman-Szymczyk, A., Szymanska-Kolba, A., Jakubik, J., Majewski, G., & Lubecka, K. (2021). Curcumin from turmeric rhizome: A potential modulator of DNA methylation machinery in breast cancer inhibition. *Nutrients*, *13*(2), 332. https://doi.org/10.3390/nu13020332.

Fattah, A., Morovati, A., Niknam, Z., Mashouri, L., Asadi, A., Tvangar Rizi, S., Abbasi, M., Shakeri, F., & Abazari, O. (2021). The synergistic combination of cisplatin and piperine induces apoptosis in MCF-7 cell line. *Iranian Journal of Public Health*. https://doi.org/10.18502/ijph.v50i5.6121.

G. Gutheil, W., Reed, G., Ray, A., Anant, S., & Dhar, A. (2012). Crocetin: An agent derived from saffron for prevention and therapy for cancer. *Current Pharmaceutical Biotechnology*, *13*(1), 173–179. https://doi.org/10.2174/138920112798868566.

Giordano & Tommonaro. (2019). Curcumin and cancer. *Nutrients, 11*(10), 2376. https://doi.org/10.3390/nu11102376.

Greenshields, A. L., Doucette, C. D., Sutton, K. M., Madera, L., Annan, H., Yaffe, P. B., Knickle, A. F., Dong, Z., & Hoskin, D. W. (2015). Piperine inhibits the growth and motility of triple-negative breast cancer cells. *Cancer Letters, 357*(1), 129–140. https://doi.org/10.1016/j.canlet.2014.11.017.

Gupta, S. C., Sung, B., Kim, J. H., Prasad, S., Li, S., & Aggarwal, B. B. (2013). Multitargeting by turmeric, the golden spice: From kitchen to clinic. *Molecular Nutrition & Food Research, 57*(9), 1510–1528. https://doi.org/10.1002/mnfr.201100741.

Gupta, S., & Shukla, S. (2022). Limitations of immunotherapy in cancer. *Cureus.* https://doi.org/10.7759/cureus.30856.

Ha, J. H., Jayaraman, M., Radhakrishnan, R., Gomathinayagam, R., Yan, M., Song, Y. S., Isidoro, C., & Dhanasekaran, D. N. (2020). Differential effects of thymoquinone on lysophosphatidic acid-induced oncogenic pathways in ovarian cancer cells. *Journal of Traditional and Complementary Medicine, 10*(3), 207–216. https://doi.org/10.1016/j.jtcme.2020.04.001.

Hao, M., Chu, Y., Lei, J., Yao, Z., Wang, P., Chen, Z., Wang, K., Sang, X., Han, X., Wang, L., & Cao, G. (2023). Pharmacological mechanisms and clinical applications of curcumin: Update. *Aging and Disease, 14*(3), 716. https://doi.org/10.14336/AD.2022.1101.

Haq, I., Imran, M., Nadeem, M., Tufail, T., Gondal, T. A., & Mubarak, M. S. (2021). Piperine: A review of its biological effects. *Phytotherapy Research, 35*(2), 680–700. https://doi.org/10.1002/ptr.6855.

Hausman, D. M. (2019). What is cancer? *Perspectives in Biology and Medicine, 62*(4), 778–784. https://doi.org/10.1353/pbm.2019.0046.

Hoshyar, R., & Mollaei, H. (2017). A comprehensive review on anticancer mechanisms of the main carotenoid of saffron, crocin. *Journal of Pharmacy and Pharmacology, 69*(11), 1419–1427. https://doi.org/10.1111/jphp.12776.

Howells, L. M., Iwuji, C. O. O., Irving, G. R. B., Barber, S., Walter, H., Sidat, Z., Griffin-Teall, N., Singh, R., Foreman, N., Patel, S. R., Morgan, B., Steward, W. P., Gescher, A., Thomas, A. L., & Brown, K. (2019). Curcumin combined with FOLFOX chemotherapy is safe and tolerable in patients with metastatic colorectal cancer in a randomized phase IIa trial. *The Journal of Nutrition, 149*(7), 1133–1139. https://doi.org/10.1093/jn/nxz029.

Hwang, Y. P., Kim, H. G., Choi, J. H., Park, B. H., Jeong, M. H., Jeong, T. C., & Jeong, H. G. (2011). Acteoside inhibits PMA-induced matrix metalloproteinase-9 expression *via* CaMK/ERK- and JNK/NF-κB-dependent signaling. *Molecular Nutrition & Food Research*, *55*(S1), S103–S116. https://doi.org/10.1002/mnfr.201000336.

Ýnce, Ý., Yýldýrým, Y., Güler, G., Medine, E. Ý., Ballýca, G., Kuþdemir, B. C., & Göker, E. (2020). Synthesis and characterization of folic acid-chitosan nanoparticles loaded with thymoquinone to target ovarian cancer cells. *Journal of Radioanalytical and Nuclear Chemistry*, *324*(1), 71–85. https://doi.org/10.1007/s10967-020-07058-z.

Iqbal, J., Abbasi, B. A., Mahmood, T., Kanwal, S., Ali, B., Shah, S. A., & Khalil, A. T. (2017). Plant-derived anticancer agents: A green anticancer approach. *Asian Pacific Journal of Tropical Biomedicine*, *7*(12), 1129–1150. https://doi.org/10.1016/j.apjtb.2017.10.016.

Islam, Md. A., Alam, F., Solayman, Md., Khalil, Md. I., Kamal, M. A., & Gan, S. H. (2016). Dietary phytochemicals: Natural swords combating inflammation and oxidation-mediated degenerative diseases. *Oxidative Medicine and Cellular Longevity*, *2016*, 1–25. https://doi.org/10.1155/2016/5137431.

Kakarala, M., Brenner, D. E., Korkaya, H., Cheng, C., Tazi, K., Ginestier, C., Liu, S., Dontu, G., & Wicha, M. S. (2010). Targeting breast stem cells with the cancer preventive compounds curcumin and piperine. *Breast Cancer Research and Treatment*, *122*(3), 777–785. https://doi.org/10.1007/s10549-009-0612-x.

Khan, M. A. (1999). Chemical composition and medicinal properties of Nigella sativa Linn. *Inflammopharmacology*, *7*(1), 15–35. https://doi.org/10.1007/s10787-999-0023-y.

Kim, D.-H., Park, K.-W., Chae, I. G., Kundu, J., Kim, E.-H., Kundu, J. K., & Chun, K.-S. (2016). Carnosic acid inhibits STAT3 signaling and induces apoptosis through generation of ROS in human colon cancer HCT116 cells: Carnosic acid induces apoptosis in HCT116 cells. *Molecular Carcinogenesis*, *55*(6), 1096–1110. https://doi.org/10.1002/mc.22353.

Kim, M. J., Ku, J. M., Choi, Y.-J., Lee, S. Y., Hong, S. H., Kim, H. I., Shin, Y. C., & Ko, S.-G. (2022). Reduced HIF-1α stability induced by 6-gingerol inhibits lung cancer growth through the induction of cell death. *Molecules*, *27*(7), 2106. https://doi.org/10.3390/molecules27072106.

Kim, M. O., Lee, M.-H., Oi, N., Kim, S.-H., Bae, K. B., Huang, Z., Kim, D. J., Reddy, K., Lee, S.-Y., Park, S. J., Kim, J. Y., Xie, H., Kundu, J. K., Ryoo,

Z. Y., Bode, A. M., Surh, Y.-J., & Dong, Z. (2014). [6]-Shogaol inhibits growth and induces apoptosis of non-small cell lung cancer cells by directly regulating Akt1/2. *Carcinogenesis, 35*(3), 683–691. https://doi.org/10.1093/carcin/bgt365.

Kim, T. W., & Lee, H. G. (2023). 6-shogaol overcomes gefitinib resistance via ER stress in ovarian cancer cells. *International Journal of Molecular Sciences, 24*(3), 2639. https://doi.org/10.3390/ijms24032639.

Lai, L., Fu, Q., Liu, Y., Jiang, K., Guo, Q., Chen, Q., Yan, B., Wang, Q., & Shen, J. (2012). Piperine suppresses tumor growth and metastasis *in vitro* and *in vivo* in a 4T1 murine breast cancer model. *Acta Pharmacologica Sinica, 33*(4), 523–530. https://doi.org/10.1038/aps.2011.209.

Lee, H., Seo, E., Kang, N., & Kim, W. (2008). [6]-Gingerol inhibits metastasis of MDA-MB-231 human breast cancer cells. *The Journal of Nutritional Biochemistry, 19*(5), 313–319. https://doi.org/10.1016/j.jnutbio.2007.05.008.

Lin, Y., Xu, J., Liao, H., Li, L., & Pan, L. (2014). Piperine induces apoptosis of lung cancer A549 cells via p53-dependent mitochondrial signaling pathway. *Tumor Biology, 35*(4), 3305–3310. https://doi.org/10.1007/s13277-013-1433-4.

Liou, G.-Y., & Storz, P. (2010). Reactive oxygen species in cancer. *Free Radical Research, 44*(5), 479–496. https://doi.org/10.3109/10715761003667554.

Loh, C.-Y., Arya, A., Naema, A. F., Wong, W. F., Sethi, G., & Looi, C. Y. (2019). Signal transducer and activator of transcription (STATs) proteins in cancer and inflammation: Functions and therapeutic implication. *Frontiers in Oncology, 9*, 48. https://doi.org/10.3389/fonc.2019.00048.

Lopresti, A. L. (2018). The problem of curcumin and its bioavailability Could its gastrointestinal influence contribute to its overall health-enhancing effects? *Advances in Nutrition, 9*(1), 41–50. https://doi.org/10.1093/advances/nmx011.

Lozon, L., Saleh, E., Menon, V., Ramadan, W. S., Amin, A., & El-Awady, R. (2022). Effect of safranal on the response of cancer cells to topoisomerase I inhibitors: Does sequence matter? *Frontiers in Pharmacology, 13*, 938471. https://doi.org/10.3389/fphar.2022.938471.

Maggi, M. A., Bisti, S., & Picco, C. (2020). Saffron: Chemical composition and neuroprotective activity. *Molecules, 25*(23), 5618. https://doi.org/10.3390/molecules25235618.

Malaekeh-Nikouei, B., Mousavi, S. H., Shahsavand, S., Mehri, S., Nassirli, H., & Moallem, S. A. (2013). Assessment of cytotoxic properties of safranal and nanoliposomal safranal in various cancer cell lines: Cytotoxicity of safranal and its liposome. *Phytotherapy Research*, *27*(12), 1868–1873. https://doi.org/10.1002/ptr.4945.

Mansingh, D. P., O. J., S., Sali, V. K., & Vasanthi, H. R. (2018). [6]-Gingerol-induced cell cycle arrest, reactive oxygen species generation, and disruption of mitochondrial membrane potential are associated with apoptosis in human gastric cancer (AGS) cells. *Journal of Biochemical and Molecular Toxicology*, *32*(10), e22206. https://doi.org/10.1002/jbt.22206.

Mao, Q.-Q., Xu, X.-Y., Cao, S.-Y., Gan, R.-Y., Corke, H., Beta, T., & Li, H.-B. (2019). Bioactive compounds and bioactivities of ginger (*Zingiber officinale* Roscoe). *Foods*, *8*(6), 185. https://doi.org/10.3390/foods8060185.

Mehta, H. J., Patel, V., & Sadikot, R. T. (2014). Curcumin and lung cancer—A review. *Targeted Oncology*, *9*(4), 295–310. https://doi.org/10.1007/s11523-014-0321-1.

Metwaly, A. M., Ghoneim, M. M., Eissa, Ibrahim. H., Elsehemy, I. A., Mostafa, A. E., Hegazy, M. M., Afifi, W. M., & Dou, D. (2021). Traditional ancient Egyptian medicine: A review. *Saudi Journal of Biological Sciences*, *28*(10), 5823–5832. https://doi.org/10.1016/j.sjbs.2021.06.044.

Michalkova, R., Mirossay, L., Gazdova, M., Kello, M., & Mojzis, J. (2021). Molecular mechanisms of antiproliferative effects of natural chalcones. *Cancers*, *13*(11), 2730. https://doi.org/10.3390/cancers13112730.

Mirzaei, H., Gharehgozlou, R., Heydarirad, G., Fahimi, S., Ghafari, S., Mosavat, S. H., Moghani, M. M., & Hajian, P. (2022). Efficacy and safety of jollab (a saffron-based beverage) on cancer-related fatigue in breast cancer patients: A double-blind randomized clinical trial. *Complementary Medicine Research*, *29*(6), 437–445. https://doi.org/10.1159/000525775.

Mohrherr, J., Uras, I. Z., Moll, H. P., & Casanova, E. (2020). STAT3: Versatile functions in non-small cell lung cancer. *Cancers*, *12*(5), 1107. https://doi.org/10.3390/cancers12051107.

Nirachonkul, W., Ogonoki, S., Thumvijit, T., Chiampanichayakul, S., Panyajai, P., Anuchapreeda, S., Tima, S., & Chiampanichayakul, S. (2021). CD123-targeted nano-curcumin molecule enhances cytotoxic efficacy in leukemic stem cells. *Nanomaterials*, *11*(11), 2974. https://doi.org/10.3390/nano11112974.

Pal, R. R., Rajpal, V., Singh, P., & Saraf, S. A. (2021). Recent findings on thymoquinone and its applications as a nanocarrier for the treatment of cancer and rheumatoid arthritis. *Pharmaceutics, 13*(6), 775. https://doi.org/10.3390/pharmaceutics13060775.

Panahi, Y., Saberi-Karimian, M., Valizadeh, O., Behnam, B., Saadat, A., Jamialahmadi, T., Majeed, M., & Sahebkar, A. (2021). Effects of curcuminoids on systemic inflammation and quality of life in patients with colorectal cancer undergoing chemotherapy: A randomized controlled trial. In A. Sahebkar & T. Sathyapalan (Eds.), *Natural Products and Human Diseases* (Vol. 1328, pp. 1–9). Springer International Publishing. https://doi.org/10.1007/978-3-030-73234-9_1.

Park, U.-H., Jeong, H.-S., Jo, E.-Y., Park, T., Yoon, S. K., Kim, E.-J., Jeong, J.-C., & Um, S.-J. (2012). Piperine, a component of black pepper, inhibits adipogenesis by antagonizing PPARγ activity in 3T3-L1 cells. *Journal of Agricultural and Food Chemistry, 60*(15), 3853–3860. https://doi.org/10.1021/jf204514a.

Prasad, S., & Tyagi, A. K. (2015). Ginger and its constituents: Role in prevention and treatment of gastrointestinal cancer. *Gastroenterology Research and Practice, 2015*, 1–11. https://doi.org/10.1155/2015/142979.

Pratheeshkumar, P., Sreekala, C., Zhang, Z., Budhraja, A., Ding, S., Son, Y.-O., Wang, X., Hitron, A., Hyun-Jung, K., Wang, L., Lee, J.-C., & Shi, X. (2012). Cancer prevention with promising natural products: Mechanisms of action and molecular targets. *Anti-Cancer Agents in Medicinal Chemistry, 12*(10), 1159–1184. https://doi.org/10.2174/187152012803833035.

Radhakrishnan, E., Bava, S. V., Narayanan, S. S., Nath, L. R., Thulasidasan, A. K. T., Soniya, E. V., & Anto, R. J. (2014). [6]-gingerol induces caspase-dependent apoptosis and prevents PMA-induced proliferation in colon cancer cells by inhibiting MAPK/AP-1 signaling. *PLoS ONE, 9*(8), e104401. https://doi.org/10.1371/journal.pone.0104401.

Ranjan, A., Ramachandran, S., Gupta, N., Kaushik, I., Wright, S., Srivastava, S., Das, H., Srivastava, S., Prasad, S., & Srivastava, S. K. (2019). Role of phytochemicals in cancer prevention. *International Journal of Molecular Sciences, 20*(20), 4981. https://doi.org/10.3390/ijms20204981.

Rasmussen, A., Murphy, K., & Hoskin, D. W. (2019). 10-gingerol inhibits ovarian cancer cell growth by inducing G2arrest. *Advanced Pharmaceutical Bulletin, 9*(4), 685–689. https://doi.org/10.15171/apb.2019.080.

Ray, A., Vasudevan, S., & Sengupta, S. (2015). 6-shogaol inhibits breast cancer cells and stem cell-like spheroids by modulation of notch signaling pathway and induction of autophagic cell death. *PLOS ONE*, *10*(9), e0137614. https://doi.org/10.1371/journal. pone.0137614.

Ribeiro-Santos, R., Andrade, M., Madella, D., Martinazzo, A. P., De Aquino Garcia Moura, L., De Melo, N. R., & Sanches-Silva, A. (2017). Revisiting an ancient spice with medicinal purposes: Cinnamon. *Trends in Food Science & Technology*, *62*, 154–169. https://doi.org/10.1016/j. tifs.2017.02.011.

Sakai, H., Kai, Y., Oguchi, A., Kimura, M., Tabata, S., Yaegashi, M., Saito, T., Sato, K., Sato, F., Yumoto, T., & Narita, M. (2016). Curcumin inhibits 5-fluorouracil-induced up-regulation of CXCL1 and CXCL2 of the colon associated with attenuation of diarrhoea development. *Basic & Clinical Pharmacology & Toxicology*, *119*(6), 540–547. https://doi. org/10.1111/bcpt.12619.

Salek, R., Dehghani, M., Mohajeri, S. A., Talaei, A., Fanipakdel, A., & Javadinia, S. A. (2021). Amelioration of anxiety, depression, and chemotherapy related toxicity after crocin administration during chemotherapy of breast cancer: A double blind, randomized clinical trial. *Phytotherapy Research*, *35*(9), 5143–5153. https://doi. org/10.1002/ptr.7180.

Samykutty, A., Shetty, A. V., Dakshinamoorthy, G., Bartik, M. M., Johnson, G. L., Webb, B., Zheng, G., Chen, A., Kalyanasundaram, R., & Munirathinam, G. (2013). Piperine, a bioactive component of pepper spice exerts therapeutic effects on androgen dependent and androgen independent prostate cancer cells. *PLoS ONE*, *8*(6), e65889. https://doi.org/10.1371/journal.pone.0065889.

Sarian, M. N., Ahmed, Q. U., Mat So'ad, S. Z., Alhassan, A. M., Murugesu, S., Perumal, V., Syed Mohamad, S. N. A., Khatib, A., & Latip, J. (2017). Antioxidant and antidiabetic effects of flavonoids: A structure-activity relationship-based study. *BioMed Research International*, *2017*, 1–14. https://doi.org/10.1155/2017/8386065.

Satoh, T., Kosaka, K., Itoh, K., Kobayashi, A., Yamamoto, M., Shimojo, Y., Kitajima, C., Cui, J., Kamins, J., Okamoto, S., Izumi, M., Shirasawa, T., & Lipton, S. A. (2008). Carnosic acid, a *catechol-type* electrophilic compound, protects neurons both *in vitro* and *in vivo* through activation of the Keap1/Nrf2 pathway via *S-* alkylation of targeted cysteines on Keap1. *Journal of Neurochemistry*, *104*(4), 1116–1131. https://doi.org/10.1111/j.1471-4159.2007.05039.x.

Schadich, E., Hlaváč, J., Volná, T., Varanasi, L., Hajdúch, M., & Džubák, P. (2016). Effects of ginger phenylpropanoids and quercetin on Nrf2-ARE pathway in human BJ fibroblasts and HaCaT keratinocytes. *BioMed Research International*, *2016*, 1–6. https://doi.org/10.1155/2016/2173275.

Selvendiran, K., Singh, J. P. V., Krishnan, K. B., & Sakthisekaran, D. (2003). Cytoprotective effect of piperine against benzo[a]pyrene induced lung cancer with reference to lipid peroxidation and antioxidant system in Swiss albino mice. *Fitoterapia*, *74*(1–2), 109–115. https://doi.org/10.1016/S0367-326X(02)00304-0.

Shanmugam, M. K., Ahn, K. S., Hsu, A., Woo, C. C., Yuan, Y., Tan, K. H. B., Chinnathambi, A., Alahmadi, T. A., Alharbi, S. A., Koh, A. P. F., Arfuso, F., Huang, R. Y.-J., Lim, L. H. K., Sethi, G., & Kumar, A. P. (2018). Thymoquinone inhibits bone metastasis of breast cancer cells through abrogation of the CXCR4 signaling axis. *Frontiers in Pharmacology*, *9*, 1294. https://doi.org/10.3389/fphar.2018.01294.

Si, L., Yang, R., Lin, R., & Yang, S. (2018). Piperine functions as a tumor suppressor for human ovarian tumor growth via activation of JNK/p38 MAPK-mediated intrinsic apoptotic pathway. *Bioscience Reports*, *38*(3), BSR20180503. https://doi.org/10.1042/BSR20180503.

Srinivasan, K. (2018). Cumin (Cuminum cyminum) and black cumin (Nigella sativa) seeds: Traditional uses, chemical constituents, and nutraceutical effects. *Food Quality and Safety*, *2*(1), 1–16. https://doi.org/10.1093/fqsafe/fyx031.

Sun, X., Zhao, P., Lin, J., Chen, K., & Shen, J. (2023). Recent advances in access to overcome cancer drug resistance by nanocarrier drug delivery system. *Cancer Drug Resistance*, *6*(2), 390–415. https://doi.org/10.20517/cdr.2023.16.

Sung, H., Ferlay, J., Siegel, R. L., Laversanne, M., Soerjomataram, I., Jemal, A., & Bray, F. (2021). Global Cancer Statistics 2020: GLOBOCAN estimates of incidence and mortality worldwide for 36 cancers in 185 countries. *CA: A Cancer Journal for Clinicians*, *71*(3), 209–249. https://doi.org/10.3322/caac.21660.

Tang, X., Ding, H., Liang, M., Chen, X., Yan, Y., Wan, N., Chen, Q., Zhang, J., & Cao, J. (2021). Curcumin induces ferroptosis in non-small-cell lung cancer via activating autophagy. *Thoracic Cancer*, *12*(8), 1219–1230. https://doi.org/10.1111/1759-7714.13904.

Targeting Breast Stem Cells with the Cancer Preventive Compounds Curcumin and Piperine—PMC. (n.d.). Retrieved 24 July 2023, from https://www.ncbi.nlm.nih.gov/pmc/articles/PMC3039120/.

Terlikowska, K., Witkowska, A., Zujko, M., Dobrzycka, B., & Terlikowski, S. (2014). Potential application of curcumin and its analogues in the treatment strategy of patients with primary epithelial ovarian cancer. *International Journal of Molecular Sciences, 15*(12), 21703–21722. https://doi.org/10.3390/ijms151221703.

Veisi, A., Akbari, G., Mard, A., Badfar, G., Zarezade, V., & Mirshekar, M. A. (2020). Role of crocin in several cancer cell lines: An updated review. *Iranian Journal of Basic Medical Sciences, 23*(1). https://doi.org/10.22038/ijbms.2019.37821.8995.

Wang, M.-Z., Gao, J., Chu, Y., Niu, J., Chen, M., Shang, Q., Peng, L.-H., & Jiang, Z.-H. (2020). Synthesis of crocetin derivatives and their potent inhibition in multiple tumor cells proliferation and inflammatory property of macrophage. *BMC Complementary Medicine and Therapies, 20*(1), 29. https://doi.org/10.1186/s12906-020-2831-y.

Weiskirchen, R. (2022). Commentary: Crocetin protected human hepatocyte LO2 cell from TGF-β-induced oxygen stress and apoptosis but promoted proliferation and autophagy via AMPK/m-TOR pathway. *Frontiers in Public Health, 10,* 1002484. https://doi.org/10.3389/fpubh.2022.1002484.

Winterhalter, P., & Straubinger, M. (2000). Saffron—Renewed interest in an ancient spice. *Food Reviews International, 16*(1), 39–59. https://doi.org/10.1081/FRI-100100281.

Wojtowicz, K., Sterzyńska, K., Świerczewska, M., Nowicki, M., Zabel, M., & Januchowski, R. (2021). Piperine targets different drug resistance mechanisms in human ovarian cancer cell lines leading to increased sensitivity to cytotoxic drugs. *International Journal of Molecular Sciences, 22*(8), 4243. https://doi.org/10.3390/ijms22084243.

Wong, S. C., Kamarudin, M. N. A., & Naidu, R. (2021). Anticancer mechanism of curcumin on human glioblastoma. *Nutrients, 13*(3), 950. https://doi.org/10.3390/nu13030950.

Xia, Y., Shen, S., & Verma, I. M. (2014). NF-κB, an active player in human cancers. *Cancer Immunology Research, 2*(9), 823–830. https://doi.org/10.1158/2326-6066.CIR-14-0112.

Xiang, Q., Liu, Z., Wang, Y., Xiao, H., Wu, W., Xiao, C., & Liu, X. (2013). Carnosic acid attenuates lipopolysaccharide-induced liver injury in rats via fortifying cellular antioxidant defense system. *Food and Chemical Toxicology, 53,* 1–9. https://doi.org/10.1016/j.fct.2012.11.001.

Yu, S.-M., & Kim, S.-J. (2015). The thymoquinone-induced production of reactive oxygen species promotes dedifferentiation through the

ERK pathway and inflammation through the p38 and PI3K pathways in rabbit articular chondrocytes. *International Journal of Molecular Medicine, 35*(2), 325–332. https://doi.org/10.3892/ijmm.2014.2014.

Zarrineh, M., Ashrafian, S., Jensen, P., Nawrocki, A., Ansari, A. M., Rezadoost, H., Ghassempour, A., & Larsen, M. R. (2022). Comprehensive proteomics and sialiomics of the anti-proliferative activity of safranal on triple negative MDA-MB-231 breast cancer cell lines. *Journal of Proteomics, 259*, 104539. https://doi.org/10.1016/j.jprot.2022.104539.

Zeng, Y., & Yang, Y. (2018). Piperine depresses the migration progression via downregulating the Akt/mTOR/MMP-9 signaling pathway in DU145 cells. *Molecular Medicine Reports.* https://doi.org/10.3892/mmr.2018.8653.

Zhang, M.-M., Wang, D., Lu, F., Zhao, R., Ye, X., He, L., Ai, L., & Wu, C.-J. (2021). Identification of the active substances and mechanisms of ginger for the treatment of colon cancer based on network pharmacology and molecular docking. *BioData Mining, 14*(1), 1. https://doi.org/10.1186/s13040-020-00232-9.

Zheng, J., Zhou, Y., Li, Y., Xu, D.-P., Li, S., & Li, H.-B. (2016). Spices for prevention and treatment of cancers. *Nutrients, 8*(8), 495. https://doi.org/10.3390/nu8080495.

Zuniga, K. E., Parma, D. L., Muñoz, E., Spaniol, M., Wargovich, M., & Ramirez, A. G. (2019). Dietary intervention among breast cancer survivors increased adherence to a Mediterranean-style, anti-inflammatory dietary pattern: The Rx for better breast health randomized controlled trial. *Breast Cancer Research and Treatment, 173*(1), 145–154. https://doi.org/10.1007/s10549-018-4982-9.

Chapter 9

Synergistic Action of Spices with Chemotherapeutics

Sakshi M. Kothawade,[a] **Saurabh Maru,**[a] **Meena Chintamaneni,**[a] **Hardeep Singh Tuli,**[b] **and Ginpreet Kaur**[a]

[a]*Shobhaben Pratapbhai Patel School of Pharmacy and Technology Management, SVKM's NMIMS, Mumbai, Maharashtra, India*
[b]*Department of Bio-Sciences and Technology, Maharishi Markandeshwar (Deemed to be University), Mullana, Haryana, India*

ginpreet.aneja@gmail.com

9.1 Introduction

Cancer therapies have several challenges such as drug resistance, toxicity, and side effects. Therefore, natural products have become popular as a substitute and adjunct therapy because of their safety and efficacy. Studies have shown that natural products, such as curcumin and resveratrol, can synergize with chemotherapeutic drugs to reduce cell proliferation and induce apoptosis, but more clinical studies are needed. Patients undergoing chemotherapy often turn to alternative therapies to alleviate symptoms, including herbal medicines [1].

Anticancer Spices: Dietary Input to Health
Edited by Hardeep Singh Tuli
Copyright © 2025 Jenny Stanford Publishing Pte. Ltd.
ISBN 978-981-5129-28-1 (Hardcover), 978-1-003-53466-2 (eBook)
www.jennystanford.com

Chemoprevention pertains to the use of pharmacological interventions to impede, postpone, or revert the progression of tumorigenesis and reduce the potential for cancer reappearance. Spices have shown efficacy as chemopreventive agents. These compounds can block carcinogenic agents, enhance DNA repair systems, and directly target cells with DNA modifications [2].

Spices are a potential alternative source of bioactive compounds that have high antioxidant activity and can trigger free radical scavenging ability at the cellular level, thus mitigating diverse metabolic syndromes. Many of these compounds, encompassing curcuminoids, limonene, allicin, cinnamic aldehyde, allyl isothiocyanate, and gingerol, have been identified as chemo-preventive agents targeting a number of malignant conditions. They work by arresting the activity of cytochrome P450 and isozymes CYP 1A1 and cyclooxygenase-2, and diminishing the activator of transcription-3 (STAT-3) and signal transducer, which is linked with tumorigenesis activated by interleukin-6 (IL-6) receptors in addition with epidermal growth factors (EGF) pertaining to a range of malignancies [3, 4].

9.2 Anticancer Therapies

9.2.1 Conventional Chemotherapy

Conventional chemotherapy drugs have severe side effects but are still widely used because they are active against all types of cancer. They work by inhibiting DNA synthesis and mitosis, averting cancer cell proliferation. Alkylating agents, antimetabolites, and topoisomerase inhibitors are the most prevalent categories of chemotherapeutic drugs. Alkylating agents such as cyclophosphamide and carmustine damage DNA. Topoisomerase inhibitors, for instance, irinotecan, doxorubicin, and etoposide, hinder the initiation of topoisomerase enzymes, causing DNA injury by overwinding the DNA. These drugs can have a substantial impact on rapidly proliferating tumors because they influence the cell cycle.

9.2.2 Hormonal Anticancer Therapy

Tamoxifen, a selective estrogen receptor modulator, has revolutionized cancer therapy by introducing targeted cancer therapy. It specifically targets tumors with estrogen receptors, but its use in hormonal therapy can have side effects due to estrogen receptor activation in other tissues. Tamoxifen leads to the progress of endometrial cancer. However, its success has inspired research into additional cancer receptors and biological markers that are addressable using drugs, leading to the destruction of cancer cells.

9.2.3 Monoclonal Antibody Therapy

Conventional chemotherapy has limitations, leading researchers to develop better-targeted chemotherapies like monoclonal antibodies (mAbs). mAbs are a type of antibody that selectively binds to cancer membrane receptors, targeting overexpressed receptors while sparing normal cells. Compared to hormonal therapy, mAbs offer greater effectiveness by specifically targeting molecular receptors and ligands. They can block the epidermal growth factor receptor (EGFR) family, which commonly exhibits excessive expression in epithelial malignant tumors. Additionally, mAbs can inhibit the vascular endothelial growth factor receptor (VEGFR), which affects tumor growth and progression. An example of a mAb-based drug is bevacizumab (Avastin), which inhibits VEGFR.

9.2.4 Tyrosine Kinase Inhibitor Therapy

Tyrosine kinase inhibitors (TKIs) are drugs that disrupt intracellular signaling, inhibiting tumor formation and growth. Unlike monoclonal antibodies (mAbs), which target specific cancer receptors, TKIs also block the enzyme involved in activating proteins in tumor signaling pathways. However, both TKIs and mAbs have limitations, as they are effective only against specific cancers expressing the target proteins and can lead to severe side effects. Upcoming cancer therapies ought to aim to treat a broader range of tumors and overcome these limitations.

9.2.5 Current Immuno-Anticancer Therapy

9.2.5.1 T cell-mediated therapy

T lymphocytes can detect cancer antigens and naturally kill cancer cells, activating the immune system to combat cancer. Cancer cells, however, have developed to evade T cell attacks by activating immune checkpoints and downregulating antigen presentation. T cell-mediated therapy aims to surmount this evasion by identifying and effectively killing cancer cells (Fig. 9.1).

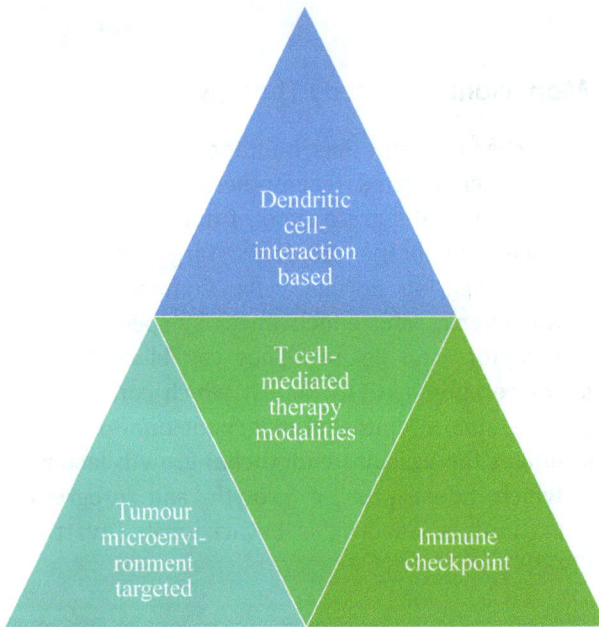

Figure 9.1 Three main T cell-mediated therapy modalities.

9.2.5.2 Immune checkpoint therapy

Cancer cells can evade immune checkpoints and are activated to boost the immune system, which stops the T cell attack. Anti-PD-1, anti-PD-L1, and anti-CTLA-4 antibodies demonstrate efficacy in the treatment of certain tumors by modulating these checkpoints. However, immune checkpoint inhibition therapy constrains its application to a specific subset of patients. Seven immune checkpoint inhibitors have received approval from the FDA. They treat various cancers but are still unsuccessful in treating solid tumors like pancreatic and brain tumors.

9.2.5.3 Tumor microenvironment-targeted therapy

The tumor microenvironment (TME) contains various cells and molecules that help cancer cells evade the immune system. Regulatory T cells (Tregs) are a crucial component of TME as they secrete immunosuppressive cytokines, halting the antitumor response of immune cells as well as activating immune checkpoints. However, immune-activating cytokines such as IL-2, IFN-α, TNF, IL-12, and GM-CSF can initiate anticancer response. Although IL-2 has been shown to inhibit metastatic melanoma, only a small percentage of patients benefit from cytokine therapy, but those who do see complete, seemingly curative outcomes.

9.2.5.4 Dendritic cell interaction-based therapy

Dendritic cells (DCs) are antigen-presenting cells that stimulate T cells and activate the adaptive immune defense system by presenting both foreign and self-antigens on their surface. The innate and adaptive immune systems are connected by DCs, and by effectively activating DCs, they encourage T cells to attack cancer cells. T cells are triggered through cell membrane-bound molecules and various secreted cytokines. Understanding the functional partnership between DCs and T cells can lead to the development of novel immunotherapies to target tumors.

9.2.5.5 Macrophage repolarization therapy

Macrophage repolarization therapy is a promising approach in cancer treatment that aims to re-educate tumor-associated macrophages (TAMs) to induce an anti-tumor response. Macrophage repolarization therapy aims to reprogram TAMs to switch from a pro-tumor phenotype to an anti-tumor phenotype, potentially aiding in cancer treatment. This therapy can utilize different agents like cytokines, small molecules, and nanomaterials. It has demonstrated potential in both ongoing clinical trials and preclinical research and assessing its safety and effectiveness.

9.3 Anticancer Spices

9.3.1 Turmeric

Source: *Curcuma longa*

Active ingredient: Curcumin

Mechanism of action: Curcumin (Fig. 9.2), a natural compound found in turmeric, is determined to inhibit the activity of NF-kappaB, a transcription factor associated with inflammation, immune response, and cell survival [5]. NF-kappaB is often overactive in cancer cells, and curcumin's inhibition of this pathway can suppress cancer cell growth and proliferation. Specifically, curcumin reduces the activity of IκB kinase, leading to the degradation of IκBα and subsequent NF-κB activation. This inhibition results in decreased expression of proteins associated with cancer progression. Curcumin can also target other signaling pathways involved in cancer, including the PI3K/Akt/mTOR pathway, which affects cell survival, proliferation, and growth. Additionally, curcumin has been shown to induce apoptosis, or programmed cell death, in cancer cells. Curcumin's effects arise from its ability to hinder activator protein-1 and focal adhesion kinase activity. Moreover, it leads to the reduction of inflammatory cytokines such as CXCL1, CXCL2, interleukins (ILs) 6, and IL-8 within different cancer cells [6, 7]. Curcumin is capable of inhibiting peroxidation by scavenging reactive free radicals. This protective ability of curcumin is due to the functional groups it contains [8]. Thus, curcumin enhances the anticancer activity of chemotherapeutic agents through a synergistic effect (Table 9.1).

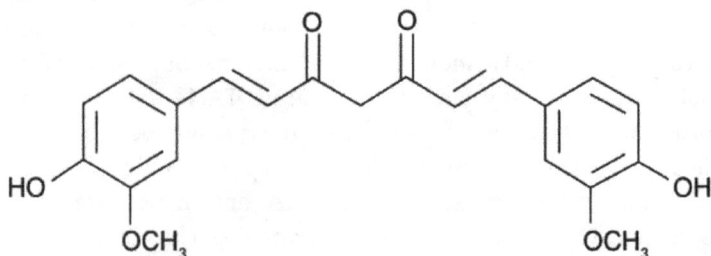

Figure 9.2 Structure of curcumin.

Table 9.1 Synergistic action of turmeric with chemotherapeutic agents [9]

Spice	Chemotherapeutic agent	Types of cancer
Turmeric	Metformin	Hepatocellular carcinoma, prostate cancer
	Docetaxel	Prostate cancer
	5-FU	Colorectal cancer, gastric cancer, breast cancer
	Cisplatin	Bladder cancer, ovarian cancer
	Celecoxib	Colorectal cancer

Curcumin exhibits various pharmacological activities, including anti-inflammatory, antioxidative, and anticancer effects. Its anticancer activity has been studied in different cancer types by targeting various signaling molecules. The study revealed that curcumin sensitized glioblastoma cells to TMZ by concurrently generating reactive oxygen species (ROS) and disrupting the AKT/mTOR signaling pathway. ROS is involved in cellular damage, while AKT/mTOR signaling regulates cell growth and survival. In the mouse model, the combination treatment of curcumin and TMZ resulted in significant tumor growth inhibition compared to individual treatments or controls. The study was conducted using U87MG cells and a U87MG xenograft mouse model. U87MG cells were resistant to TMZ treatment alone, but when combined with CUM, the combination showed a synergistic antitumor effect. In the U87MG xenograft mouse model, both CUM and TMZ alone decreased tumor volume and weight compared to the control group. When given in combination form, it enhances tumor growth inhibition [10].

9.3.2 Capsicum

Source: Chili pepper extract

Active ingredient: Capsaicin

Mechanism of action: Capsaicin (Fig. 9.3), found in chili pepper, exhibits several mechanisms that can potentially aid in cancer treatment. It can induce apoptosis, or programmed cell death, in cancer cells by activating caspase enzymes. This selective killing of cancer cells spares healthy cells. Capsaicin also inhibits angiogenesis, the growth of new blood vessels that nourish tumors, by blocking the activity of VEGF. This hampers the tumor's access to nutrients and oxygen. Additionally, capsaicin possesses anti-inflammatory properties, which can help mitigate chronic inflammation, a risk factor for cancer development and tumor growth. These effects of capsaicin may contribute to slowing down cancer progression [7].

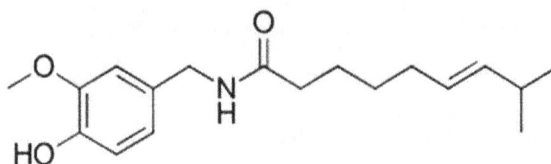

Figure 9.3 Structure of capsaicin.

9.3.3 Ginger Source: *Zingiber officinale*

Active ingredients: Gingerols (Fig. 9.4) and shogaols, zingerone, paradols, and sesquiterpenes

Mechanism of action: Ginger has been found to potentially inhibit cancer by inducing apoptosis, or programmed cell death, in cancer cells. Compounds like gingerols and shogaols found in ginger have demonstrated this effect in various types of cancer cells, such as those found in the colon, ovaries, and lungs. Additionally, ginger may impact cancer cell signaling pathways by inhibiting the activation of NF-κB. By preventing NF-κB activation, ginger has the potential to hinder cancer cell proliferation and metastasis [11].

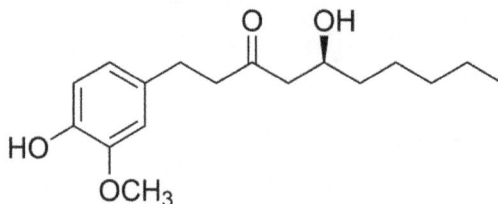

Figure 9.4 Structure of gingerol.

9.3.4 Cumin

Source: *Cuminum cyminum*

Active ingredients: Cuminaldehyde (Fig. 9.5), thymol, and beta carotene

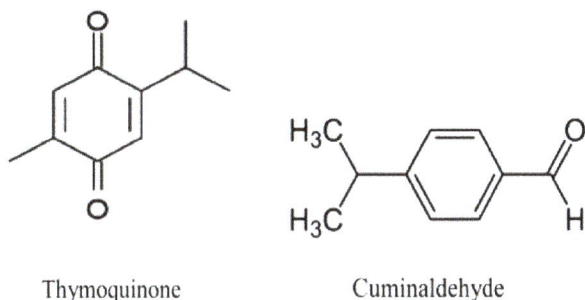

Thymoquinone   Cuminaldehyde

Figure 9.5 Structure of thymoquinone and cuminaldehyde.

Mechanism of action: Cumin (Fig. 9.6) has shown potential in inducing apoptosis and cell cycle arrest in cancer cells, thereby impeding their growth and spread. It contains compounds that can modulate signaling pathways involved in cancer development, including MAPK/ERK and NF-κB [12]. Thymoquinone, a component

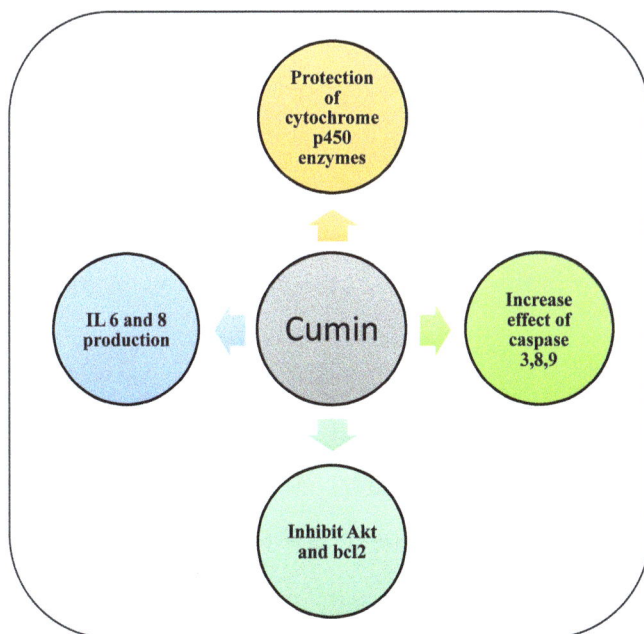

Figure 9.6 Mechanism of action of cumin.

of cumin, inhibits the JAK/STAT pathway by reducing STAT3 phosphorylation, leading to decreased cyclin levels and inhibiting the growth of various cancer cells. It also hinders the Wnt/β-catenin pathway, reducing β-catenin nuclear accumulation and suppressing target gene expression, thus inhibiting metastasis and growth in bladder and colorectal cancer. Thymoquinone induces auto-ubiquitination of UHRF1, enhancing p73 expression and inducing apoptosis [13]. It may also inhibit tumor angiogenesis and restrain prostate tumor growth [14].

9.3.5 Cardamom

Source: *Elettaria cardamomum*

Active ingredients: 1,8-cineole (Fig. 9.7), limonene, alpha-terpinyl acetate, and eugenol

Mechanism of action: Research studies have indicated that cardamom exhibits potential anticancer properties by triggering apoptosis, a process that induces programmed cell death in cancer cells, thereby inhibiting their growth. Additionally, cardamom has been observed to halt the cell cycle progression in cancer cells, effectively preventing their division and subsequent growth. Moreover, it may also hinder angiogenesis, the formation of new blood vessels, which is vital for tumor growth and metastasis, thereby impeding the proliferation and dissemination of cancer cells [15].

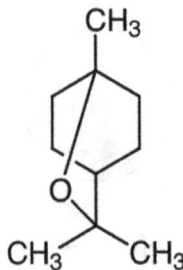

Figure 9.7 Structure of 1,8-cineole.

9.3.6 Garlic

Source: *Allium sativum*

Active ingredient: Allicin (Fig. 9.8)

Mechanism of action: Garlic compounds have been shown to induce programmed cell death, or apoptosis, in cancer cells. Garlic's alleged potential anticancer effects are organosulfur components and metabolic byproducts. These natural compounds, including diallyl sulfide, diallyl disulfide, diallyl trisulfide, diallyl tetrasulfide, S-allyl mercaptocysteine, and allicin, possess antioxidant properties and demonstrate chemo-sensitization effects. These organosulfur compounds have gained significant attention for their potential in cancer research [16]. Garlic compounds have also been shown to inhibit the growth and division of cancer cells. This can help slow down the progression of cancer. Garlic can also modulate the immune system, helping it to identify and attack cancer cells. Chronic inflammation is connected with an increased risk of cancer. Garlic contains compounds that have anti-inflammatory properties, which may help reduce cancer risk [17].

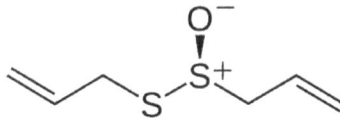

Figure 9.8 Structure of allicin.

9.3.7 Cinnamon

Source: *Cinnamomum verum*

Active ingredients: Cinnamaldehyde (Fig. 9.9), eugenol, coumarin, proanthocyanidins, and cinnamic acid

Mechanism of action: Cinnamon extracts can activate certain proteins, such as caspase-3, -8, and -9, which play important roles in initiating the apoptotic process. These proteins can cleave specific substrates within the cell and lead to cell death. Cinnamon has also been found to downregulate certain anti-apoptotic proteins, such as Bcl-2 and Bcl-xl, which can avert apoptosis from occurring. Chronic inflammation is recognized to accelerate the development and spread of cancer, and cinnamon has been discovered to inhibit the production of pro-inflammatory cytokines, such as TNF-α and IL-6. This may help reduce the inflammation associated with cancer and slow down its progression. Cinnamon has been found to exhibit anti-angiogenic properties [18].

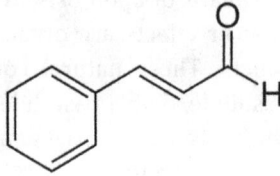

Figure 9.9 Structure of cinnamaldehyde.

9.3.8 Fenugreek

Source: *Trigonella foenum-graecum*

Active ingredients: Alkaloids, saponins, diosgenin (Fig. 9.10) and flavonoids

Mechanism of action: Oxidative stress and chronic inflammation are known to make an impact on the development and progression of cancer, so reducing these factors may aid in preventing or slowing down the growth of cancer cells. Another potential mechanism is through the modulation of hormone levels. Some studies have found that fenugreek extracts can reduce levels of certain hormones, such as estrogen and testosterone, which are a part of the advancement of certain types of cancer, including breast and prostate cancer. Studies have suggested that fenugreek extracts can increase the activity of immune cells, such as natural killer cells, which are accountable for recognizing and attacking cancer cells [19].

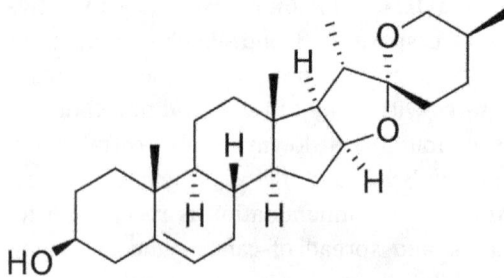

Figure 9.10 Structure of diosgenin.

9.3.9 Black Pepper

Source: *Piper nigrum*

Active ingredients: Piperine (Fig. 9.11) and other alkaloids [20]

Mechanism of action: Numerous laboratory experiments indicate that black pepper's piperine may have anticancer effects. Piperine has been shown in test-tube research to reduce the replication of breast, prostate, and colon cancer cells and promote cancer cell death, despite the lack of human trials in this regard. Piperine suppresses the nuclear localization of β-catenin in HCT116 cells and inhibits the canonical Wnt pathway caused by the overexpression of β-catenin, β-catenin S33A, or dnTCF4 VP16. Using the HeLa, SiHa, and CaSki *in vitro* cervical cancer model, piperine altered the cyclooxygenase 2 (PTGS2) pathway.

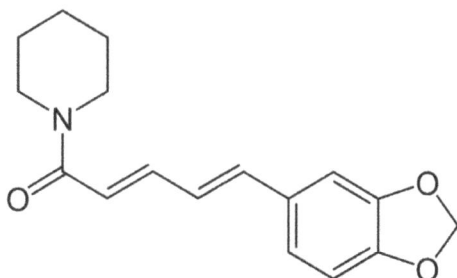

Figure 9.11 Structure of piperine.

9.4 Mechanism of Action of Spices

Phytochemicals exhibit anticancer activities through several mechanisms, such as DNA damage, cell cycle arrest, activation of apoptosis, suppression of epigenetic alterations, and regulation of cell signaling pathways (Table 9.2). Phytochemicals can suppress MAPK/ERK signaling pathways, inhibit the proliferation of cancer cells, and reduce invasiveness. Phytochemicals can also induce apoptosis in cancer cells by enhancing caspase activities and inhibiting Bcl-2. Examples of phytochemicals that induce apoptosis in cancer cells include 5-methoxyangenylalkannin, punicalagin, esculetin, diosgenin, artabotryside A, and caffeic acid. Apoptosis

Table 9.2 Spices and their anticancer mechanism

Spices	Active ingredient	Anticancer: Mechanism of action	Refs.
Turmeric	Curcumin	Regulates cell signaling and gene expression regulatory pathways	[21]
		DNA damage and fragmentation; chromatin condensation	[2]
Capsicum	Capsaicin	Downregulation of survival, angiogenesis, and metastasis gene expression	[22]
Ginger	6-Shogaol	Akt and STAT signaling pathway	[23]
	Gingerol	Intrinsic apoptosis pathway	
Cumin	Thymoquinone	Regulation of the JAK/STAT and Wnt/β-catenin signaling pathways by thymoquinone	[13]
Garlic	Allicin	STAT3 signaling pathway	[24]
Fenugreek	Diosgenin, flavonoids, alkaloids	Inhibition of angiogenesis, cell signaling pathways, and tumor cell metastasis and invasion	[25]
Black pepper	Piperine	Suppressing cancer stem cell (CSC) self-renewal and variation of ER stress and autophagy	[26]

plays a crucial role in eliminating tumor cells, and the modulation of signaling pathways and induction of apoptosis serve as rational bases for the use of various medications in the prevention and treatment of carcinogenesis. Several phytochemicals have shown potential as anticancer agents through different mechanisms. For example, some compounds induce apoptosis, such as falcarindiol-3-acetate, lutein, and rhein. Others inhibit cell cycle progression, including ferulic acid, withaferin A, and kaempferol. Additionally, some phytochemicals can inhibit epigenetic variations that contribute to cancer development, such as sulforaphane. These compounds may have inhibitory effects on cyclin-dependent kinases (CDKs) or DNA methyltransferases (DNMTs) and histone deacetylases (HDACs), among other mechanisms. Phytochemicals have potential anticancer effects by inducing apoptosis, inhibiting cell cycle progression, and preventing epigenetic variations and DNA damage. Various phytochemicals have been shown to inhibit DNMTs, HDACs, and onco-miRNA while upregulating tumor-inhibitory genes to prevent cancer growth and invasion. In addition, phytochemicals have been found to exhibit anti-mutagenic and anti-oxidant activities to prevent DNA damage and mutations, which are the main causes of carcinogenesis. Some examples of chemopreventive phytochemicals with anti-mutagenic and anti-oxidant activities include turmeric, capsaicin, ginger, cumin, cardamom, garlic, and cinnamon [1].

9.5 Synergistic Effect of Spices with Chemotherapeutics against Various Cancers

Phytochemicals are known to enhance the therapeutic effects of conventional anticancer drugs through various mechanisms such as increased bioavailability, target blockage, and drug stabilization (Table 9.3). The rising use of herbal medicines in conjunction with conventional drugs is attributed to factors like high treatment costs, multidrug resistance, and treatment inefficacy. The complex cell signaling network requires multiple modulating strategies for effective treatment, and the combined use of phytomedicines and conventional drugs can produce additive or synergistic effects through the action of multiple chemical compounds on single or multiple target sites [1]. Table 9.4 shows spices in preclinical and clinical studies [34].

9.6 Discussion and Future Directions

The induction of cancer requires multiple factors, including the formation of phlegm. Herbal medicine has the potential to eliminate phlegm and regulate qi in the blood, which can enhance the effectiveness of chemotherapy. Certain herbal medicines can regulate the P450 system or phase-II metabolism, thus enhancing chemotherapy. Many natural compounds activate or inhibit the enzyme system responsible for the metabolism or elimination of carcinogens. The interaction between herbal medicine and chemotherapy affects the efficacy of chemotherapeutic agents, and

Table 9.3 Studies conducted for combination of spices and chemotherapeutic agents

Cancer type	Treatment	Findings	Refs
Pancreatic cancer	Curcumin (2000 mg/die continuously (4 capsules, each of 500 mg, every day) + gemcitabine (10 mg/m^2)	Medium progression-free survival and overall survival were 8.4 and 10.2 months, respectively	[27]
Colorectal cancer	FOLFOX (5-fluorouracil and oxaliplatin) + Curcumin	Inhibition of growth by downregulating EGFR and IGF-1R expression and activation, attenuating NF-κB activity	[28]
Hepatocellular carcinoma	Sorafenib + capsaicin	Suppression of proliferation, attaining a high-level synergism result (reticence rates over 50%), and stimulating HCC apoptotic cell death	[29]
Colorectal cancer	Ginger + 5-FU	Combination therapy of ginger extract and Gelam honey shows synergistic suppression of colon cancer cell growth and enhanced effect when combined with 5-FU chemotherapy	[30]
Lung and colorectal carcinoma cells	Allicin + 5 FU	The combination induced higher levels of apoptosis and promoted cell cycle arrest, leading to reduced tumor growth	[31]
Colorectal cancer	Cinnamaldehyde + 5 FU and oxaliplatin	Enhanced apoptosis and downregulated chemotherapeutic agent-associated genes. It had antagonistic effects when combined with irinotecan	[32]
Breast cancer cell line	Piperine + cisplatin	The combination induced apoptosis and reduced Bcl-2 while increasing caspase 3, p53, caspase 9, and Bax	[33]

Table 9.4 Spices in preclinical and clinical studiesClick or tap here to enter text.

Spice	Active component	Animal model for preclinical trials	Findings
Zingiber officinale	6-Shogaol	Nude mice model of non-small cell lung cancer	Suppressed lung cancer and prostate cancer cells. Inhibition of Akt pathways and downregulated STAT3
Allium sativum	Allicin	Nude mice model of cholangiocarcinoma	Inhibition of STAT3 pathway and suppressed metastasis, and epithelial-mesenchymal transition of cancer cells
Zingiber officinale	Gingerol	Syngenic mouse model of spontaneous breast cancer metastasis	Activated caspase-3 initiation and suppressed the orthotopic cancer growth of mouse brain metastatic 4T1Br4 mammary tumor cells to multiple organs such as lung, bone, and brain
Thymol	Thyme (*Thymus vulgaris*)	Oral squamous cell carcinoma Cal27- & HeLa-derived mouse xenografts	Reduced tumor volume, decreased cell proliferation, induced apoptosis
Thymoquinone	Black cumin (*Nigella sativa*)	Athymic nude mice	Reduced tumor weight and size, induced apoptosis, inhibited STAT3 phosphorylation
Curcumin	Turmeric (*Curcuma longa*)	Various cancer cells	Chemopreventive and chemotherapeutic role, efficacy shown in clinical trials against different cancers

an appropriate appraisal system should be in place for cancer patients undergoing chemotherapy. The positive interactions between herbal medicine and chemotherapy should be incorporated into integrative chemotherapy for the management of diverse cancer forms. They continue to be a valuable resource for discovering new therapeutic agents, but their transition from preclinical efficacy to clinical trials poses challenges. Identifying appropriate *in vitro* and *in vivo* models to demonstrate effectiveness and facilitate inclusion in clinical trials remains difficult. To address these challenges, alternative *in vitro* and in silico methods should be proposed to reduce the time and costs associated with *in vivo* studies. Emphasizing drug delivery systems and exploring derivatives can enhance the bioavailability and efficacy of natural compounds [1, 2].

9.7   Concluding Remarks

In order to mitigate the side effects and economic burden associated with conventional cancer treatments, there is a growing interest in the discovery of anticancer phytochemicals and combinations of these compounds with chemotherapeutic agents. The combination of phytochemicals with chemotherapy has been discovered to mediate effective antitumor outcomes by altering different signaling pathways through modulation. Therefore, further research is necessary to identify and discover more useful synergistic anticancer phytochemicals, while also providing patients with proper counseling about the consumption of natural products. This will aid researchers in avoiding harmful combinations of phytochemicals and chemotherapy.

Conflict of Interest

The authors declare that the study was conducted in the absence of any commercial or financial relationships that could be construed as a potential conflict of interest.

Ethical Approval

Not applicable

Competing Interests

Authors declare no competing interest.

Authors' Contributions

GK visualized the presented idea and contributed to the manuscript writing. SK contributed to literature searches and the preparation of the manuscript. HT supervised and contributed to the final manuscript revision and approval. GK revised and approved the manuscript.

Funding

Not applicable

Availability of Data and Materials

The data used and analyzed during the present study are available from the corresponding author on reasonable request.

References

1. Ayaz M, Nawaz A, Ahmad S, et al. Underlying anticancer mechanisms and synergistic combinations of phytochemicals with cancer chemotherapeutics: Potential benefits and risks. *J Food Qual.* 2022, 2022.

2. Dehelean CA, Marcovici I, Soica C, et al. Plant-derived anticancer compounds as new perspectives in drug discovery and alternative therapy. *Molecules.* 2021, 26.

3. Mughal MH. Spices: A mechanistic anticancer treatise. *Journal of Nutrition, Food Research and Technology.* 2019, 2:14–19.

4. Kim K, Khang D. Past, present, and future of anticancer nanomedicine. *Int J Nanomedicine.* Dove Medical Press Ltd. 2020, p. 5719–5743.

5. Pezzani R, Salehi B, Vitalini S, et al. Synergistic effects of plant derivatives and conventional chemotherapeutic agents: An update on the cancer perspective. *Medicina (Lithuania).* MDPI AG. 2019.

6. Younes M, Mardirossian R, Rizk L, et al. The synergistic effects of curcumin and chemotherapeutic drugs in inhibiting metastatic, invasive and proliferative pathways. *Plants.* MDPI. 2022.

7. Zhang S, Wang D, Huang J, et al. Application of capsaicin as a potential new therapeutic drug in human cancers. *J Clin Pharm Ther.* Blackwell Publishing Ltd. 2020, p. 16–28.

8. Stanić Z. Curcumin, a compound from natural sources, a true scientific challenge – A review. *Plant Foods for Human Nutrition.* Springer, New York LLC. 2017.

9. Tan BL, Norhaizan ME. Curcumin combination chemotherapy: The implication and efficacy in cancer. *Molecules.* MDPI AG. 2019.

10. Yin H, Zhou Y, Wen C, et al. Curcumin sensitizes glioblastoma to temozolomide by simultaneously generating ROS and disrupting AKT/mTOR signaling. *Oncol Rep.* 2014, 32:1610–1616.

11. Prasad S, Tyagi AK. Ginger and its constituents: Role in prevention and treatment of gastrointestinal cancer. *Gastroenterol Res Pract.* Hindawi Publishing Corporation. 2015.

12. Khan MA, Chen HC, Tania M, et al. Anticancer activities of Nigella sativa (Black Cumin). *African Journal of Traditional, Complementary and Alternative Medicines.* 2011, 8:226–232.

13. Farooqi AA, Attar R, Xu B. Anticancer and anti-metastatic role of thymoquinone: Regulation of oncogenic signaling cascades by thymoquinone. *Int J Mol Sci.* MDPI. 2022.

14. Yi T, Cho SG, Yi Z, et al. Thymoquinone inhibits tumor angiogenesis and tumor growth through suppressing AKT and extracellular signal-regulated kinase signaling pathways. *Mol Cancer Ther.* 2008, 7:1789–1796.

15. Elguindy NM, Yacout GA, El Azab EF, et al. Chemoprotective effect of Elettaria cardamomum against chemically induced hepatocellular carcinoma in rats by inhibiting NF-κB, oxidative stress, and activity of ornithine decarboxylase. *South African Journal of Botany.* 2016, 105:251–258.

16. Zheng J, Zhou Y, Li Y, et al. Spices for prevention and treatment of cancers. *Nutrients.* MDPI AG. 2016.

17. Karmakar S, Choudhury SR, Banik NL, et al. *Anti-Cancer Agents in Medicinal Chemistry.* 2011.

18. Liu Y, An T, Wan D, et al. Targets and mechanism used by cinnamaldehyde, the main active ingredient in cinnamon, in the treatment of breast cancer. *Front Pharmacol.* 2020, 11.

19. Alsemari A, Alkhodairy F, Aldakan A, et al. The selective cytotoxic anti-cancer properties and proteomic analysis of Trigonella Foenum-Graecum. *BMC Complement Altern Med.* 2014, 14.

20. Turrini E, Sestili P, Fimognari C. Overview of the anticancer potential of the "King of Spices" piper nigrum and its main constituent piperine. *Toxins (Basel)*. MDPI. 2020.

21. Kunnumakkara AB, Bordoloi D, Harsha C, et al. Curcumin mediates anticancer effects by modulating multiple cell signaling pathways. *Clin Sci*. Portland Press Ltd. 2017, p. 1781–1799.

22. Aggarwal BB, Kunnumakkara AB, Harlkumar KB, et al. Potential of spice-derived phytochemicals for cancer prevention. *Planta Med*. 2008, p. 1560–1569.

23. Saha A, Blando J, Silver E, et al. 6-Shogaol from dried ginger inhibits growth of prostate cancer cells both *in vitro* and *in vivo* through inhibition of STAT3 and NF-κB signaling. *Cancer Prevention Research*. 2014, 7:627–638.

24. Huang L, Song Y, Lian J, et al. Allicin inhibits the invasion of lung adenocarcinoma cells by altering tissue inhibitor of metalloproteinase/matrix metalloproteinase balance via reducing the activity of phosphoinositide 3-kinase/AKT signaling. *Oncol Lett*. 2017, 14:468–474.

25. Ren Q li, Wang Q, Zhang X Qun, et al. Anticancer activity of diosgenin and its molecular mechanism. *Chin J Integr Med*. Springer Science and Business Media Deutschland GmbH. 2023.

26. Rather RA, Bhagat M. Cancer chemoprevention and piperine: Molecular mechanisms and therapeutic opportunities. *Front Cell Dev Biol*. Frontiers Media S.A. 2018.

27. Pastorelli D, Fabricio ASC, Giovanis P, et al. Phytosome complex of curcumin as complementary therapy of advanced pancreatic cancer improves safety and efficacy of gemcitabine: Results of a prospective phase II trial. *Pharmacol Res*. 2018, 132:72–79.

28. Patel BB, Majumdar APN. Synergistic role of curcumin with current therapeutics in colorectal cancer: Minireview. *Nutr Cancer*. 2009, p. 842–846.

29. Zhang SS, Ni YH, Zhao CR, et al. Capsaicin enhances the antitumor activity of sorafenib in hepatocellular carcinoma cells and mouse xenograft tumors through increased ERK signaling. *Acta Pharmacol Sin*. 2018, 39:438–448.

30. Hakim L, Alias E, Makpol S, et al. Gelam honey and ginger potentiate the anti cancer effect of 5-FU against HCT 116 colorectal cancer cells. *Asian Pacific Journal of Cancer Prevention*. 2014, 15:4651–4657.

31. Țigu AB, Toma VA, Mot AC, et al. The synergistic antitumor effect of 5-fluorouracil combined with allicin against lung and colorectal carcinoma cells. *Molecules*. 2020, 25.

32. Yu C, Liu SL, Qi MH, et al. Cinnamaldehyde/ chemotherapeutic agents interaction and drug-metabolizing genes in colorectal cancer. *Mol Med Rep*. 2014, 9:669–676.

33. Fattah A, Morovati A, Niknam Z, et al. The synergistic combination of cisplatin and piperine induces apoptosis in MCF-7 cell line [internet]. *Iran J Public Health*. 2021. Available from: http://ijph.tums.ac.ir.

34. Choudhari AS, Mandave PC, Deshpande M, et al. Phytochemicals in cancer treatment: From preclinical studies to clinical practice. *Front Pharmacol*. Frontiers Media S.A. 2020.

Chapter 10

Role of Spices in Bioprotection and Clinical Trials: A Review

Mokshi Pathania,[a] **Koshika Sharma,**[a] **Munish Sharma,**[b]
Gurpreet Kaur,[c] **Deepak Sharma,**[d] **and Sakshi Bhushan**[a]

[a]*Department of Botany, Central University of Jammu,*
Bagla Suchani, Jammu & Kashmir, India
[b]*Department of Plant Science, Central University of Himachal Pradesh,*
Shahpur Parisar, Kangra, Himachal Pradesh, India
[c]*Department of Biotechnology, Thapar Institute of Engineering and Technology,*
Patiala, Punjab, India
[d]*Department of Plant Science, University of Manitoba, Winnipeg, Canada*

bhushan.sakshi8@gmail.com, deepak180001@gmail.com

10.1 Introduction

Since ancient times, mankind has looked upon to mother nature, as a source of natural drugs (Petrovska, et al., 2012). Traditional medicines are still regarded as the best healthcare system for the treatment of various diseases and it is one of the most effective methods of healthcare in over 60% of the world's total population. Interestingly, about 80% of people in developing countries depend directly on medicinal plants for therapeutic purposes, owing to their affordability, easy availability, and

Anticancer Spices: Dietary Input to Health
Edited by Hardeep Singh Tuli
Copyright © 2025 Jenny Stanford Publishing Pte. Ltd.
ISBN 978-981-5129-28-1 (Hardcover), 978-1-003-53466-2 (eBook)
www.jennystanford.com

accessibility (Shrestha, et al., 2003). Owing to the bioprotective activities of herbs, modern research has shifted toward the demonstration of the role of crucial phytoconstituents/ phytochemicals against various deleterious ailments including pancreatic, colon, breast, and lung cancer (Bhagat, et al., 2016).

Spices have been widely used as condiments for thousands of years because of their flavor, taste, and color. Due to the pandemic, people have started showing huge interest in exploring their medicinal properties. In spite of the fact that many medicinal plants have been reported to date, which play a key role in curing diseases, still there are major lacunas in their standardization and human usage at proper dosages (Fig. 10.1). Therefore, many clinical trials are now being conducted on certain important spices of therapeutic interest due to the presence of bioactive compounds such as alkaloids, terpenes, flavonoids, phenylpropanoids, and anthocyanins (Table 10.1) (Zheng, et al., 2016).

Interestingly, spices like black pepper, fenugreek, curcumin, ginger, garlic, clove, coriander, basil, saffron, black cumin, and many more are still under clinical trials to prevent and cure cancer conditions. Not only for cancer treatment, all these spices play an important role in fighting indigestion, skin diseases, viral/bacterial infections, inflammation, and neurodegenerative disorders (Kaefer, et al., 2008). This is because bioactive compounds present in these spices show action through different modes of action. The main mechanisms include inducing apoptosis, inhibiting proliferation, migration, and invasion of tumors, and sensitizing tumors to radiotherapy and chemotherapy (Wani, et al., 2022).

During the past few years, mounting healthcare expenditures and an increased desire to maintain good health and quality of life have shifted researchers' attention to diet, phytonutrients, disease prevention, and health promotion. Importantly, biomolecules in plants regulate key mechanisms in the therapeutic properties of spices/herbs (Wani, et al., 2022). Therefore, in Asian countries, including India, China, Japan, and Korea, there is an ancient tradition and cultural practice of attributing healing properties to herbs/plants/spices, which are extensively used in food

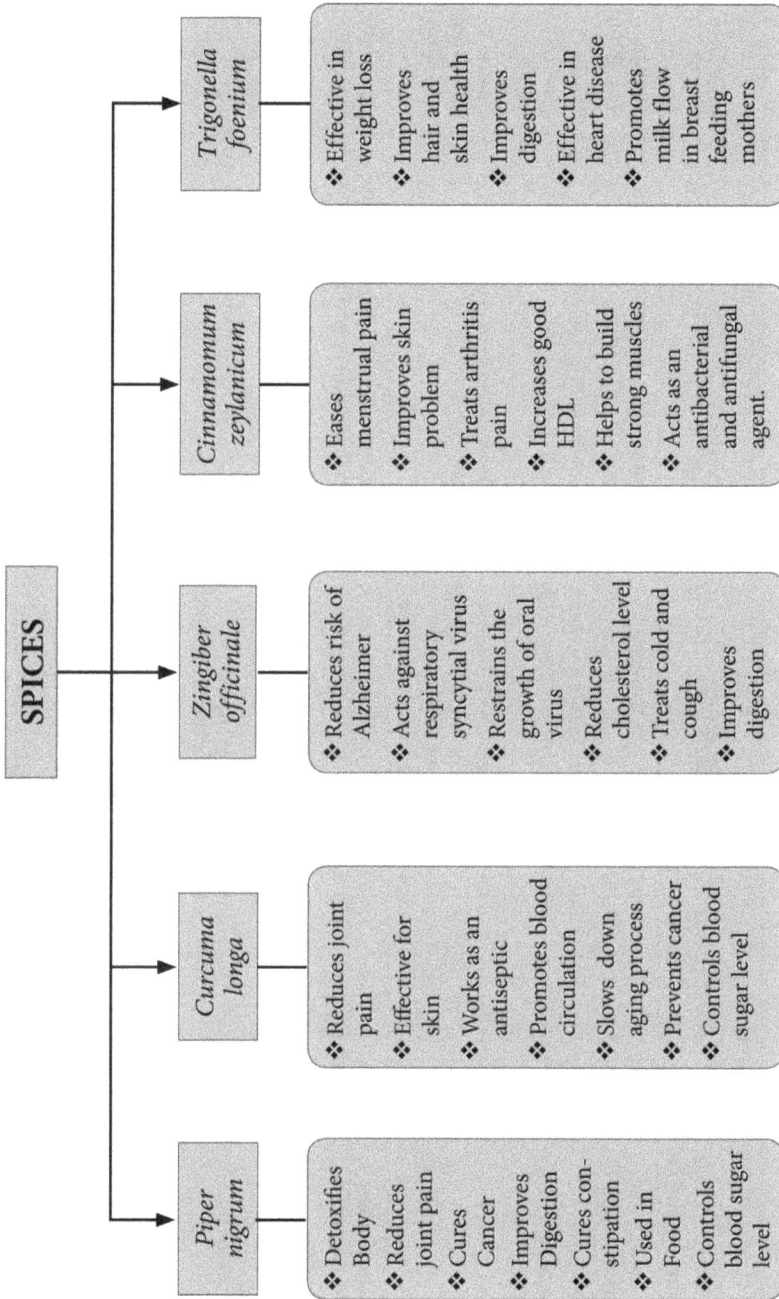

Figure 10.1 Uses of various spices.

Table 10.1 Clinical trials with different spices

Disorder	Type of trial/ duration/phase	Dose/treatment group	Observation	Reference
Curcuma longa (Turmeric)				
Pancreatic cancer (advanced stage)	Phase II, open-label trial	8 g curcumin; $n = 25$ patients; 2 months	No treatment-related toxicities were observed	(Dhillon, et al., 2008)
Breast cancer (advanced & metastatic)	Phase I, dose-escalation trial	500 mg/day curcumin + docetaxel for seven consecutive days, $n = 14$	Three dose-limiting toxicities were observed	(Bayet-Robert, et al., 2010)
Prostate cancer	Randomized, phase II	6 g/day for 7 days every 3 weeks, $n = 50$; 24 patients received placebo and docetaxel and 26 patients received docetaxel and curcumin	No difference between groups was reported	(Passildas-Jahanmohans, et al., 2021)
Pancreatic cancer (locally advanced & metastatic	Phase II, open-label trial	$n = 44$; 13 locally advanced and 34 metastatic	Partial response in 27.3% of patients and stable disease in 34.1% of patients	(Pastorelli, et al., 2018)
Pancreatic cancer (locally advanced & metastatic)	Phase II, open-label trial	8,000 mg of curcumin by mouth daily, concurrently with gemcitabine 1,000 mg/m (2) IV; $n = 17$; 4 locally advanced and 11 metastatic	The median time to tumor progression was 2.5 months	(Epelbaums, et al., 2010)
Gemcitabine-resistant pancreatic cancer	Phase I/II trial	8 g oral curcumin daily in combination with gemcitabine; $n = 21$; 19 patients received combination therapy and 2 patients received gemcitabine monotherapy	Phase I study outcome showed the safety of oral curcumin-containing products. Additionally, no patients withdrew from this study because of curcumin-containing product intolerability, thus meeting the primary endpoint of the phase II study	(Kanai, et al., 2011)

Disorder	Type of trial/duration/phase	Dose/treatment group	Observation	Reference
Colorectal cancer with inoperable liver metastases	Phase I, dose-escalation trial	$n = 12500$ mg, 1,000 mg, or 2,000 mg of curcumin-containing products + FOLFOX	This study revealed curcumin-containing products to be safe and tolerable adjuncts to FOLFOX chemotherapy in patients with CRLM at doses up to 2 g	(James, et al., 2015)
Colorectal cancer, liver metastases	Phase IIA	$n = 28$; 9 received FOLFOX alone and 18 received FOLFOX + curcumin-containing product	Daily oral curcumin-containing product combined with FOLFOX chemotherapy was safe and tolerable	(Irving, et al., 2015)
Colorectal treatment	For 12 weeks	1500 mg curcumin; $n = 44$ patients were given orally 2 times per day	No significant action of the concerned cancer	(Cruz-Core, et al., 2017)
Oral leucoplakia	Randomized trial for six months	4000 mg of curcumin, $n = 223$	It was concluded that 75 patients exhibited complete or partial responses and 62 patients from the placebo group showed a significant difference	(Golombick, et al., 2012)
Non-alcoholic fatty liver disease	8 weeks	1000 mg; $n = 50$ patients were given divided dose	It was reported that curcumin-containing product was well-tolerated and safe during the whole trial	(Panahi, et al., 2017)
Zingiber officinale (Ginger)				
Chemotherapy	5 days	1.2 g of ginger extract	After 3 consecutive cycles, it was found that the effect of vomiting was less than nausea	(Marx, et al., 2017)

(continued)

Table 10.1 *(continued)*

Disorder	Type of trial/ duration/phase	Dose/treatment group	Observation	Reference
Prostate cancer	Phase 1 for 2 weeks	100 mg of ginger extract	Suppressed the growth of the PC-3 xenograft, confirming its anti-prostate effects	(Karna, et al., 2017)
Migraine	Controlled trial	400 mg; $n = 60$	Potential to cure acute migraine	(Martins, et al., 2019)
Apoptotic and inhibitory effects on cell proliferation	Phase 2 for 24 hours	Concentration range = 50/100 or 200 µg/ml	Down-regulation of anti-apoptotic genes (Bcl-2), growth factor receptors (EBFR family) and downstream of signaling partners (PI3k, Ras/Raf/MAPK), cell cycle machinery (CDKs, TERT, TOP2A, TOP2B)	(Nair, et al., 2014)
Colorectal cancer	For 3/7 days	250 mg of ginger extract or capsules, $n = 10$	Reduced colonic COX-1 protein levels	(Jiang, et al., 2013)
Increased risk for colorectal cancer	Pilot trial for 28 days	Pilot trial with 250 g of ginger extract powder	Reduced Bax expression, P21, Bcl-2, while increasing apoptosis and differentiation	(Citronberg, et al., 2013)
***Cinnamomum* (Cinnamon)**				
Risk for the glycemic amounts	Triple-blind placebo-controlled randomized clinical trial, for 3 months	$n = 147$ 500 mg of capsules twice daily for 3 months	Capacity to regulate BMI, lipid profile, and glycemic amounts	(Roghayeh Zare, et al., 2019)
Role of cinnamon in decreasing glycemic level	Phase 1 for 90 days	$n = 160$	Reduced glycemic measures in a person with type-2 diabetes	(Jose, et al., 2022)

Disorder	Type of trial/ duration/phase	Dose/treatment group	Observation	Reference
Type-2 diabetes	For 12 weeks	500 mg of cinnamon or placebo thrice daily having $n = 27$/group	Results showed an improved response of fasting plasma glucose (FPG)	[Romeo, et al., 2020]
Type-2 diabetes	Controlled trial	$n = 44$ patients	The administration has very little beneficial effect on the reduction of ICAM-1 and VCAM-1 in patients with type-2 diabetes	[Bruno, et al., 2008]
Piper nigrum (Black Pepper)				
Non-alcoholic fatty liver disease	Randomized double-blind	$n = 65$, Phospholipidated curcumin 250 mg/day equivalent to 50 mg/day pure curcumin	Alteration in serum adipokines levels. Curcumin efficacy increased with long-term use at a higher dose	[Mirhafez, et al., 2019]
Metabolic syndrome	Randomized control trial for 8 weeks	1 g/day; $N = 117$ with ($n = 59$) or placebo ($n = 58$) groups	Significantly attenuates the systemic oxidative stress in such patients	[Panahi, et al., 2016]
Non-alcoholic fatty liver disease	Randomized controlled parallel-group trial	500 mg curcuminoids; $n = 70$; 5 mg piperine	Reduces the severity of the disease	[Panahi, et al., 2019]
Type-2 diabetes	Randomized double-blind placebo-controlled trial	A daily dose of 500 mg/day co-administered with piperine 5 mg/day	Glycemic and hepatic studies reported regulation of type-2 and the therapeutic potential of BP	[Panahi, et al., 2018]

(continued)

Table 10.1 *(continued)*

Trigonella foenum-graecum (Fenugreek)

Disorder	Type of trial/ duration/phase	Dose/treatment group	Observation	Reference
Type-2 diabetes mellitus (T2DM)	8 weeks	15 g; n = 48 patients	Fenugreek seed consumption significantly decreased high-sensitivity C-reactive protein, increased superoxide dismutase activity, and did not affect GPX, TAC, IL-6, or TNF-α levels	[Tavakoly, et al., 2018]
Younger male symptoms of aging	30–60 days	57 patients of 26 years of age were given 400 mg of curcumin	The fenugreek male groups significantly reported the improvement in males showing aged symptoms thus establishing effective nutritional intervention for improving aging male symptoms, anxiety levels, and grip strength	[Hausenblas, et al., 2021]
Hyperglycemia	10 days	3 g; n = 60 patients administered fenugreek powder	This resulted in a significant fall in mean glucose levels suggesting that a daily diet with fenugreek seeds can be explored as an add-on therapy along with other medications	[Kooshki, et al., 2020]
Sexual cycle and its behavioral response in females	42 days	250 mg; n = 48 women	The results showed an enhancement in estradiol, free testosterone, and, total testosterone, hormones. But there was no improvement shown in the level of progesterone and FSH	[Khanna, et al., 2021]

preparations (Sahoo, et al., 2021). Moreover, phytochemicals/ constituents in spices, which primarily serve in plant protection, are vitamins of the 21st century. Considering the above facts, it is important to explore the local knowledge, in order to establish a scientific basis for its benefits and utilization, especially through clinical trials and a few of the spices are still undergoing extensive clinical trials for establishing their authentication. Keeping this in view, the present review is focused on important spices, which are presently being studied via such studies in the following sections.

10.1.1 *Piper nigrum* (Black Pepper)

One of the most widely used spices, *P. nigrum* has significant ethnobotanical importance. It is cultivated in over 26 countries, with overall production of 315–320 000 tons of pepper (black and white). The important growing locations are India, Indonesia, Malaysia, Brazil, Thailand, Sri Lanka, Vietnam, and China (Krishnamoorthy, et al., 2010). Black pepper is often considered as a traditional remedy against various diseases including cough, sore throat, and many more common conditions. It is added to food to enhance flavors. Black pepper is characterized by its pungent smell contributed by the alkaloid piperine and flavor due to volatile oil. Piperine is found in 2–7.4% of both black and white peppers, with higher amounts observed in black pepper fruits. It has radiation-protective effects and may help lower blood cholesterol, triglycerides, and glucose levels. Other alkaloids in pepper extracts, such as piperanine, piperettine, piperylin A, piperolein B, and pipericine, also exhibit some pungency, but their overall contribution to pepper pungency is minor (Ekor, et al., 2014).

   A literature survey reveals that black pepper is well-known for its anti-inflammatory, anti-cancerous, antioxidant, antinociceptive, and bio-stimulating activities (Fig. 10.2) (Srinivasan, et al., 2007). It is also very effective in various gastrointestinal problems. Among several studies, many observations have provided evidence of its role in the modulation of critical checkpoints that can result in cancer if not inhibited or arrested. Studies show that piperine, a chemical constituent found in black pepper, shows synergistic

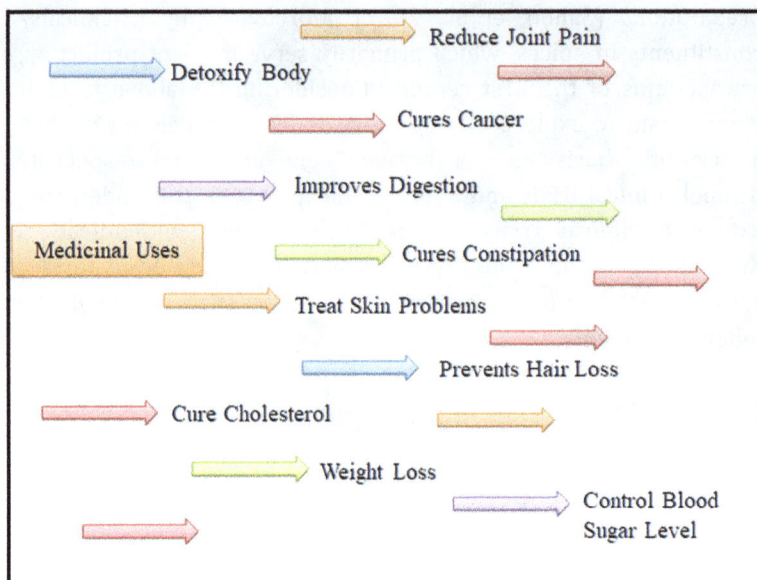

Figure 10.2 Schematic representation of different roles of black pepper.

antiproliferative action against the MCF7 cell line, further is also synergizes tamoxifen in combination with hesperidin (Khamis, et al., 2018). In some cases, in the MDA MB-231 cell line model, it is known to lower the LC50 of paclitaxel and during the paclitaxel action time, it reduces the lag phase. An experiment was performed in mice, in an *in vivo* model, EMT6/P cells inoculation in Balb/C, where piperine with thymoquinone inhibits the angiogenesis process and induces apoptosis. The results showed that black pepper reduces the proliferation of cells and induces apoptosis by activating caspase-3 and inhibiting the cleavage of PARP (poly(ADP-ribose) polymerase) (Khamis, et al., 2018). Mt, et al. (2013) showed that piperine pretreatment has a tendency to accelerate paclitaxel-mediated killing in breast cancer cells. The results of the treatment with black pepper showed the regulation of the cell cycle and arrest at the G1 phase and apoptosis was observed in SK-MEL and B16-F0 cell lines because of the activation of checkpoint kinase-1 followed by cleavage of Caspase-3 and downregulation of XIAP (Moorthi, et al., 2013). One of the studies reveals cancer inhibition by giving curcumin–piperine dual drug-loaded nanoparticles during multidrug-resistant cancer trials (Rajagopalan, et al., 2020). In the same way, the extrication of BP showed anti-cancer effects during the study of a cholangiocarcinoma cell line. Piperine effectively suppressed the proliferation of affected cells in prostate cancer cell lines by lowering the overall levels of phosphorylated STAT-3 and nuclear factor-kB (NF-kB) (Sedeky, et al., 2018). When BP-based nanoparticles containing piperine were compared to free medicines, their cytotoxicity increased significantly, raising the G2/M and pre-GI populations. Due to the presence of piperine, inhibition of cell-cycle progression in rectal cancer cells was observed resulting in ROS-mediated apoptosis (Yaffe, et al., 2013).

A lot of clinical trials were conducted on black pepper to know about its effective role against various diseases. Piperine (PIP), the most important ingredient found in both black and white pepper, was considered and focused on these investigations. Because of the aforementioned facts, the effect of BP supple-mentation with turmeric extract and ginger on prostaglandin E2 (PGE2) in patients with chronic knee osteoarthritis was detected, in which 60 patients with two distinct levels of knee osteoarthritis (Grades 2 and 3) were evaluated for four weeks. It was observed that the intake of selected herbs twice improved PGE_2 levels in patients with chronic knee osteoarthritis (Heidari-Beni, et al., 2020). Similarly, PIP was studied for its effect on the metabolism and pharmacokinetics of Carbamazepine (CBZ) in 12 volunteers/patients, which showed the presence of potential pharmacokinetic interaction between PP and CBZ (Chashmniam, et al., 2019) conducted a double-blind placebo-controlled trial with 55 subjects who received curcumin (500 mg) in combination with piperine (5 mg) for 8 weeks. Interestingly, PIP and curcumin modulated PAB values in studied patients. In a study, supplementing PIP in 40 oropharyngeal dysphagia (OP) patients indicated strong improvement in safety, after swallowing with a maximal therapeutic effect at 1 mM (Rofes, et al., 2013). It was inferenced that short-term treatment of patients suffering from knee osteoarthritis with PIP, significantly attenuates systemic oxidative stress in such patients, thus overall relieving them from osteoarthritis symptoms (Panahi, et al., 2016). A similar clinical trial by (Panahi, et al., 2019) in non-alcoholic fatty liver disease (NAFLD) in a randomized controlled, parallel-group trial with 70 subjects for 12 weeks, established that BP results in beneficial effects if administered as PIP along with curcuminoids on disease severity in patients with NAFLD. A trial involving patients suffering from type-2 were supplemented with BP as PIP in addition to curcuminoids and were assessed for their glycemic and hepatic biomarkers. Interestingly, this study also reported the regulation of both parameters indicating the therapeutic potential of BP (Panahi, et al., 2018).

10.1.2 *Curcuma longa* (Turmeric)

Curcuma longa, also known as turmeric, is a South and Southeast Asian native. It has traditionally been used in a variety of food preparations as well as women's cosmetic formulas. It originated in the tropical forests of South India's west coast and has been propagated vegetatively for thousands of years in the Indian subcontinent. It belongs to the Zingiberaceae family and comprises hundreds of rhizomatous herbs found in India, China, Indonesia, Siam, the Malay Archipelago, and Northern Australia. The chemistry or physiological effect of extracts and ingredients of distinct curcuma species is unclear in the literature, and proper verification of the source plant is still missing (Govindrajan, et al., 1980). Approximately 235 compounds have been reported to date, including phenolic, terpenoids, diarylheptanoids, diarylpentanoids, phenylpropene, monoterpenes, sesquiterpenes, diterpenes, triterpenoids, sterols, alkaloids, and others. Apart from these, curcuminoids and essential oils have been discovered to be key bioactive components, contributing to a variety of bioactivities in *in vitro* and *in vivo* bioassays, and are reported to be abundant in rhizomes. Curcuminoids in turmeric rhizomes vary greatly depending on variety, location, source, growth method, and environmental conditions. Furthermore, differences in the composition of essential oils of turmeric rhizomes have been observed depending on variety and geographical region (Li, et al., 2011). Among the many phytoconstituents, curcumin has been identified as the most important component in the rhizomes of *Curcuma longa L.*, which has also been isolated in a pure crystalline form from the turmeric plant for investigation as an effective anti-cancer drug (Laabbar, et al., 1990).

Extensive research over the past decades has shown that curcuminoids, which belong to the diferuloylmethane class of natural compounds, interfere with several cell signaling pathways, lending evidence to curcumin's possible function in cancer prevention. It has been observed that curcumin modulates the balance in the mitochondrial membrane potential, which, in turn, suppresses the Bcl-xL protein (Wang, et al., 2008). Since the extrinsic apoptotic pathway depends upon death receptors on cells, it further triggers tumor necrosis factor (TNF)-related apoptosis. Several *in vitro* investigations have established the significance of curcumin in the stimulation of the expression of death receptors DR 4 and DR 5 (Braga, et al., 2003). Interestingly, numerous studies have demonstrated turmeric's and its phytoconstituents' exceptional ability to trigger apoptosis in various cell lines by blocking or downregulating intracellular transcription factors (Tfs). These factors include NF-κB, activator protein-1 (AP-1), cyclooxygenase-II (COX-2), nitric oxide synthase, matrix metalloproteinase-9 (MMP-9), and STAT3, which are involved in many cell survival processes. Curcumin, according to Siddiqui, et al. (2018), follows a new anti-cancer strategy by reducing/decreasing glucose absorption and lactate generation in cancer cells via the process of downregulation of pyruvate kinase M2 (PKM2). Furthermore, several studies have investigated curcumin and its derivatives for its capacity to decrease numerous cancers by targeting cells (Fig. 10.3).

Owing to the anti-cancerous potential of *C. longa,* at least six phase-I clinical trials have been investigated, which were based upon investigations of the pharmacokinetics and dynamics of pure curcumin in human subjects. These experiment trials reported systemic exposure of curcumin and curcumin-containing products at the dose level of 8000 mg/day, which was safe and tolerable. Furthermore, the peak serum values/concentrations ranged from 47 ng/ml to 1389 ng/ml daily. Interestingly, five clinical studies have been done in order to evaluate curcumin supplementation

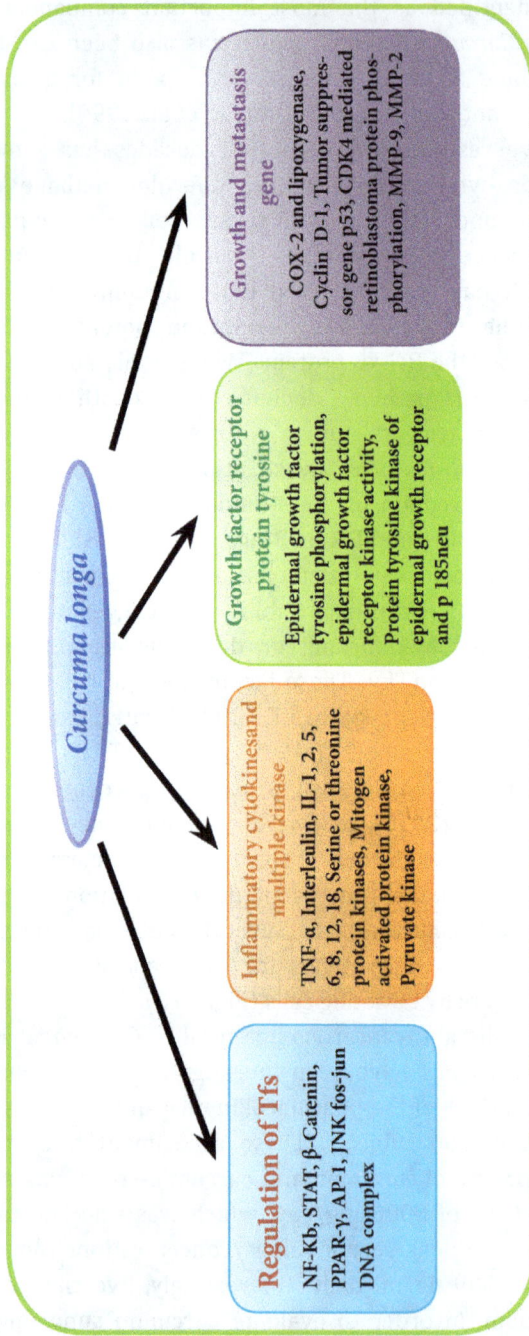

Figure 10.3 Schematic representation of molecular targets of curcumin.

on biomarkers of different types of cancer in such patients. The range of dose was between 20 mg/day and 3,000 mg/day. It was observed that there was an association between alteration in biomarkers and patient outcome, as a result, obtained pointed toward increased TAC and decreased SOD (Hejazi, et al., 2016), enhanced p53 expression and reduction in TNF-alpha (Panahi, et al., 2014), decreased TGF-beta and IL-6 (Panahi, et al., 2014), and nitric oxide reduction (Ghahaulat, et al., 2012). A study conducted by Cruz-Corre, et al. (2017) in patients with corectal condition (n = 44 patients), at a dose of 1500 mg oral, 2 times/day using pure curcumin indicated no significant change in the action of concerned CUR.

Similarly, patients suffering from oral leucoplakia introduced with curcumin-based products were investigated in a randomized study/trial in 223 patients. It was concluded that 75 patients exhibited complete or partial responses and 62 patients from the placebo group showed significant differences. In a double-blind placebo study, 36 multiple myeloma patients receiving 4000 mg curcumin-containing product for three months were considered. The results obtained indicated a decrease in the free light chain ratio (rFLC) (Golombick, et al., 2012). Curcumin is also known to be effective in non-alcoholic fatty liver disease (NAFLD). A study used subjects that were divided into two parts, and further, these two divided doses (1000 mg) were administered for 8 weeks in n = 50 and the placebo with n = 50. The results showed that during the whole trial, the curcumin-containing products were quite effective (Panahi, et al., 2017). Similarly, a trial focused on 228 patients also established favorable results regarding curcumin-containing products on subjects when administered at higher doses, which efficiently decreased liver marker enzymes (Mansour-Ghanaei, et al., 2019). A few case reports have suggested that curcumin-containing products may have an anti-cancer impact after 60 months of testing, as the patient's tumor remained stable with minor variations in paraprotein levels (Zaidi, et al., 2017). Another case report published used imatinib and a curcumin-containing product in a patient suffering from a c-kit–positive metastatic ACC, who was administered 225 mg/month of a curcumin-containing product indicated significant results (Demiray, et al., 2016). In a randomized phase-II clinical trial, docetaxel and curcumin were compared to docetaxel and placebo in patients with metastatic castration-resistant prostate cancer (Passildas-Jahanmohan, et al., 2021). This study concluded that there is no significant difference in progression-free survival, responsiveness to prostate-specific antigen, or overall survival rate between the groups tested. Furthermore, three clinical trials were conducted to evaluate different formulations and curcumin-based products in combination with gemcitabine at a dose of 1000 mg weekly for 3–4 weeks (Kanai, et al., 2011). In patients utilizing this combination of a curcumin-containing medication and gemcitabine, the overall disease control rate was 61.4%, with lower-than-expected hepatological damage. Furthermore, in patients with metastatic colorectal cancer, a combination phase-I dose escalation experiment/study and phase-II trial including oral consumption of curcumin-containing products with folinic acid, fluorouracil, and oxaliplatin (FOLFOX) (CUFOX) was done. Curcumin was proven to be safe and well tolerated by FOLFOX in phase I, but no complete response was recorded in phase II (Howells, et al., 2015).

10.1.3   *Zingiber officinale* (Ginger)

Zingiber officinale belonging to the family Zingiberacae is often called "ginger". It is a perennial plant with having long cultivation history. Among various spices, it is one of the most popular spices with an enriched and long history of cultivation for more than 2000 years. Moreover, it has been extensively used as a flavoring agent for its pungency and is well described in Indian Ayurveda and traditional Chinese and complementary medicine. Till now, almost 160 phytoconstituents have been reported that include volatile oils, gingerol and its analogues, phenylalkanoids, sulfonates, diarylheptanoids steroids, and monoterpenoid glycoside compounds (Imtiyaz, et al., 2013). There is strong evidence that ginger has the ability to act against various disorders such as gastrointestinal, cancer, obesity, nervous conditions, cardiovascular diseases, liver and kidney disorders, and diabetes (Zhang, et al., 2021). It has been used medicinally since antiquity, having considerable records in Sanskrit, Chinese, Arabic, and Greek ethnomedicine. The primary medicinal component is pale yellow or taupe brown in color, with an irregular mass of thick, figure-branched, fleshy, and scaly structures, and an aromatic and spicy scent.

Jiang, et al. (2013) looked into ginger's potential as an anti-inflammatory agent in the prevention of colorectal cancer. A randomized controlled trial on 10 participants with a higher likelihood of colon cancer was induced with 250 mg of ginger extract or capsules for 3/7 days, which dramatically lowered colonic COX-1 protein levels. Ginger had no effect on 15-PGDH protein expression in either high- or low-risk subjects. Citronberg, et al. (2013) conducted a pilot study on 20 persons at high risk for colorectal cancer who were given 250 g of ginger extract powder (5% gingerols/8 capsules) or a placebo daily for 28 days. Ginger was found to inhibit Bax, p21, Bcl-2, and hTERT expression while enhancing apoptosis and differentiation. The findings suggested that ginger may inhibit proliferation in normal-appearing colonic epithelium and support a bigger investigation to test these effects further. Zick, et al. (2014) conducted a study with 20 volunteers who were randomly randomized to either a placebo or 2.0 g/d ginger for 28 days. Patients receiving ginger therapy showed considerably lower levels of AA and greater levels of LTB4 when compared to placebo. Ginger, a COX and PGE2 inhibitor, has been shown in one research to reduce the incidence of adenomas and PGE2 levels in persons at high risk of colon cancer. A study by Marx, et al. (2017) was carried out to overcome serious methodological flaws in their earlier studies. During the first three cycles of chemotherapy, patients were randomly assigned to 1.2 g of standardized ginger extract as a medication, and the functional living index emesis (FLIE) questionnaire was used to measure the outcomes with the quality of life (QOL). After the three consecutive cycles, vomiting was less often than nausea only for the ginger extract as compared to that of placebo in which the effect of vomiting and nausea is greater. In a research project, carried out in the US (Karna, et al., 2019), the daily oral treatment of ginger at a dose of 100 mg/kg body weight; on the other hand, reduced the growth of the PC-3 xenograft, demonstrating its anti-prostate properties, both *in vitro* and *in vivo*. Furthermore, the same dose reduced the enhanced activity of tumor necrosis factor-alpha (TNF-alpha) in another trial. Gunathilake, et al. (2015) and Rupasinghe, et al. (2015) studied that ginger has been shown to inhibit tumor growth through a variety of molecular pathways, including the upregulation of suppressor genes, apoptosis, and the induction and inactivation of vascular endothelial growth factor (VEGF), a tumor angiogenic factor that promotes tumor growth and progression (Gunathilake, et al., 2015).

Martins, et al. (2019) conducted a study in which 60 patients were given a 400-mg dose of ginger extract to test the potential of ginger to improve acute migraine as a standard treatment. According to Nair, et al. (2014), fatty acid esters of phloridzin promote apoptosis in human liver cancer cells via altered gene expression. He investigated the antiproliferative action of fatty acid esters in HepG2 and normal cells. Hepatic cancer cells and normal human hepatocytes (HP-F) were treated for 24 hours with varied doses of fatty acids at 1, 10, 50, and 100. This was thought to be due to the downregulation of anti-apoptotic genes (Bcl-2), growth factor receptors (EBFR family), signaling partners (PI3k, Ras/Raf/MAPK), and cell cycle machinery (CDKs, TERT, TOP2A, TOP2B). As a result, phloridzin fatty esters have the ability to reduce the expression of several critical proteins involved in cell cycle regulation, cell cycle regulation, and apoptosis. Treatment with ginger extract increased apoptosis by lowering the expression of genes implicated in the Ras/ERK and PI3K/Akt pathways. It also boosted caspase-9 expression, which induced apoptosis in HT-29 colorectal cancer cells (Fig. 10.4).

6-Shogaol from dried ginger suppresses prostate cancer cell growth both *in vitro* and *in vivo* by inhibiting STAT3 and NF-κB signaling (Saha, et al., 2014). The investigations found that the effect of ginger derivatives SHO on the proliferation of prostate cancer cells was evaluated when prostrate cells were treated with ginger extract. By lowering constitutive and interleukin (IL) levels, 6-SHO successfully triggered apoptosis in cultured human cells (LNCaP, DU145, and PC3), which activated STAT3 and reduced both constitutive and TNF-induced NF-κB activity in these cells.

It also reduced the expression of several STAT3 and NF-κB target genes, including cyclin D1, cell cycle, and apoptosis regulatory genes. 6-SHO was found to be more effective at fighting cancer than two other chemicals present in ginger, 6-gingerol, and 6-paradol. Ginger's cytotoxic effects and underlying mechanisms in prostate cancer were investigated both *in vivo* and *in vitro*. 6-gingerol, 10-gingerol, 6-shogaol, and 10-shogaol were discovered to have an antiproliferative effect on human prostate cancer cells by downregulating the protein expression of multidrug resistance-related protein 1 (MRP1) and glutathione-S-transferase (GST) (Saha, et al., 2014). In a similar study, 6-gingerol inhibited the development of HeLa human cervical cancer cells and triggered cell cycle arrest in the G0/G1 phase by lowering cyclin A and cyclin D1 protein levels (Liu, et al., 2012).

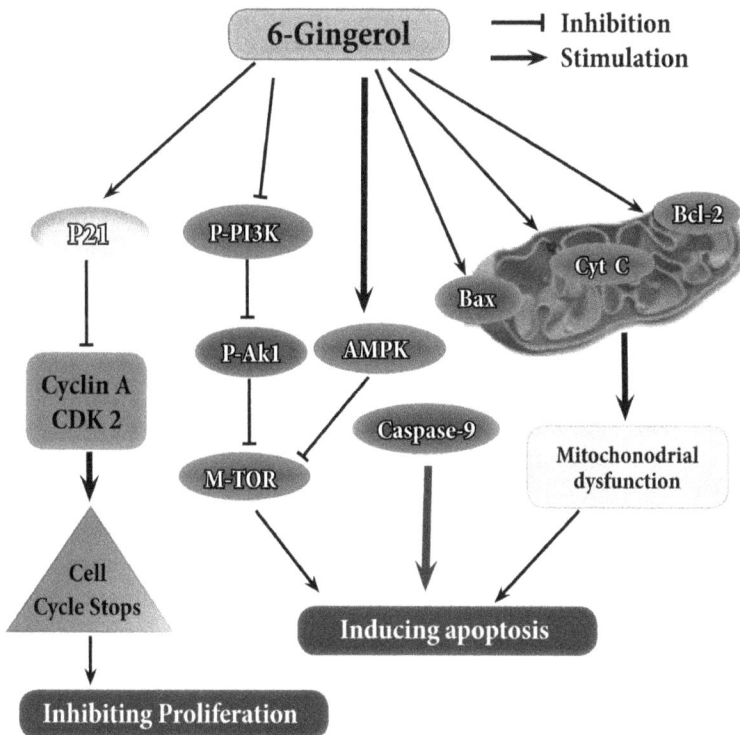

Figure 10.4 Factors affecting inhibition and stimulation of apoptosis.

10.1.4 *Cinnamomum zeylanicum*

Cinnamon is an ancient spice derived from the bark of numerous kinds of evergreen trees of the *Cinnamomum genus*. Cinnamon is native to Sri Lanka and China, while it is also native to southern China and mainland Southeast Asia, including west Myanmar. *Cinnamomum zeylanicum*, often called "true cinnamon" or "Ceylon cinnamon," is principally used for its aromatic bark, which is used as a spice under the culinary name "cinnamon." The buds are also used as a spice, particularly in India and Asia, as well as in Europe and North America. According to a review of the literature, cinnamon aqueous extract may be effective as an anti-inflammatory and antioxidant agent. Sri Lankan medicine has traditionally used its extract to cure/treat detrimental disorders such as cancer, diabetes, allergies, inflammations, and microbial and parasite infections due to its wide range of uses, including as a flavoring agent and spice (Gruenwald, et al., 2010).

Cinnamon contains many resinous compounds like cinnamaldehyde, cinnamate, cinnamic acid, and many essential oils. According to Singh, et al. (2014), the spicy taste and scent are caused by the presence of cinnamaldehyde and occur as a result of oxygen absorption. Cinnamon darkens in color as it ages, improving the resinous components. Several studies indicate that cinnamon has a variety of physiochemical qualities. Cinnamon contains a variety of essential oils, including trans-cinnamaldehyde, cinnamyl acetate, eugenol, L-borneol, caryophyllene oxide, b-caryophyllene, L-bornyl acetate, E-nerolidol, -cubebene, -terpineol, -terpinolene, and -thujene (Singh, et al., 2007). Due to the presence of these compounds, the aqueous extract of cinnamon has been known to act against cancerous cells and also inhibit cell growth (Wahab, et al., 2017; Ariaee-Nasab, et al., 2014). The observation made it clear that cinnamon aqueous extract is more potent as compared to individual phytoconstituent (Sing, et al., 2009). An *in vitro* study also reported toxicity of cinnamon against oral squamous carcinoma cells (OSCC) reaching almost 90% within 48 hours. Moreover, OSCC along with saffron showed cytotoxicity at lower concentrations (Dehghani Nazhvani, et al., 2020). It has been also observed to downregulate proangiogenic factors leading to antiangiogenic properties via modulating

VEGF expression, which, in turn, inhibits Cox-2, HIF-1α, STAT3, and protein kinase B (AKT) in *in vitro* as well as *in vivo* systems of the experiment (Luo, et al., 2017). Yun, et al. (2009) reported the presence of cinnamon increased the cytolytic activity of CD8+ T lymphocytes via increased production of perforin and granzymes. Cinnamon extracts have been studied to see if they can decrease the production of proapoptotic genes, including Bcl-2, Bcl-xL, and survivin, via NFkB and activator protein AP-1 signaling, which was supported by molecular docking study done by Kwon, et al. (2010) and Varalakshmi, et al. (2017). The Histone deacetylase family member-8 (HDAC8) played a crucial role in the progression of many cancer types such as human colon, lung, and cervical. Therefore, the knockdown of HDAC8 showed the attenuation of cancer conditions, which was reported during the use of cinnamon, cinnamic acid, cinnamyl alcohol, and cinnamaldehyde *in vitro* and *in vivo* systems of study (Patil, et al., 2017). Similarly, enhanced activity of 26S proteasome is positively associated with the transformed cancerous cells. Procyanidine, one of the active phytoconstituents of cinnamon, is reported to have antiprotease activity against 26S, thus regulating cancer cell survival and proliferation (Gopalakrishnan, et al., 2018). Abeysekera, et al. (2022) analyzed leaf extracts of Ceylon cinnamon against MCF7, HePG2, and AN3CA carcinoma cell lines and evaluated cytotoxicity, which was significant against these cell lines.

Several clinical trials on the bioactivities of cinnamon have been conducted. A randomized experiment with 147 individuals was done to investigate BMI, glycemic indices, and lipid profile using a triple-blind response. Cinnamon was discovered to have the ability to regulate all parameters (Zare, et al., 2019). In a similar investigation, a triple-blind clinical trial was designed to assess the efficacy of cinnamon as an adjuvant treatment in lowering glycemic levels in 160 persons with type-2 diabetes by monitoring different glycated hemoglobin levels for 90 days. Cinnamon lowered glycemic measurements in those with type-2 diabetes, albeit only slightly (Lira, et al., 2022). In a similar study, individuals with prediabetes were considered for a double-blind placebo-controlled clinical investigation in which randomly assigned patients received 500 mg of cinnamon or placebo thrice daily for 12 weeks (n = 27/group). The results showed that those patients who were given cinnamon had a better response to fasting plasma glucose (FPG) (Romeo, et al., 2020). Another trial was conducted to investigate the benefit and utilization of cinnamon for 44 patients who were screened for type-2 diabetes based on ICAM-1 and VCAM-1 levels. Cinnamon supplementation appears to have a negligible effect on the reduction of ICAM-1 and VCAM-1 in type-2 diabetes patients for the development of atherogenesis.

10.1.5 *Trigonella foenum* (Fenugreek)

Fenugreek (*Trigonella foenum-graecum L.*), because of its yellowish-white triangular blossoms, is also known as Trigonella, which means 'small triangle' in Latin (Hiles, et al., 2021). According to historical studies, it is believed that fenugreek is efficiently used in both Chinese and Ayurvedic medicine to cure diseases in humans (Smith, et al., 2003). One of the important constituents of fenugreek is sapogenin whose content varies during its developmental stages. It is also believed that the sapogenin content of fenugreek plants in Ethiopia is much more than that of those in Palestine. Since it is a legume crop, it also plays an important role in fixing nitrogen as well as serving as a source of fertilizer for many crops. Fenugreek is believed to be very essential for soothing and relaxing inflamed tissues. This is because of its natural constituents including mucilagins. Apart from this, it is also a natural source of iron, thiamine, sodium, and sulfate (Arivalagan, et al., 2013). Trigonella's entire plant body contains many elements, but its seeds contain alkaloids such as trigonelline, gentianine, and carpine chemicals. Fiber, 4-hydroxyisoleucine, and fenugreekine are also found in the seeds, respectively. By enhancing insulin receptors and boosting insulin secretion, fenugreek seeds may increase glucose utilization and insulin secretion, thereby lowering diabetes (Pandian, et al., 2022). Sethi, et al. (2018) conducted a clinical trial on the pro-apoptotic and anti-cancer properties of diosgenin, a naturally occurring compound in fenugreek seeds. This sapogenin chemical contained in fenugreek seeds has anti-cancer effects. It has been shown to reverse multi-drug resistance in cancer cells, making them more receptive to standard chemotherapy. There is no prior evidence to support the use of fenugreek in diabetic patients, but a study was undertaken in which fenugreek was studied and investigated for its effects on oxidative stress and inflammation in persons with type-2 diabetes mellitus (T2DM) (Tavakoly, et al., 2018). 48 T2DM patients were randomly assigned to one of two groups: intervention or control. Patients in the intervention group were given 15 gm of fenugreek seed powder each day and conducted physical tests to determine the optimum nutritional intake. Fenugreek seed consumption reduced high-sensitivity C-reactive protein, enhanced superoxide dismutase activity, and had no effect on GPX, TAC, IL-6, or TNF- levels (Tavakoly, et al., 2018). In research with 12 patients divided into two groups, fenugreek was compared to glibenclamide for managing blood glucose in patients with uncontrolled type-II DM on standard medication. The patients were divided into two groups and given 2 g of fenugreek per day, where fenugreek was able to act as an anti-diabetic medicine to reduce blood glucose levels (Najdi, et al., 2019). A study was conducted to investigate the effect of Trigonella on the male symptoms of aging in healthy younger males. A randomized controlled experiment was conducted with volunteers (n = 57; age = 26) who were given 400 mg of fenugreek (n = 19). The fenugreek male groups considerably improved in males, demonstrating aged symptoms and establishing an effective dietary intervention for improving aging male symptoms, anxiety levels, and grip strength (Hausenblas, et al., 2021). Nowadays, stress-induced hyperglycemia is found to be associated with critically ill patients. A study was focused on a randomized controlled clinical trial that consisted of 60 patients (n = 30), and about 3 g of fenugreek powder was administered. It was seen that treatment for 10 days resulted in a significant fall in mean glucose levels, the results laid a proposal that fenugreek seeds if taken along with a daily diet can be explored as an add-on therapy along with other medications (Kooshki, et al., 2020). Since fenugreek seeds have been shown to possess high fiber content, therefore a short-term investigation was designed in patients with diabetes. Interestingly, these seeds were able to exert hypocholesterolemic and hypoglycaemic effects in studied patients. Similarly, a long-term study determined hypolipidemic regulation of fenugreek (25 g). This trial indicated selective action of fenugreek to reduce LDL and VLDL that can prevent atherosclerosis (Sharma, et al., 1996). There was a study conducted on healthy menstruating women to observe benefits in their sexual cycle and their behavioral response, like irritability. 48 women were selected for this trial and 250 mg of fenugreek was given to them as a supplement. The results showed an enhancement in estradiol, free testosterone, and total testosterone, hormones. However, there was no improvement shown in the level of progesterone and FSH. Therefore, the study concluded that FSH can be used as a natural alternative for women with sexual issues (Khanna, et al., 2021).

10.2 Conclusion

Since ancient times, spices have been used not only to flavor food but are also well-known for their medicinal power. India is well-known for its spices and medicinal herbs, which possess a wide range of physiological and pharmacological qualities. Importantly, the anti-inflammatory, anti-cancer, and anti-diabetic properties of cinnamon, ginger, turmeric, and curcumin have been extensively researched. Today, there is enough scientific evidence that plants can help in alleviating the conditions associated with specific diseases and can prevent or reduce risks associated with degenerative diseases including diabetes, obesity, cardiovascular diseases, and cancer. This fact is itself supported by many experimental findings in a meta-analysis of more than 1.5 million healthy adults. Scientific research has proven that spices/herbs possess phytochemicals that can act as strong bioprotective agents in both *in vitro* and *in vivo*, and in clinical studies, establishing their crucial role in future drug discovery and medicinal solutions. One of the difficulties in understanding the value of herbs for health is a lack of nomenclature, standardized extracts, heterogeneity in studies, and a lack of knowledge of chemical profiles. Nonetheless, the evidence is intriguing and warrants more investigation. It is critical to conduct more clinical trials in order to determine which will benefit the most from these natural medicines.

References

Abeysekera, W. P. K. M., Premakumara, G. A. S., Ratnasooriya, W. D., & Abeysekera, W. K. S. M. (2022). Anti-inflammatory, cytotoxicity and antilipidemic properties: Novel bioactivities of true cinnamon (Cinnamomum zeylanicum Blume) leaf. *BMC Complementary Medicine and Therapies, 22*(1), 1–15.

Ahmad, A., Alghamdi, S. S., Mahmood, K., & Afzal, M. (2016). Fenugreek a multipurpose crop: Potentialities and improvements. *Saudi Journal of Biological Sciences, 23*(2), 300–310. https://doi.org/10.1016/j.sjbs.2015.09.015.

Arivalagan, M. Gangopadhyay, K. K., & Kumar, G. (2013). Determination of steroidal saponins and fixed oil content in fenugreek (Trigonella foenum-graecum) genotypes. *Indian Journal Pharmaceutical Science, 75*(1), 110–113.

Banerjee, S., & Banerjee, S. (2023). Anticancer potential and molecular mechanisms of cinnamaldehyde and its congeners present in the cinnamon. *Plant Physiologia, 3*(2), 173–207. http://dx.doi.org/10.3390/physiologia3020013.

Basch, E., Ulbricht, C., Kuo, G., Szapary, P., & Smith, M. (2003). Therapeutic applications of fenugreek. *Alternative Medicine Review: A Journal of Clinical Therapeutic, 8*(1), 20–27.

Bhagat, N., & Chaturvedi, A. (2016). Spices as an alternative therapy for cancer treatment. *Systematic Reviews in Pharmacy, 7*(1), 46–56.

Braga, M. E., Leal, P. F., Carvalho, J. E., & Meireles, M. A. A. (2003). Comparison of yield, composition, and antioxidant activity of turmeric (Curcuma longa L.) extracts obtained using various techniques. *Journal of Agricultural and Food Chemistry, 51*(22), 6604–6611.

Chashmniam, S., Mirhafez, S. R., Dehabeh, M., Hariri, M., Azimi Nezhad, M., Nobakht M., & Gh, B. F. (2019). A pilot study of the effect of phospholipid curcumin on serum metabolomic profile in patients with non-alcoholic fatty liver disease: A randomized, double-blind, placebo-controlled trial. *European Journal of Clinical Nutrition, 73*(9), 1224–1235.

Cruz-Correa, M., Hylind, L. M., Marrero, J. H., Zahurak, M. L., Murray-Stewart, T., Casero Jr, R. A., ... & Giardiello, F. M. (2018). Efficacy and safety of curcumin in treatment of intestinal adenomas in patients with familial adenomatous polyposis. *Gastroenterology, 155*(3), 668–673.

Dehghani Nazhvani, A., Sarafraz, N., Askari, F., Heidari, F., & Razmkhah, M. (2020). Anti-cancer effects of traditional medicinal herbs on oral squamous cell carcinoma. *Asian Pacific Journal of Cancer Prevention (APJCP), 21*(2), 479–484. https://doi.org/10.31557/APJCP.2020.21.2.479.

Deol, P. K., & Kaur, I. P. (2013). Improving the therapeutic efficiency of ginger extract for treatment of colon cancer using a suitably designed multiparticulate system. *Journal of Drug Targeting, 21*(9), 855–865. https://doi.org/10.3109/1061186X.2013.829076.

Do, M. T., Kim, H. G., Choi, J. H., Khanal, T., Park, B. H., Tran, T. P., & Jeong, H. G. (2013). Antitumor efficacy of piperine in the treatment of human HER2-overexpressing breast cancer cells. *Food Chemistry, 141*(3), 2591–2599.

Ekor, M. (2014). The growing use of herbal medicines: Issues relating to adverse reactions and challenges in monitoring safety. *Frontiers in Pharmacology, 4*, 177.

El-Ashmawy, N. E., Khedr, N. F., El-Bahrawy, H. A., & Abo Mansour, H. E. (2018). Ginger extract adjuvant to doxorubicin in mammary carcinoma: Study of some molecular mechanisms. *European Journal of Nutrition, 57*(3), 981–989. https://doi.org/10.1007/s00394-017-1382-6.

Golombick, T., Diamond, T. H., Manoharan, A., & Ramakrishna, R. (2012). Monoclonal gammopathy of undetermined significance, smoldering multiple myeloma, and curcumin: A randomized, double-blind placebo-controlled cross-over 4g study and an open-label 8g extension study. *American Journal of Hematology, 87*(5), 455–460.

Gopalakrishnan, S., Ediga, H. H., Reddy, S. S., Reddy, G. B., & Ismail, A. (2018). Procyanidin-B2 enriched fraction of cinnamon acts as a proteasome inhibitor and anti-proliferative agent in human prostate cancer cells. *IUBMB life, 70*(5), 445–457. https://doi.org/10.1002/iub.1735.

Govindarajan, V. S., & Stahl, W. H. (1980). Turmeric—Chemistry, technology, and quality. *Critical Reviews in Food Science & Nutrition, 12*(3), 199–301.

Gundala, S. R., Mukkavilli, R., Yang, C., Yadav, P., Tandon, V., Vangala, S., & Aneja, R. (2014). Enterohepatic recirculation of bioactive ginger phytochemicals is associated with enhanced tumor growth-inhibitory activity of ginger extract. *Carcinogenesis, 35*(6), 1320–1329.

Heidari-Beni, M., Moravejolahkami, A. R., Gorgian, P., Askari, G., Tarrahi, M. J., & Bahreini-Esfahani, N. (2020). Herbal formulation "turmeric extract, black pepper, and ginger" versus Naproxen for chronic knee osteoarthritis: A randomized, double-blind, controlled clinical trial. *Phytotherapy Research, 34*(8), 2067–2073.

Housenblas. H., Conway, K., Coyle, K., Barton, E., Smith, L., Esposito, M., Harvey, C., Oakes, D., & Hooper, D. (2021). Efficiency of fenugreek seed extract on psychological and physical health: A randomized placebo-controlled double-blind clinical trial. *Journal of Complementary and Integrative Medicine, 18*(2), 445–448.

Howells, L. M., Iwuji, C. O. O., Irving, G. R. B., Barber, S., Walter, H., Sidat, Z., Griffin-Teall, N., Singh, R., Foreman, N., Patel, S. R., Morgan, B., Steward, W. P., Gescher, A., Thomas, A. L., & Brown, K. (2019). Curcumin combined with FOLFOX chemotherapy is safe and tolerable in patients with metastatic colorectal cancer in a randomized phase IIa trial. *The Journal of Nutrition, 149*(7), 1133–1139. https://doi.org/10.1093/jn/nxz029.

Imtiyaz, S., Rahman, K., Sultana, A., Tariq, M., & Chaudhary, S. S. (2013). Zingiber officinale Rosc.: A traditional herb with medicinal properties. *CELLMED, 3*(4), 26–1.

Jafarirad, S., Mansoori, A., Adineh, A., Panahi, Y., Hadi, A., & Goodarzi, R. (2019). Does turmeric/curcumin supplementation change anthropometric indices in patients with non-alcoholic fatty liver disease? A systematic review and meta-analysis of randomized controlled trials. *Clinical Nutrition Research, 8*(3), 196–208.

Kaefer, C. M., & Milner, J. A. (2008). The role of herbs and spices in cancer prevention. *The Journal of Nutritional Biochemistry, 19*(6), 347–361.

Kanai, M., Yoshimura, K., Asada, M., Imaizumi, A., Suzuki, C., Matsumoto, S., ... & Aggarwal, B. B. (2011). A phase I/II study of gemcitabine-based chemotherapy plus curcumin for patients with gemcitabine-resistant pancreatic cancer. *Cancer Chemotherapy and Pharmacology, 68*, 157–164.

Karna, P., Chagani, S., Gundala, S. R., Rida, P. C., Asif, G., Sharma, V., ... & Aneja, R. (2012). Benefits of whole ginger extract in prostate cancer. *British Journal of Nutrition, 107*(4), 473–484.

Khamis, A. A., Ali, E. M., Abd El-Moneim, M. A., Abd-Alhaseeb, M. M., El-Magd, M. A., & Salim, E. I. (2018). Hesperidin, piperine and bee venom synergistically potentiate the anticancer effect of tamoxifen against breast cancer cells. *Biomedicine & Pharmacotherapy, 105*, 1335–1343.

Khanna, A., Thomas, J., John, F., et al. (2021). Safety and influence of a novel extract of fenugreek on healthy young women: A randomized, double-blinded, placebo-controlled study. *Clinical Phytoscience 7,* 63. https://doi.org/10.1186/s40816-021-00296-y.

Kooshki, A., Khazaei, Z., Rad, M., Zarghi, A., & Chanbari Mogaddam, A. (2018). Effects of fenugreek seed powder on stress-induces hyperglycemia and clinical outcomes in critically ill patients: A randomized clinical trial. *Biomedical Research and Therapy, 5*(9), 2664–2670.

Krishnamoorthy, B., & Parthasarathy, V. A. (2010). Improvement of black pepper. *CABI Reviews, 2010,* 1–12.

Kwon, H. K., Hwang, J. S., So, J. S., Lee, C. G., Sahoo, A., Ryu, J. H., ... & Im, S. H. (2010). Cinnamon extract induces tumor cell death through inhibition of NFκB and AP1. *BMC Cancer, 10,* 1–10.

Laabbar, W., Abbaoui, A., Elgot, A., Mokni, M., Amri, M., Masmoudi-Kouki, O., & Gamrani, H. (2021). Aluminum induced oxidative stress, astrogliosis and cell death in rat astrocytes, is prevented by curcumin. *Journal of Chemical Neuroanatomy, 112,* 101915.

Li, S., Yuan, W., Deng, G., Wang, P., Yang, P., & Aggarwal, B. (2011). Chemical composition and product quality control of turmeric (Curcuma longa L.). *Pharmaceutical Crops, 2,* 28–54.

Lira Neto, J. C. G., Damasceno, M. M. C., Ciol, M. A., de Freitas, R. W. J. F., de Araújo, M. F. M., Teixeira, C. R. S., Carvalho, G. C. N., Lisboa, K. W. S. C., Marques, R. L. L., Alencar, A. M. P. G., & Zanetti, M. L. (2022). Efficacy of cinnamon as an adjuvant in reducing the glycemic biomarkers of type 2 diabetes mellitus: A three-month, randomized, triple-blind, placebo-controlled clinical trial. *Journal of the American Nutrition Association, 41*(3), 266–274. https://doi.org/10.1 080/07315724.2021.1878967.

Lira Neto, J. C. G., Damasceno, M. M. C., Ciol, M. A., de Freitas, R. W. J. F., de Araújo, M. F. M., Teixeira, C. R. S., Carvalho, G. C. N., Lisboa, K. W. S. C., Marques, R. L. L., Alencar, A. M. P. G., & Zanetti, M. L. (2022). Efficacy of cinnamon as an adjuvant in reducing the glycemic biomarkers of type 2 diabetes mellitus: A three-month, randomized, triple-blind, placebo-controlled clinical trial. *Journal of the American Nutrition Association, 41*(3), 266–274. https://doi.org/10.1080/07315724.202 1.1878967.

Liu, Q., Peng, Y. B., Qi, L. W., Cheng, X. L., Xu, X. J., Liu, L. L., Liu, E, H., & Li, P. (2012). The cytotoxicity mechanism of 6-shogaol-treated Hela human cervical cancer cells revealed by label-free shotgun proteomics and bioinformatics analysis. *Evidence-Based Complementary and Alternative Medicine, 2012*, 278652.

Luo, M., Lin, H., He, Y., & Zhang, Y. (2020). The influence of corncob-based biochar on remediation of arsenic and cadmium in yellow soil and cinnamon soil. *Science of The Total Environment, 7*, 137014.

Maurya, A., Dubey, B., & Dwivedi, A. (2016). A review of ethnobotanical and pharmacological approaches of Fenugreek (*Trigonellafoenum-graecum*). *Evidence-Based Complementary and Alternative Medicine, 21*(1), 53–62.

Mirmiran, P., Davari, M., Hashemi, R., Hedayati, M., Sahranavard, S., Bahreini, S., Tavakoly, R., & Talaei, B. (2019). A randomized controlled trial to determining the effect of cinnamon on the plasma levels of soluble forms of vascular adhesion molecules in type 2 diabetes mellitus. *European Journal of Clinical Nutrition, 73*(12), 1605–1612. https://doi.org/10.1038/s41430-019-0523-9.

Moorthi, C., & Kathiresan, K. (2013). Curcumin–piperine/curcumin–quercetin/curcumin–silibinin dual drug-loaded nanoparticulate combination therapy: A novel approach to target and treat multidrug-resistant cancers. *Journal of Medical Hypotheses and Ideas, 7*(1), 15–20.

Nachvak, S. M., Soleimani, D., Rahimi, M., Azizi, A., Moradinazar, M., Rouhani, M. H., Halashi, B., Abbasi, A., & Miryan, M. (2022). Ginger as an anticolorectal cancer spice: A systematic review of *in vitro* to clinical evidence. *Food Science & Nutrition, 11*(2), 651–660. https://doi.org/10.1002/fsn3.3153.

Najdi, R. A., Hagras, M. M., Kamel, F. O., & Magadmi, R. M. (2019). A randomized controlled clinical trial evaluating the effect of *Trigonella foenum-graecum* (fenugreek) versus glibenclamide in patients with diabetes. *African Health Sciences, 19*(1), 1594–1601. https://doi.org/10.4314/ahs.v19i1.34.

Neelakantan, N., Narayanan, M., de Souza, R. J., & van Dam, R. M. (2014). Effect of fenugreek (Trigonella foenum-graecum L.) intake on glycemia: A meta-analysis of clinical trials. *Nutrition Journal, 13*, 1–11.

Nerkar, Amit & Ghadge, Srushti. (2022). Ethnopharmacological review of ginger for anticancer activity. *Current Trends in Pharmacy and Pharmaceutical Chemistry, 4*, 158–164. 10.18231/j.ctppc.2022.028.

Ohshiro, M., Kuroyanagi, M., & Ueno, A. (1990). Structures of sesquiterpenes from Curcuma longa. *Phytochemistry, 29*(7), 2201–2205.

Oladunni Balogun, F., Tayo AdeyeOluwa, E., & Omotayo Tom Ashafa, A. (2020). Pharmacological potentials of ginger. *IntechOpen*. DOI: 10.5772/intechopen.88848.

Panahi, Y., Kianpour, P., Mohtashami, R., Jafari, R., Simental-Mendía, L. E., & Sahebkar, A. (2016). Curcumin lowers serum lipids and uric acid in subjects with nonalcoholic fatty liver disease: A randomized controlled trial. *Journal of Cardiovascular Pharmacology*, *68*(3), 223–229.

Panahi, Y., Rahimnia, A. R., Sharafi, M., Alishiri, G., Saburi, A., & Sahebkar, A. (2014). Curcuminoid treatment for knee osteoarthritis: A randomized double-blind placebo-controlled trial. *Phytotherapy Research*, *28*(11), 1625–1631.

Pandian, R. S., Anuradha, C. V., & Viswanathan, P. (2002). Gastroprotective effect of fenugreek seeds (Trigonella foenum graecum) on experimental gastric ulcer in rats. *Journal of Ethnopharmacology*, *81*(3), 393–397.

Patil, M., Choudhari, A. S., Pandita, S., Islam, M. A., Raina, P., & Kaul-Ghanekar, R. (2017). Cinnamaldehyde, cinnamic acid, and cinnamyl alcohol, the bioactives of cinnamomum cassia exhibit hdac8 inhibitory activity: An *in vitro* and in silico study. *Pharmacognosy Magazine, 13*(3), S645–S651. https://doi.org/10.4103/pm.pm_389_16.

Petrovska, B. B. (2012). Historical review of medicinal plants' usage. *Pharmacognosy Reviews*, *6*(11), 1.

Rajagopalan, P., Wahab, S., Dera, A. A., Chandramoorthy, H. C., Irfan, S., Patel, A. A., & Ahmad, I. (2020). Anti-cancer activity of ethanolic leaf extract of Salvia officinalis against oral squamous carcinoma cells *in vitro* via caspase mediated mitochondrial apoptosis. *Pharmacognosy Magazine, 16*(3), S546–S552.

Romeo, G. R., Lee, J., Mulla, C. M., Noh, Y., Holden, C., & Lee, B. C. (2020). Influence of cinnamon on glycemic control in individuals with prediabetes: A randomized controlled trial. *Journal of the Endocrine Society*, *4*(11), bvaa094. https://doi.org/10.1210/jendso/bvaa094.

Saha, A., Blando, J., Silver, E., Beltran, L., Sessler, J., & DiGiovanni, J. (2014). 6-Shogaol from dried ginger inhibits growth of prostate cancer cells both *in vitro* and *in vivo* through inhibition of STAT3 and NF-κB signaling. *Cancer Prevention Research (Philadelphia, Pa.), 7*(6), 627–638. https://doi.org/10.1158/1940-6207.CAPR-13-0420.

Sahoo, H., Govil, D., James, K. S., & Prasad, R. D. (2021). Health issues, health care utilization and health care expenditure among elderly in India: Thematic review of literature. *Aging and Health Research*, *1*(2), 100012.

Samykutty, A., Shetty, A. V., Dakshinamoorthy, G., Bartik, M. M., Johnson, G. L., Webb, B., ... & Munirathinam, G. (2013). Piperine, a bioactive component of pepper spice exerts therapeutic effects on androgen dependent and androgen independent prostate cancer cells. *PLoS One, 8*(6), e65889.

Sedeky, A. S., Khalil, I. A., Hefnawy, A., & El-Sherbiny, I. M. (2018). Development of core-shell nanocarrier system for augmenting piperine cytotoxic activity against human brain cancer cell line. *European Journal of Pharmaceutical Sciences, 118*, 103–112.

Sharma, R. D., Sarkar, A., Hazra, D. K., Misra, B., Singh, J. B., Maheshwari, B. B., & Sharma, S. K. (1996). Hypolipidaemic effect of fenugreek seeds: A chronic study in non-insulin dependent diabetic patients. *Phytotherapy Research, 10*, 332–334.

Singh, S., Chaurasia, P. K., & Bharati, S. L. (2023). Hypoglycemic and hypocholesterolemic properties of fenugreek: A comprehensive assessment. *Applied Food Research, 100311.*

Srinivasan, K. (2007). Black pepper and its pungent principle-piperine: A review of diverse physiological effects. *Critical Reviews in Food Science and Nutrition, 47*(8), 735–748.

Takooree, H., Aumeeruddy, M. Z., Rengasamy, K. R., Venugopala, K. N., Jeewon, R., Zengin, G., & Mahomoodally, M. F. (2019). A systematic review on black pepper (Piper nigrum L.): From folk uses to pharmacological applications. *Critical Reviews in Food Science and Nutrition, 59*(1), S210–S243.

Varalakshmi, B., Anand, V., Karpagam, T., Shanmugapriya, A., Gomathi, S., Sugunabai, J., & Sathianachiyar, S. (2017). Phytochemical analysis of cinnamomum zeylanicum bark and molecular docking of procyanidin B2 against the transcription factor NF-κB. *Free Radicals and Antioxidants, 7*(2), 195–199.

Varshney, H., & Siddique, Y. H. (2023). Medicinal properties of fenugreek: A review. *The Open Biology Journal, 11*(1).

Wang, L. Y., Zhang, M., Zhang, C. F., & Wang, Z. T. (2008). Alkaloid and sesquiterpenes from the root tuber of Curcuma longa. *Acta Pharmaceutica Sinica, 43*(7), 724–727.

Wani, S. A., Singh, A., & Kumar, P. (Eds.). (2022). *Spice Bioactive Compounds: Properties, Applications, and Health Benefits.* CRC Press.

Wu, J., Sun, X., Guo, X., Ge, S., & Zhang, Q. (2017). Physicochemical properties, antimicrobial activity and oil release of fish gelatin films incorporated with cinnamon essential oil. *Aquaculture and Fisheries, 2*(4), 185–192.

Yaffe, P. B., Doucette, C. D., Walsh, M., & Hoskin, D. W. (2013). Piperine impairs cell cycle progression and causes reactive oxygen species-dependent apoptosis in rectal cancer cells. *Experimental and Molecular Pathology, 94*(1), 109–114.

Yun, J. W., You, J. R., Kim, Y. S., Kim, S. H., Cho, E. Y., Yoon, J. H., ... & Kang, B. C. (2018). *In vitro* and *in vivo* safety studies of cinnamon extract (Cinnamomum cassia) on general and genetic toxicology. *Regulatory Toxicology and Pharmacology, 95*, 115–123.

Zadorozhna, M., & Mangieri, D. (2019). Mechanisms of chemopreventive and therapeutic proprieties of ginger extracts in cancer. *International Journal of Molecular Sciences, 22*(12), 6599. https://doi.org/10.3390/ijms22126599.

Zare, R., Nadjarzadeh, A., Zarshenas, M. M., Shams, M., & Heydari, M. (2019). Efficacy of cinnamon in patients with type II diabetes mellitus: A randomized controlled clinical trial. *Clinical Nutrition (Edinburgh, Scotland), 38*(2). https://doi.org/10.1016/j.clnu.2018.03.003.

Zhang, B., Liu, Y., Wang, H., Liu, W., Cheong, K. L., & Teng, B. (2021). Effect of sodium alginate-agar coating containing ginger essential oil on the shelf life and quality of beef. *Food Control, 130*, 108216.

Zheng, J., Zhou, Y., Li, Y., Xu, D. P., Li, S., & Li, H. B. (2016). Spices for prevention and treatment of cancers. *Nutrients, 8*(8), 495.

Index

ultra-performance liquid
chromatography (UPLC) 25
UPLC, *see* ultra-performance liquid
chromatography
urolithiasis 13

very low-density lipoprotein
(VLDL) 15, 270
vitamins 2–3, 5, 9, 28, 31, 199,
255
VLDL, *see* very low-density
lipoprotein

vascular endothelial growth factor
(VEGF) 59, 62, 70, 154,
156–158, 166, 204, 227, 232,
264
vascular endothelial growth factor
receptor (VEGFR) 166, 227
VEGF, *see* vascular endothelial
growth factor
VEGFR, *see* vascular endothelial
growth factor receptor

Wurzburg cells 140

Zingiber officinale 3, 30, 34, 43,
160, 196, 232, 251
zingiberene 30–31, 61, 196